Out of Sight, Into Mind

OUT OF SIGHT, INTO MIND

The History and Philosophy of Yogic Perception

JED FORMAN

COLUMBIA UNIVERSITY PRESS *NEW YORK*

Columbia University Press
Publishers Since 1893
New York   Chichester, West Sussex

Library of Congress Cataloging-in-Publication Data
Names: Forman, Jed, author.
Title: Out of sight, into mind : the history and philosophy of yogic perception / Jed Forman.
Other titles: Yogic perception across Indo-Tibetan traditions
Description: New York : Columbia University Press, [2025] | Revision of the author's thesis (PhD, University of California, Santa Barbara, 2021) under the title: Yogic perception across Indo-Tibetan traditions. | Includes bibliographical references and index.
Identifiers: LCCN 2024024135 (print) | LCCN 2024024136 (ebook) | ISBN 9780231215527 (hardback) | ISBN 9780231215534 (trade paperback) | ISBN 9780231560801 (ebook)
Subjects: LCSH: Yoga. | Perception (Philosophy)
Classification: LCC BL1238.52 .F67 2025 (print) | LCC BL1238.52 (ebook) | DDC 181/.45—dc23/eng/20240828

Cover design: Milenda Nan Ok Lee
Cover art: Veronique G / Shutterstock

Contents

Acknowledgments vii

Introduction 1

PART ONE: Hindu Traditions and Epistemology

ONE Extramission, Remote Seeing, and Intuitions 13

TWO The Epistemology of Authority and Testimony 38

PART TWO: Indian Buddhism and Phenomenology

THREE Pragmatism and Coherentism 75

FOUR Omniphenomenology 107

PART THREE: Tibetan Buddhism and Language

FIVE Gelug Representationalism 139

SIX Sakya Antirepresentationalism 169

Conclusion 203

Acknowledgments

While normally said of child rearing, the adage is no less applicable to writing: it takes a village. There are countless people I would like to acknowledge in helping me bring this book to fruition. My sincere gratitude goes to the Fulbright Commission, the United States–India Educational Foundation, as well as the American Institute of Indian Studies for generous grants supporting fifteen months of continuous research in India. I am also grateful to my host institution in India, the Central Institute for Higher Tibetan Studies (CIHTS) in Sarnath, which became my intellectual home abroad, especially Ven. Dr. Wangchuk Dorjee Negi, Dr. Penpa Dorjee, and Ven. Dr. Tashi Tsering for their advisership during my tenure there.

There are several incredible experts at CIHTS whom I had the great fortune to consult for my research. I am indebted to Dr. Pradeep Gokhale for his help with several Sanskrit texts, as well as the late Dr. Ramshankar Tripathi, who was unfailingly kind and generous with his expertise and welcome. I was also blessed to work with Ven. Dawa Sherpa, a rising Sanskrit and Tibetan scholar at CIHTS. I greatly appreciate both Ngawang Thogmed's and Geshe Losang Tsultrim's taking the time to clarify some hard to interpret passages. In Dharamshala, I was grateful for input from Khenpo Kaḥdrag on Sakya texts.

Fond memories and gratitude also extend to Sera Jey Monastery in Bylakuppe, including the Sera Jey Secondary School, where I had the rewarding opportunity to volunteer as an English instructor. Without Ven. Jampa Chöphel and Ven. Losang Donyö, I would have had no introductions to some of the fantastic Geshes with whom I worked. My thanks to them. The late Geshe Chime Tsering embodied both wisdom and compassion in taking so much time with me during my study of *Dgongs pa rab gsal*. He is dearly missed. Geshe Ngawang Gyeltsen was equally generous in his review of various sections of the major Gelug epistemology commentaries concerning yogic perception. I am further grateful to Geshe Ngawang Sangye and Geshe Yama Rinchen for their conversations on key difficult points.

There are several scholars stateside who were instrumental in completing my monograph. Congruent with researching for this book, I had the fortune to work on a coauthored book project with José Cabezón, Jay Garfield, Sonam Thakchoe, John Powers, Douglas Duckworth, Thomas Doctor, Ven. Tashi Tsering, and Ryan Conlon. I thank them for their colleagueship and ongoing conversations about Buddhist philosophy. I am especially grateful to Jay, whose philosophical eye on previous drafts greatly improved the project. A special thank you also goes to José, my advisor and constant mentor. I am also grateful to Vesna Wallace and Ann Taves, who have been equally indispensable.

I had the fortunate support of the Shinjo Ito Postdoctoral Fellowship at the Numata Center for Buddhist Studies at University of California, Berkeley, to transform my dissertation research into this monograph. During my time in Berkeley, Robert Sharf and Jacob Dalton were wonderful conversation partners about much of its content. My thanks also to Robert and Sally Sutherland Goldman, who expanded my Sanskrit world and broadened my thinking about the contents of this book. I am also indebted to Elisa Freschi, Alessandro Graheli, Bhikṣu Hejung, Parimal Patil, and Davey Tomlinson with whom I translated Jñānaśrīmitra's *Yoginirṇayaprakaraṇa* during a workshop at the University of Toronto in June 2024. They were instrumental in helping me correct my previous errors in translating this text. I am also thankful to Naomi Worth and Anil Mundra, who lent their expertise in personal communications, as well as to Daniel Wyche for his editorial work.

Continued work on this monograph was also generously supported by The Robert H. N. Ho Family Foundation, which helped fund the workshop in Toronto and seed funds my position at Simpson College. I am grateful for their ongoing support. Finally, I am unrequitedly indebted to my family. My parents, George and Marion, have shown unflinching support throughout this wild journey. And last and most certainly most, I owe everything to my wife Kelli Forman, my true sine qua non. Without you, nothing. With you, everything. Anything good about this book is to this village's credit. Anything lacking is my fault only.

Introduction

> Superstition is a considerable ingredient in almost all religions, . . . there being nothing but philosophy able entirely to conquer these unaccountable terrors.
>
> —DAVID HUME, *ESSAYS, MORAL, POLITICAL, AND LITERARY*

> Superstition sets the world on fire; philosophy snuffs it out.
>
> —VOLTAIRE, *DICTIONNAIRE PHILOSOPHIQUE*

> Superstitions are, for the most part, but the shadows of great truths.
>
> —TRYON EDWARDS, *A DICTIONARY OF THOUGHTS, BEING A CYCLOPEDIA OF LACONIC QUOTATIONS FROM THE BEST AUTHORS, BOTH ANCIENT AND MODERN*

ENLIGHTENMENT FIGURES SAW themselves as saviors against the evils of superstition. Rationality, they argued, was the antithesis of superstition, and only it could wrest muddled minds from the grips of spurious notions. As Hume suggests, these falsities were largely the sin of religion. The Enlightenment thus set the stage for an ongoing confrontation between religion and philosophy. The conviction in this dichotomy has persisted. It continues to inform contemporary philosophy, determining what subjects, authors, and traditions, among other sources, we deem deserving of philosophical attention—what gets to be considered "philosophy" at all.

This prejudice is especially prevalent in comparative philosophy, biasing the selection of its non-Western counterparts. A favoritism for what appears secular or "analytical" haunts the philosophical analysis of Buddhism,[1] as well as the analysis of Indian and Tibetan (Indo-Tibetan)[2] thought more generally. The result is a "Buddhist Exceptionalism" in the Western gaze that ignores those elements prejudiced as superstitious or religious.[3]

One goal of this book is to complicate these divisions. It takes what, at first topical blush, may seem wholly religious, yogic perception, and reveals it to be deeply philosophical. True, proponents of yogic perception embrace some superstitious notions. But this does not vitiate profound truths in their discussion. As Tryon Edwards attests, "Superstitions are, for the most part, but the shadows of great truths." This is not to say that superstitions *are true*. Rather, we can discover philosophical truths through the exploration of superstitious topics.

In fact, despite its antagonism toward religion, Euro-American philosophy has long afforded its own seminal figures this charity. Philosophers do not discount the epistemological value of the *Meditations* despite Descartes's obvious theological apologetics. Similarly, Kant's religious inflection of noumena does not dissuade philosophers from taking his account seriously. We can repeat this ad nauseum: Plato's theory of ideal forms, Rousseau's theory of human rights,[4] Wollstonecraft's feminism,[5] and so on. Yet there seems to be a certain amnesia of this fact toward foreign traditions. When confronted with unfamiliar religious elements, philosophers of the Western academy often balk. They keep non-Western works and their topics at a philosophical distance, as if their religious elements poison the well. Or, at most, they stick to the rivers and lakes that they're used to, selectively picking elements seemingly sanitized of religious trappings.[6]

I contend that yogic perception is one such topic that has been kept at arm's length for these reasons. Yet there is a wealth of extractable philosophical sophistication mixed into these debates—in fact, philosophy is their essence. This fact remains veiled to Euro-American philosophers, who, despite their own traditions being equally embedded in a religious genealogy, find the religious base of Indo-Tibetan philosophy unfamiliar, and therefore prejudice Indo-Tibetan as unphilosophical. To extract this essence, we need an eluent, a substance that separates the parts of a mixture. This is provided by a comparison to that same Euro-American philosophical tradition, through which we can churn yogic perception's philosophical import to the surface. But this requires care, since we neither want to confuse that essence for the eluent, nor think that essence is a *product* of interaction with the eluent. To do so would be to misrepresent Indo-Tibetan traditions, either projecting on them what is not there, or thinking that they are philosophically impotent without Euro-American intervention.

Overview

Main Arguments

To perform this extraction responsibly thus demands that two processes be kept separate. The first is that I represent the intellectual history of yogic perception accurately. This descriptive enterprise must be sequestered from the second requirement, its comparative interpretation.[7] Indeed, the first is a prerequisite for the second, since Indo-Tibetan texts are highly reader responsible and thus replete with ellipsis. A lot of groundwork must be done to make amble sense of the concepts discussed in these texts before they can be felicitously compared with their Euro-American counterparts. This requires immersion in their intellectual milieu, which itself is a diachronic phenomenon evolving over the centuries.

On the descriptive front, it is difficult to give an all-encompassing definition of "yogic perception" across traditions and time, given its polysemy. But we can attempt a polythetic one. To begin, we must consider the word "yoga," of which "yogic" is an adjective. Rather than denoting difficult, contorted postures, "yoga" in both Indian and Tibetan traditions describes a range of spiritual practices. The word "yoga" comes from the Sanskrit root *yuj*, meaning to yoke, to join, to unite, or to absorb with. This etymology is revealing, since most Indo-Tibetan traditions agree that yogic perception involves a type of mental absorption, where the mind directly joins with whatever it is cognizing. This distinguishes *yogic* perception from normal perception. In the latter, the external sense faculties (the eyes, ears, nose, etc.) function as intermediaries. And because normal perception is filtered through these faculties, its grasp of reality is skewed and limited. Yogic perception, by contrast, is said to afford special insight into its object, since the mind directly unites with its object without sensory mediation.

The ability for yogis to perceive objects directly is said to afford them a host of perceptual feats. These fall into two categories. The first I dub "enumerative knowledge." Yogis are said to possess acute abilities—much like Superman's X-ray vision—that allow them to perceive distant, subtle, and occluded objects. This includes peering into heaven, witnessing all its celestial beings, as well as observing individuals' transmigrations through realms from death to rebirth—a capacity that makes yogis uniquely authoritative in postmortem matters. The other category is "spiritual knowledge." Yogis perceive metaphysical entities as well, such as the cosmic soul (*ātman*) or the nature of reality. Such knowledge helps the yogis as well as their disciples progress toward liberation, freedom from the cycle of transmigration. Most theories of yogic perception encompass both forms of knowledge, albeit in varying degrees. And much of the debate around yogic perception concerns how it affords both.[8]

This question is intimately connected to theories concerning how yogic perception is cultivated. Among the available explanations, meditation is key. Here, the root *yuj* is again relevant in its valence as "absorption:" "yoga" is often synonymous with meditative concentration in Indo-Tibetan traditions. The sort of meditation used to gain yogic perception, however, might appear alien to those acquainted with more popular forms. The goal of yogic meditation is to hold an object in the mind's eye with unwavering focus. Eventually, with sustained effort, that object becomes as vivid as a hallucination, as if it were right before oneself. Is this, then, a type of delusion? It would seem so. But many of the authors explored in this book go to great lengths to demonstrate that it is not.

As I have suggested, however, yogic perception is not a monolith. Its theory is diachronic, changing over time. To recreate this intellectual development, then, I proceed somewhat chronologically across a millennium of development—from the fifth until the sixteenth centuries and from India through Tibet—in three parts with two chapters each. Part I focuses (though not exclusively) on Indian non-Buddhist, or "Hindu," theories of yogic perception, whereas part II focuses squarely on Indian Buddhist materials through the end of the first millennium CE.[9] At the turn of the millennium, Buddhism was waning in India and flourishing in Tibet. Part III is thus exclusivity devoted to Tibetan debates during the second millennium and ends roughly in the sixteenth century. Although by no means the end of Tibetan Buddhist scholastic development (which continues to this day), this century was undoubtedly one of its creative zeniths.[10]

I argue that the intellectual development of yogic perception is a product of attempts to synthesize its two purported affordances: (1) enumerative knowledge of discrete objects and (2) spiritual knowledge of metaphysical truths required for liberation. Part I focuses on how these two elements functioned in non-Buddhist theories of yogic perception. In these traditions, there is no tension inherent in yogic perception's capacity to grant both.

But Buddhist antirealism creates just such an epistemological tension. The Buddhists I examine argue that external objects do not ultimately exist. Thus, these Buddhists must explain how yogic perception provides knowledge of these discreet objects, while also revealing that those objects are not real. This tension is explored in part II. Indian Buddhists seemed reluctant to abandon either of these prongs, since the loss of either would put their tradition's authority in jeopardy. They thus had to be creative in explaining how enumerative knowledge of objects could coincide with metaphysical insight into their nonexistence. As a result, a combination of pragmatic, representationalist, and antirepresentationalist approaches became possible solutions.

Part III analyzes how this tension manifested in Tibetan sources. I argue that while the Gelug (*Dge lugs*) school eschews pragmatism and maintains representationalism, the Sakya (*Sa skya*) school doubles down on pragmatism and eschews representationalism. Each school thus favors one approach over the other and disproportionately uses that framework as a hermeneutic to interpret their Indian predecessors.

The book's conclusion gives a more detailed rundown of this intellectual history. I encourage readers unfamiliar with Indo-Tibetan philosophy to read it first as a précis, so that they can better follow this development chapter to chapter. Fulfilment of the second requirement, the comparative explanation, occurs on a more granular level, within each chapter. Each chapter is organized around a synchronic philosophical theme in comparison with a Euro-American counterpart. Readers less interested in yogic perception's intellectual development over the *longue durée* can also read this book modularly, skipping from chapter to chapter as philosophical topics interest them. I provide a philosophical synopsis of each chapter in the next subsection.

The title of this monograph, *Out of Sight, Into Mind*, captures both the synchronically interpretive and diachronically descriptive goals of this work. The phrase "out of sight, out of mind" denotes a lack of attention on something not immediately apparent. By focusing on yogic perception, whose philosophical import may not be immediately obvious, my goal is to bring attention to those aspects of Indo-Tibetan thought whose philosophical relevance has been overlooked. That is, to bring them from out of sight back into mind. The titular phrase also summarizes the historical story this book tells. The earliest theories of yogic perception that I explore describe it as a function of vision. The word "out" is key, since these theories subscribe to a projective understanding of yogic perception as literally coming out from the eyes, "out of sight." Later, yogic perception was theorized not just as a type of special vision but as a product of a mental capacity. With time, its objects also became more mental, increasingly focused on abstract concepts over tangible entities. Historically, therefore, theories of yogic perception transitioned away from sight as the explanatory mechanism toward the mind as its primary instrument. That is, they moved "out of sight, into mind."

Chapter Synopses

Chapter 1 is the most intellectual-historical chapter of the book. It explores the earliest textual articulations of yogic perception, with particular focus on Patañjali's (fourth century CE) *Yogasūtras.* In this text, yogic perception is described as a type of projective vision or extramission able to perceive objects that are distant, occluded, or subtle. The chapter considers how this extramissive theory was formalized by Naiyāyikas and Vaiśeṣikas and how vestiges of it are found even in Buddhist materials. With an appeal to cognitive science, I argue that descriptions of yogic perception as projective owe their historical longevity to their intuitiveness. Philosophically, I argue that this insight gives us an important hermeneutic for philosophical exegesis. Intuitions can exert a powerful influence on philosophical thinking, even overriding an author's desire for logical consistency. Interpreters should thus be cautious to assume that sound hermeneutics invariably elides contradictions. I take Hegel (1770–1831) as an example.

Chapter 2 examines questions of testimony and scriptural authority. The Pūrva-Mīmāṃsā tradition argues that the Vedas—the authoritative scripture for Hindu traditions—articulate divine truths that no individual can corroborate. They thus reject yogic perception. Most other Indian traditions argue that this supposition is a contradiction, contending that authoritative scripture is by definition a *record* of spiritual insight. I relate this debate to Robert Audi's (1941–) critique of David Hume (1711–1776), according to which sound testimony requires an epistemological chain anchored in experience. Like Audi, many Indian theorists who advocate yogic perception argue a foundationalist epistemology, according to which sound testimony must reduce to some direct experience that serves as its warrant. But others opt for a coherentist picture, where testimonial authority and direct experience mutually corroborate each other, neither taking precedent over the other.

Chapter 3 sets the groundwork for subsequent chapters. I explore the Buddhist understanding of yogic perception as a product of meditative fixation. The problem for Buddhists is to explain how meditation—as a type of imagination—can afford knowledge of the world. I discuss how Buddhists rely on a form of pragmatism to address this conundrum, drawing parallels to Charles S. Peirce (1839–1914). This pragmatism becomes the polemical target of later Mīmāṃsaka interlocutors. Buddhist attempts to parry these attacks force them to nuance their understanding of yogic perception in interesting ways. I demonstrate that their rebuttals again reveal a certain coherentist strain.

Chapter 4 concerns yogic perception and omniscience. On this point, Buddhists face another challenge. How can yogic perception grant omniscience of all objects if it also realizes that those objects do not exist? Buddhists answer that yogic perception perceives these objects without reifying them as distinct from the perceiver. I draw parallels here to the phenomenological reduction proposed by Edmund Husserl (1859–1938), which similarly brackets subject-object dichotomies. But I argue that Husserl's phenomenology (and many of those phenomenologists that followed him) gives an axiomatic primacy to first-person experience. A phenomenological analysis of Buddhist theories of omniscient yogic perception, however, suggests a further deconstruction of this first-person perspective. I draw on some anecdotal data and psychological studies to demonstrate that this non-first-person state may indeed comprise our most fundamental phenomenology, what I dub "omniphenomenology."

Chapter 5 begins a foray into Tibetan materials, focusing on the Gelug school and its intellectual precursors. I argue that in contrast to an Indian Buddhist pedigree that described yogic perception pragmatically, the Gelug school opts for a much more representationalist view. In other words, yogic perception is warranted because its appearances represent real things in the world. I draw parallels between their view and Bertrand Russell's (1872–1970) representative realism. But Gelugpas must tread lightly here. In contrast to naive realists, they must also explain why *normal*, nonyogic appearances obscure reality. Otherwise, there would be no reason to cultivate yogic perception as a corrective. These constraints force Gelugpas to hedge in creative ways. Their synthesis offers an intriguing alternative to naive realism, something I dub "quasirepresentationalism."

Chapter 6 explores another Tibetan strategy, advocated by the Sakya school, that eschews representationalism. They interpret the earlier Buddhist appeal to pragmatism as evidence that reality per se is inexpressible. Yogic perception thus cannot be described as representing reality, since the reality that it perceives transcends representation. I understand the Sakya position here as a rejection of metaphysics, realist or otherwise. I compare this point of view to that of Ludwig Wittgenstein (1889–1951), who takes a similar stance. But this engenders a paradox: the rejection of metaphysics itself expresses a metaphysical stance. Similarly, Sakya scholars argue that language is instrumental in realizing what is beyond language in yogic perception, despite maintaining that language has no capacity to so refer. While Wittgenstein is elliptical about this conundrum, Sakyapas probe it with zeal, since it is the key link between yogic practice and realization. Putting these traditions in conversation reveals some enticing solutions to the problem.

A Note on Conventions

This work abides by some conventions that are common to other scholarly volumes and others that are idiosyncratic. Sanskrit proper nouns, unless they are the names of works, are left untranslated but are transliterated. Some Sanskrit titles are left untranslated if they convey names rather than meanings. Tibetan proper nouns are phoneticized and parenthetically transliterated in their first instance. Because I have translated the names of texts, I do not abide by the common convention of using abbreviations for titles, though I always supply the Sanskrit equivalent in parentheses after their first occurrence, opting for a shortened title thereafter.

All translations are my own, unless otherwise noted. For translations of Sanskrit, Pāli, Tibetan, and Hindi works, I have bracketed additional, conjectural language that I supply for clarity not found in the text proper. Italics in translations are used to various ends. Most often, they indicate when an author ventriloquizes a hypothetical interlocutor contradicting the author's own position. These are also tagged with "Objection" in brackets.

Elsewhere, I use italics to indicate when the original material was in verse rather than prose.

As per scholarly convention, asterisks precede reconstructions of a word in the text's original language from translation, usually from Tibetan back into Sanskrit. Citations are in the format of page, period, and line number (e.g., 5.12) for specificity, unless a verse is cited, which is prefaced with "v." after the page number, when available. In such cases, the chapter and or volume number precedes the verse with periods (e.g., v. 7.3.456 for volume 7, chapter 3, verse 456). Any other typeset conventions are not universal and explained ad hoc.

I have attempted to make the language inclusive. That is, wherever possible I have used "they" and its variants as a third-person singular pronoun in place of gendered pronouns such as "she" and "he." I have not opted for this convention, however, in translations of works with gendered pronouns. Although I aim to present the philosophical sophistication of these Indo-Tibetan works, I do not wish to elide their flaws. Indo-Tibetan philosophy was largely and unfortunately written by men and for men exclusively. I think it is important not to erase this historical blight.

PART ONE

Hindu Traditions and Epistemology

ONE

Extramission, Remote Seeing, and Intuitions

Introduction: Feeling Truthy

Until recently, the notion of learning styles was all but dogma in education. The theory is intuitive. Because we are all individual, with different aptitudes and preferences, it makes sense that everyone would have their own optimal learning style. This notion was formalized in the VARK model. The theory claims that each person is either a visual (V), auditory (A), reading-based (R), or physical, kinesthetic (K) learner. Those who first hear about this theory (including myself) often immediately identify with one of these four over the others. I often find reading tedious. But give me a good visual depiction of the same information and it clicks. My partner, with equal confidence, claims, "Oh, I'm much more of a kinesthetic learner." She must do something physical to integrate new information.

But this *feeling* that something aptly describes our experience can be deceiving. Astrologers, soothsayers, and fortune tellers, for example, exploit a similar feeling, dressing up well-informed guesses in the guise of clairvoyance.[1] In fact, VARK appears to amount to just as much woo-woo. The model has continually failed to identify any consistent psychological trait. Research reveals that *everyone* uses all four learning styles; there is no evidence (barring disabilities) that people intrinsically favor one more than the other. Rather, style inclination varies with the topic that one is studying.[2]

Although VARK fails as a psychological model for *learning,* the investigation of VARK was not psychologically fruitless. For example, that VARK seems obvious reveals limitations in our ability to self-assess our own learning patterns. This itself is a profound psychological insight. Analysis of inaccurate theories can thus reveal important truths.

I take this as a particularly important lesson for the discipline of philosophy. Often, philosophical analysis focuses squarely on whether some position, proposition, theory, or hypothesis is true.[3] And if it is found untrue, the philosophical analysis stops. But it need not. Truths can be found orthogonally, as it were, by looking deeply into flawed ideas.

In this chapter I discuss what is perhaps the earliest theories of yogic perception. These propose that vision works extramissively, where the eyes, instead of receiving light, see objects by protectively shooting out "rays" (*raśmi*). Extramission is, of course, optically inaccurate. Nevertheless, extramission's theoretical prevalence in Indian literature reveals psychological and philosophical truths, each of which influence the other.

Consider the psychological component. Even Indian traditions that formally *reject* extramission harbor implicit, extramissive descriptions of yogic perception. This incongruity reveals two things: (1) extramission marks an intuitive understanding of perception; and (2) these intuitions can resurface even when one holds reflective beliefs to the contrary. Point 2 must be considered when reading others' philosophical works, and this constitutes the philosophical component. Namely, our interpretation of philosophy must anticipate this natural human tendency toward incongruity; we must resist the assumption that the soundest account of authorial intent categorically offers the greatest systematic consistency. To put it simply, we need better delineation between philosophical exegesis and rational reconstruction.

This chapter explores this tolerance for incongruity and its ramifications for philosophical hermeneutics in turn. The examination of this incongruity parallels another tension found in the Indian literature concerning yogic perception's two purported roles: enumerative knowledge of discrete objects and spiritual insight. I demonstrate the genesis of these two understandings of yogic perception, as well as their relationship both to extramissive theories and the rejection of those theories, as the chapter proceeds in two parts. The first considers the intellectual history of Hindu and Buddhist notions of yogic perception, including its capacity for enumerative knowledge—usually in the form of a type of remote seeing—as well as for spiritual insight. Hindu authors theorize the former capacity extramissively. But in the second part of this chapter I explore how, despite their formal rejection of extramission, Buddhists retain these vestiges. In the conclusion, I consider what lessons this affords philosophy.

Extramission and Remote Seeing

Extramission

The earliest theorizations of yogic perception comprises the confluence of two precursors, the first being extramission. Extramission was a common theory of perception among Indian philosophical traditions. It describes some of the senses not as receptive but projective. In the case of vision, the eyes are said to see objects by emitting a ray that touches them. In Sanskrit literature, this was eventually dubbed *prāpyakārin,* literally, "acting having reached [the object]."[4] The earliest textual evidence for *prāpyakārin* theory traces to the *Bṛhadāraṇyaka Upaniṣad* in the eighth century BCE.[5] Verse 4.3.6 reads: "'When the sun and the moon have both set, the fire has gone out, and speech has stopped, Yājñavalkya, what serves as the light for a man?' 'The soul serves as his light. It is through the light of the soul that he sits, goes out, works, and returns.' 'Just so, Yājñavalkya.'"[6]

The text argues that in the absence of an external light source, the soul (*ātman*) projects its own inner light, allowing the individual to find their way in the dark. Similar passages occur even in the *Ṛg Veda,* perhaps the oldest surviving Indian text (ca. 1500–1000 BCE).[7] Indeed, night vision is an ongoing conundrum for Indian authors, who repeatedly theorize that the ability to see (even if faintly) at night must be the product of some inner projective light. This projective light is also often said to be transmitted through the gaze. For example, the *Śiva Purāṇa* (ca. fourth century BCE) describes the gaze (*darśan*) of Śiva, one of the most important gods of the Hindu pantheon: "[The seeker] will gain the gaze (*darśana*) of Śiva and even self-contentedness. That gaze will remove impurities, just like the rays of the sun."[8] Here, the gaze of the deity projects sun-like rays that rid the worshipper of impurities.

The salvific power of the deity's projective gaze is a central component of modern-day Hindu practice. Contemporary Hindus still engage in the practice of *darśan* or "seeing" where one receives blessings from sacred images through the power of their gaze. The *rāj yog* practice of modern-day Radhasoamis is predicated on a similar concept. During *rāj yog*, the disciple and guru stare intensely at each other. It is believed that the projective substance of the guru's sight mingles with the disciple's, affording the adherent's direct insight into the soul.[9] If we remember that the source of this light (as transmitted through the eyes) is itself the soul, then this is intuitive.

But these rays can also be deadly. A famed story from the *Matsyapurāṇa* recounts Śiva burning the god Kāma to ashes with his blazing third eye.[10] Contemporary practitioners also believe in the potential danger of Śiva's gaze, since it can emit such a powerful "force" that it may kill an unwitting bystander.[11] The analogy of Śiva's gaze to the rays of the sun thus bespeaks a long tradition of understanding sight as a projective beam, one that can impart spiritual blessings and harm.

The Buddhist Pāli canon contains a similar understanding of luminous spiritual beams. Descriptions of consciousness, in lieu of the soul, as an extending light were prevalent in Buddhist literature. In the *Sutta on the State of Lust* (*Atthirāgasutta*), the mind of enlightenment is analogized to a sunbeam that does not land anywhere but extends forever. The light of normal minds, by contrast, is obstructed by objects.[12] There is, in fact, a longstanding history of Buddhist sources describing the mind luminally, where consciousness is characterized as a luminous entity that extends outward to cognize objects.[13] I argue that Buddhists in these texts are participating in a shared Indian cultural milieu, within which seeing objects was understood to occur through projective light. But it is also clear that Buddhists largely, unlike other Indian schools, explicitly rejected projective light as a literal theory of vision, as we will see.

Other Hindu philosophical traditions, however, took these connotations literally. It was these authors who eventually used the moniker *prāpyakārin* to describe the eye reaching out to sense its object. For example, the Nyāya or "Logician" tradition was one of the earliest codifiers of Indian epistemology. As such, they were highly invested in explaining perceptual function. Thus, Akṣapāda Gautama's *Nyāyasūtras* (third century CE), the root text for Naiyāyikas, argues that perception "apprehends its object through a special contact (*sannikarṣa-viśeṣa*) between the object and a ray (*raśmi*)."[14] This is perhaps the earliest explicit articulation of *prāpyakārin* theory—describing a literal ray that is projected from the eyes to reach and cognize its object.

Remote Seeing

The second precursor to yogic perception is the notion of remote seeing. This is an equally ancient Indian idea. It suggests that certain beings have the capacity to perceive objects over far distances, or even perceive occluded objects. In modern parlance, this paranormal ability is called "tel-esthesia." The oldest Indian reference to remote seeing I have found hails from the *Rāmāyaṇa*. This famed epic recounting the adventures of King Rāma has existed in various forms from at least the seventh century BCE. The section below recounts how Sampāti, a vulture, was able to see Sītā, Rāma's kidnapped wife, and Rāvaṇa, her captor and demon-king of (modern-day) Sri Lanka, across the sea over a hundred leagues[15] away.

You will see the daughter of King Janaka of Maithila, Sītā, there
In Laṇkā, concealed on all sides by the sea.
Reaching the end of the sea, situated a full hundred leagues beyond,
You will see Rāvaṇa on the southern bank.
. . .
Standing here, I behold Rāvaṇa and Sītā alike.
Just like the divine visual prowess of the eagle, Suparṇa,
So too naturally and because of the virility of our food
Can we always see more than a hundred leagues away, O Monkeys.[16]

The attribution of remote seeing (*dūra-darśin*) to vultures is also found in the *Narasiṁha Purāṇa*[17] as well as the *Hitopedaśa*,[18] a medieval collection of maxims and sayings. In the discussions of yogic perception I examine throughout this book, vultures and eagles are repeatedly referenced as examples of remote seeing.

These protoyogic perception elements—remote seeing and extramissive light—were incorporated into a type of yogic supersensory power in the *Yogasūtras* of Patañjali. This text hails from around the fourth century CE. Nevertheless, it will become clear that its aphorisms record much older ideas, particularly with reference to yogic perception. I focus especially on verse 3.25.[19] Here, Patañjali describes yogis' unique capacity to see distant objects. I have added Vyāsa's fifth- or six-century commentary (*Bhāṣya*) for clarity.

> *There is the knowledge of subtle, occluded, and distant objects by casting the light* (āloka-nyāsa) *of [mental] activity.*
>
> It is said that this mental activity is luminous (*jyotis*). The mind's light belongs to that activity; when it is cast toward a subtle (*sūkṣma*), occluded (*vyavahita*), or distant (*viprakṛṣṭa*) object, the yogi discovers that object.[20]

Patañjali describes perception of those objects that are hidden for most but accessible to the yogic gaze. "Subtle" (*sūkṣma*) denotes objects that may be too small or ephemeral for most to see. "Occluded" (*vyavahita*) denotes objects that are obstructed from view by visual impediments (such as walls, clouds, darkness). "Distant" (*viprakṛṣṭa*) denotes objects that are far-off, removed by a long distance. These three terms form a leitmotif that recurs throughout Hindu and Buddhist sources. Although extensive scholarship demonstrates that the *Yogasūtras* are deeply indebted to Buddhist thought,[21] this terminological triad appears to have its genesis in the *Yogasūtras*, since I have found it in no earlier text, Buddhist or otherwise. It thus marks an instance where the *Yogasūtras* were influential on Buddhist writers in turn.[22]

The term *āloka* here is ambiguous. It can mean "light" or "sight." Both possibilities appear in popular translation.[23] It is unclear if either reading is necessitated by the sutra, but Vyāsa's commentary glosses it as "light," specifically referring to this higher sense capacity as "luminous." If *āloka* does denote "light," Patañjali intends a type of *prāpyakārin*, where yogis cast their light to see these objects.[24] On this assumption, Patañjali suggests that these perceptual abilities are due to especially powerful visual rays that allow yogis to focus in on subtle objects, penetrate obstructions (like X-ray vision) to see occluded ones, and project their visual rays over great distances to apprehend distant objects. It is also worth noting, however, that Vyāsa describes this ability as a *mental* (*manas*) light. Remote seeing as a *mental* rather than strictly visual capacity is a common theme among subsequent commentators. It may be, then, that Vyāsa's addition marks a transition from a purely visual description of remote seeing toward a mental one—out of sight, into mind.

Another *Yogasūtra* that recurs throughout my book is 3.16, which reads, "Meditation (*saṃyama*) on the three types of transformation (*pariṇāma*) brings knowledge of the past and future,"[25] where Patañjali identifies change as coming in three varieties.[26] By meditating on the nature of change, the yogi gains clairvoyant retrocognition and precognition. While *Yogasūtra* 3.25

is of particular importance and is oft cited in textual discussions of yogic perception, 3.16 makes several appearances as well.

Remote Seeing Codified

The Vaiśeṣika Tradition

Projective remote seeing would not be codified under the moniker "yogic perception" until about the ninth century CE. This culmination occurs within the Vaiśeṣika tradition, which was highly preoccupied with metaphysical taxonomies interpreted through Nyāya epistemology. There was thus a high degree of exchange between Vaiśeṣika and Nyāya, and they eventually became folded into a singular tradition under neo-Nyāya in the tenth century. But even before this amalgam, the two traditions were highly, mutually influential. To begin the discussion, I first trace the intellectual precursors within Vaiśeṣika leading to its codification of projective yogic perception.

The Vaiśeṣika root text, the *Vaiśeṣikasūtras*, does not use the word "yogic perception" proper. But its earliest commentary, Praśastapāda's sixth-century *Digest on Phenomena and Meanings* (*Padārthadharmasaṃgraha*), directly incorporates Patañjali's theory in its articulation of yogic perception: "Absorbed yogis, who are different from us, have a vision of things' essential nature (*svarūpa*) . . . which arises from a mind honed by yogic practice. . . . Unabsorbed yogis, on the other hand, perceive subtle (*sukṣma*), occluded (*vyavahita*), and distant (*viprakṛṣṭa*) objects through the power of their yogic practice involving fourfold contact."[27]

Praśastapāda describes two tiers of yogis, those who are unabsorbed (*viyukta*) and those who are absorbed (*yukta*)—in other words, those yogis *not* engaged in meditation and those who are. Praśastapāda argues that unabsorbed yogic perception can perceive the subtle, occluded, and distant objects described in *Yogasūtra* 3.25 through "fourfold contact." This term denotes cognitions where four components are involved: a connection between the soul, the mind, the senses, and the object.[28]

Absorbed yogis, on the other hand, see more subtle phenomena still, such as atoms and the soul (*ātman*), but without fourfold contact. In absorbed perception, these are seen directly with the mind.[29] Interestingly, however, Vyāsa's commentary on *Yogasūtra* 3.25 argues that it is with a light belonging to "mental activity" that yogis see subtle, occluded, and distant objects. Thus, Praśastapāda seems to bifurcate Vyāsa's theory into two categories: (1) unabsorbed yogic perception sees those three objects with the eye (but not the mind), whereas (2) absorbed yogic perception sees more refined metaphysical objects with the mind directly.

Śrīdhara's ninth- or tenth-century *Kandala Flower of Logic* (*Nyāyakandalī*), a commentary on Praśastapāda's own commentary, marks the first use of "yogic perception" as a term of art within Vaiśeṣika. He explains, "When Praśastapāda's text says, 'the yogi is different from us,' it is talking about yogic perception."[30] Interestingly, Śrīdhara does not discuss unabsorbed yogic perception specifically. On the assumption that he accepts, like Praśastapāda, that unabsorbed yogic perception occurs through fourfold contact, then he would concur that it is *prāpyakārin*, since he agrees that the eyes emit rays to perceive their objects.[31] Still, he appears to preserve this projective notion even when explaining *absorbed* yogic perception. Discussing the absorbed type, he writes:

> At that time, they have not destroyed the obstructive stains and so have no vision of supersensible (*atīndriya*) objects. They are thus said to be "absorbed." "Absorbed" means unwavering concentration "with a mind developed by yogic generated practice" on one's own soul . . . as it exists within oneself as well as others.[32]

First, Śrīdhara argues that absorbed yogic perception is unable to perceive objects that are supersensible (*atīndriya*), since it is focused on the soul (but presumably, those who have destroyed the stains can do so). He elsewhere makes clear that this occurs because "the yogi restrains (*pratyāhṛtya*) the mind from the external senses."[33] Thus, we see Śrīdhara recapitulate Praśastapāda's argument that absorbed yogic perception perceives via the mind without fourfold contact. But then, Śrīdhara appears to walk back this restriction on absorbed yogic perception. He suggests that absorbed yogis not only perceive their own soul, but that of others. Explaining further, he argues:

> But when one practices continuous meditation on the spatiotemporal location, etc., of another's soul with a desire to know it, then they amass a practice of inconceivable (*acintya*) power, which has the quality of knowing the reality of

another's soul, etc. And through that power, consciousness *comes out of the body* [emphasis added] to join with others' souls.[34]

So, yogic perception not only allows one to apprehend the cosmic soul, but the soul of other individuals. This latter ability is an extension of *prāpyakārin*. Just as sight must extend rays to see an object in visual perception, consciousness itself leaves the body to apprehend another's individual soul via yogic perception.[35] Thus, though Śrīdhara maintains that absorbed yogic perception occurs without fourfold contact, he retains *prāpyakārin* connotations in its description, citing the mind in place of visual rays as extending out to perceive objects.[36]

But if Śrīdhara here intends a type of mental *prāpyakārin*, this would run counter to his tradition's taxonomy. *Prāpyakārin* theory, across both Nyāya and Vaiśeṣika, only concerns the external senses—the eyes, ears, nose, mouth, and touch. The mind (*manas*) is not considered an external sense organ in these traditions.[37] Therefore, absorbed yogic perception cannot technically be *prāpyakārin*, since it only occurs via the mind. On the other hand, the notion of a nonphysical *prāpyakārin* outside of the physical senses is not unheard of in the larger Indian milieu. Though a later example, the Digambara Jain Amṛtacandra (tenth century) seems to take this position. Little is known about this figure, except from his commentaries. Below is an excerpt from his commentary on the *Pith Instructions* (*Pravacanasāra*) (second century), the *Light on Reality* (*Tattvapradīpika*): "Because it is beyond the eyes (*akṣātītatva*), the soul that obtains a remoteness beyond the discursive scope of the *prāpyakārin* [senses] knows and sees . . . all objects. So too does the knowing yogi, with their miraculous powers, achieve such an ability . . . toward objects."[38]

Amṛtacandra describes absorbed yogic perception of the soul. Nevertheless, he argues it reaches farther and is more remote than the *prāpyakārin* senses, working beyond them (*akṣātītatva*). It is thus not impossible that Śrīdhara also intends a type of *prāpyakārin* in the case of absorbed yogic perception. On the other hand, Amṛtacandra's framework may be idiosyncratic and thus not applicable to that of Śrīdhara, who is working with the presuppositions of a different philosophical tradition. At the very least, however, this demonstrates that the extramissive connotations of *prāpyakārin* can bleed into the analysis of absorbed yogic perception via the mind or soul, even when *prāpyakārin* theory is not strictly applicable.

The Nyāya Tradition

The Nyāya school builds their theory of yogic perception from the *Vaiśeṣikasūtras*. Interestingly, however, they appear to use the appellation "yogic perception" before known Vaiśeṣika commentators. The Nyāya theory of yogic perception resembles Vaiśeṣika's, but with some notable differences. This earliest Naiyāyika mention hails from the oldest surviving commentary available on the *Nyāyasūtras* by Pakṣilasvāmin Vātsyāyana (ca. 450 CE, hereafter Vātsyāyana). Here we see Vātsyāyana cite the *Vaiśeṣikasūtras* as evidence for his description:

> Do the epistemic instruments converge on one epistemic object? Or do they distinguish their own object separately? We observe both. That the soul exists is based on a credible teaching. Inferentially, one understands that "the mark of the soul is desire, hatred, effort, pleasure, pain, and consciousness" (verse 1.1.10). However, the yogi (*yuñjāna*) has a perception born from yogic concentration. And thus, Vaiśeṣikasūtra 9.1.13 says,
>
> *The soul is perceptible through a special connection between the soul and the mind.*[39]

Vātsyāyana's introductory question concerns the relationship between epistemic instruments (*pramāṇas*) and their objects (*prameyas*). Specifically, he contrasts perception (*pratyakṣa*) with inference (*anumāna*). Are all objects that are inferable also perceptible, and vice versa? Or are some types of objects only perceptible and others only inferable? Vātsyāyana argues that it depends on the object. We can both see a fire perceptually when we approach it or infer its presence by seeing smoke in the distance. The soul, however, can only be inferred by normal people—it can't be perceived by normal sensory perception. But it can be perceived by *yogic* perception. Thus, perception of the soul requires the development of a special kind of perception, whereas fire can be perceived with the senses.[40] Again, drawing on *Vaiśeṣikasūtra* 9.1.13, Vātsyāyana argues that this perception eschews fourfold contact and is accomplished directly by the mind.

It would be much later before the Nyāya tradition would make use of *Yogāsūtra* 3.25. The earliest evidence I have found for this citation hails from Jayanta Bhaṭṭa's (fl. 880–890) *Bouquet of Reasons* (*Nyāyamañjarī*). In this text, Jayanta offers evidence for the possibility of remote seeing within a section on proofs for the existence of yogic perception (*yogi-pratyakṣa-sādhana*). As in texts I previously examined, he draws from *Yogasūtra* 3.25 for his description of yogic perception as a type of remote seeing (*viprakṛṣṭa-jñāna*):

> Superior seeing is an authentic cognition. Cats (lit. the enemy of mice) can see a multitude of objects deposited in a place where a veil of thick darkness has descended, just as we, dependent on light, see that multitude situated close to us. It is also said in the *Rāmāyaṇa* that Sampāti, King of the Vultures, saw the beautiful daughter in law of Daśaratha, Sītā, even though she was a hundred leagues away. . . . When this is perfected, they become yogis. This vision is excellent because it has subtle (*sūkṣma*), occluded (*vyavahita*), and distant (*viprakṛṣṭa*) things, as well the past and the future, as its objects.[41]

Jayanta's interpretation is in the lineage of the *Yogasūtras*. First, in addition to the three objects described in *Yogasūtra* 3.25—subtle, occluded, and distant objects—Jayanta references 3.16, seeing the past and future. He cites both as instances of yogic perception. He adds, "Just as a normal people like us might perceive their brother who is yet to arrive, so will yogis perceive a future phenomenon."[42] This trope of a girl having a premonition that her brother would return home is a pervasive example of clairvoyance in Indian literature. Interestingly, it also traces back to Praśastapāda.[43] Furthermore, we see Jayanta reference the *Rāmāyaṇa* when discussing Sampāti, the vulture who was able to see Rāvaṇa and Sītā across the sea a hundred leagues away. Here, this example's connection to yogic perception is made explicit.

Our next key Naiyāyika figure, Bhāsarvajña (ca. 950), offers perhaps the clearest synthesis of the components of yogic perception discussed so far. His *Ornament for Logic* (*Nyāyabhūṣaṇa*) contains references to *Yogasūtra* 3.25 and incorporates Praśastapāda's distinction between absorbed and unabsorbed yogic perception. He also includes Jayanta Bhaṭṭa's assessment that yogic perception includes cognition of past and future objects, à la *Yogasūtra* 3.16.

> The perception that grasps three different types of distant (*viprakṛṣṭa*) objects either altogether or separately is said to be yogic perception. These are: (1) distant places, such as the True-World Heaven (*satyaloka*), etc., or far-off realms that

> are occluded (*vyavahita*), such as that of the Nāgas,[44] etc.; (2) distant times, such as the past and the future; and (3) distant natures, such as atoms or space, etc. That yogi exists in two states: the absorbed state (*yukta*) and the unabsorbed state (*ayukta*). In the absorbed state, since one is united with phenomena, etc., which is just a connection between the soul and the mind, that yogi grasps all objects (*aśeṣa-artha-grahaṇa*). This is said intending supreme yogis. But the mere yogi does not grasp all objects.[45]

While Bhāsarvajña mentions both distant (*viprakṛṣṭa*) and occluded (*vyavahita*) objects reminiscent of *Yogasūtra* 3.25, he does not make any explicit mention of subtle (*sūkṣma*) objects. Notably, Bhāsarvajña expands the provenance of absorbed yogic perception to include not just "spiritual" objects, but enumerative knowledge of "all objects." This suggests an omniscient type of yogic perception held by "supreme yogis" (*paramayogi*), perhaps Śrīdhara's absorbed yogi with the stains destroyed, who perceive discrete, distant objects in addition to the soul.[46]

A theory of omniscient yogic perception was also held by Bhāsarvajña's Buddhist juniors, Śāntarakṣita and Kamalaśīla, as we see in chapter 4. Interestingly, like those Buddhist authors, Bhāsarvajña argues absorbed yogic perception gains this enumerative knowledge exactly because it *bypasses* the senses, grasping those objects directly via the mind.

> When the object is grasped by taste, the eyes, or the skin, there is fourfold contact, meaning a connection between four things: the soul is joined with the mind, the mind with the senses, and the senses with the object. When the object is grasped by the ears, there is contact between three things: the soul, the mind, and the ears. When the object is grasped by the mind, there is contact between the mind and soul. Seer cognition (*ārṣa*) is included in this. It is not another type of epistemic instrument, since it is subsumed under the characteristics of yogic perception, which is the complete experience of imperceptibles (*aparokṣa*) when those objects are distant, such as [the aforementioned] places.[47]

Here, we see Bhāsarvajña draw on *Vaiśeṣikasūtra* 9.1.13: "With regard to the soul, it is perceived through a special connection between the soul and the mind." Bhāsarvajña is thus in line with Praśastapāda and subsequent Vaiśeṣika theories of absorbed yogic perception. But Bhāsarvajña's formulation also departs from Praśastapāda's in an important respect. According to the latter, absorbed and unabsorbed yogic perception perceived different types of phenomena. While absorbed yogic perception perceived metaphysical objects, like soul, time, and wind, unabsorbed yogic perception perceived those discrete entities described by *Yogasūtra* 3.25—subtle (*sukṣma*), occluded (*vyavahita*), and distant (*viprakṛṣṭa*) objects.

Bhāsarvajña, on the other hand, does not stratify metaphysical and discrete objects between absorbed and unabsorbed types. Even though absorbed yogic perception is focused exclusively on the soul, this does not preclude its cognition of discrete objects or distant places. Thus, although, as per *Vaiśeṣikasūtra* 9.1.13, absorbed yogic perception only involves a twofold (as opposed to fourfold) connection between the soul and the mind, it is still able to cognize objects other than the soul. Here, then, we see Bhāsarvajña combine yogic perception's warrant of both enumerative knowledge and metaphysical knowledge into the absorbed type, whereas before these warrants were separated between unabsorbed and absorbed yogic perception.

Thus we see a continuation of yogic perception's growing role as an umbrella term. First, in the *Yogasūtras*, remote seeing and spiritual insight remained conceptually distinct. Then, the Vaiśeṣika tradition folded them into two types of yogic perception—unabsorbed and absorbed. Here, Bhāsarvajña accommodates *both* under absorbed yogic perception only, as if this type is not just epistemically distinct, but epistemically superior. But as yogic perception increases its semantic range, the epistemic issues become increasingly thorny. Bhāsarvajña uses phrases—which his epistemic commitments should reject—to explain absorbed yogic perception's clairvoyant feats, such as the soul's being "joined" (*sahita*) with distant, physical objects, reminiscent of Śrīdhara's explanation that consciousness exits the body. As yogic perception subsumes an increasing range of epistemological functions, its theorization tends toward epistemological incongruity. This feature manifests in Buddhist sources as well.

The Buddhist Tradition

The earliest Buddhist figure to mention "yogic perception" explicitly was the famed founder of Buddhism's own brand of epistemology, Dignāga (ca. 480–540), who drew much of his innovation from Nyāya sources. But neither extramission nor remote seeing figure into his presentation of yogic perception. These elements would not enter the Buddhist analysis of yogic perception at least until the works of Dignāga's most famed commentator, Dharmakīrti (b. 660). Nevertheless, there is an abundance of Buddhist literature predating Dignāga that describe the remote-seeing feats associated with yogic perception in Nyāya and Vaśeṣika sources, though without the appellation. These include the perception of distant objects, times, places (like heaven), and even other minds. In these earlier Buddhist sources, all these abilities are said to be afforded by the divine eye (Pāli *dibbacakkhu*).[48]

My discussion of the divine eye centers the works of the famed fifth-century Theravādin master Buddhaghoṣa, whose *Path of Purification* (*Visuddhimagga*) is a vast compendium of meditation techniques. The *Path of Purification* discusses the divine eye at several points, including its ability to perceive the transmigration of beings from death to rebirth, the future, and distant realms.[49]

Each of the seven times the divine eye is described in the *Path of Purification*, it is said to be afforded by "extending light" (Pāli *ālokaṃ vaḍḍhetvā*). For example, describing its ability to perceive distant worlds, Buddhaghoṣa writes, "Through the divine eye, someone standing in one place extends light and sees the form of Brahmā."[50] Buddhaghoṣa also mentions light when giving an etymology of the "divine eye," playing off the polysemy of *dibba* as both divine and light: "Because it possesses light, the divine eye is exceedingly bright. Thus, it is divine. Because it has a great range—able to see forms behind walls, etc.—it is divine."[51] Extending light also affords the divine eye's telepathic ability. Buddhaghoṣa writes: "How is it this ability culminates in knowledge of others' minds? It occurs through the power of the divine eye. Therefore, the monk extends light, and through the divine eye, they see the color of the blood that moves in the heart of another, and thus investigate their mind."[52]

Buddhaghoṣa's description is reminiscent of both Śrīdhara and Amṛtacandra, who described yogic perception as the ability to perceive another's soul (*ātman*).[53] In place of knowing another's soul, Buddhaghoṣa discusses the ability to know another's mind. In ancient India, the heart was considered the corporeal residence of both the soul and mind. Buddhaghoṣa's description of the divine eye's ability to literally peer into the heart of another thus may draw on older theories of soul-reading through the heart. Buddhaghoṣa's substitution of the mind for the soul makes sense, given his rejection of the soul's existence (*anātman*).[54]

It is tempting to read Buddhaghoṣa here as subscribing to a type of *prāpyakārin*. After all, Buddhaghoṣa states the divine eye "extends light" and "possesses light." But there is some ambiguity. Buddhaghoṣa's phrase "because it possesses (*pariggaha*) light (*āloka*), the divine eye is exceedingly bright (*mahāggaha*)" could be read in different ways. "*Pariggaha*" may mean grasping, as in receiving light, or encapsulating, as in containing (and thus projecting?) light.[55] It is also not entirely clear whether "extending light" (*ālokaṃ vaḍḍhetvā*) suggests something extramissive. Extending light refers to a mediation method known as *kasiṇa,* where one constructs—either physically or meditatively—a disk (*kasiṇa*) made from some element and meditates on it in order to control that element. In the case of the divine eye, one meditates on the light element or *kasiṇa*, affording the ability to see distant external objects. The range of that sight is said to increase with the distance one can extend that light meditatively.[56]

Extending the light *kasiṇa* thus may not denote literal *prāpyakārin*. Because this process is meditative, it is not clear whether the meditator literally casts light (*aloka-nyāsa*) in the way suggested by *Yogasūtra* 3.25 or projects a ray (*raśmi*) in the manner suggested by *Nyāyasūtra* 3.1.34. On the other hand, *kasiṇa* is not a *merely* meditative method. Eventually, the elements on which one meditates are said to literally manifest; this is the goal of *kasiṇa* practice. At the very least, the isomorphism between extending the light *kasiṇa* (*ālokaṃ vaḍḍhetvā*) and the *prāpyakārin* notion of projective light, both to see distant objects, may be operating with similar cultural intuitions about vision.[57]

These extramissive connotations are even more interesting given that Buddhists by and large explicitly reject *prāpyakārin* as a theory of visual perception.[58] Buddhaghoṣa is one such example. He states, "The eye and ear, among others, grasp their objects without reaching them (*asampatta*)."[59] Buddhaghoṣa's rough contemporary, Vasubandhu (fl. fourth or fifth century), agrees, arguing, "The eyes, ears, and mind do not reach (*aprāpta*) their objects." Furthermore, he excludes the possibility that *prāpyakārin* could be mental, "Because the mind is not a type of physical form, it cannot reach (*prāptum*) anything."[60] By the tenth century, Buddhist opponents understood Buddhists to reject *prāpyakārin* categorically.[61] Nevertheless, there is evidence that fourth- and fifth-century Buddhist positions on *prāpyakārin* may have not been so uniform.[62] And whether Buddhaghoṣa would argue that the *divine* eye is, like the physical eye, non-*prāpyakārin* remains unclear.

Other Buddhists, however, were reticent to discuss remote seeing at all. For example, Dharmakīrti references vulture's remote seeing with a heavy dose of sarcasm. He quips, "If you are concerned with the instruments for remote seeing, come, we will seek out the vultures!"[63] Being able to spot objects from afar, Dharmakīrti jests, is literally something for the birds. Dharmakīrti is also one of the earliest Buddhists (besides Dignāga) to give an explicit account of yogic perception. Thus, while both the Vaiśeṣika and Nyāya schools explicitly accommodate two types of yogic perception—unabsorbed as remote seeing and absorbed a spiritual insight—Dharmakīrti is reluctant to admit the former. His strategy is to downplay yogic perception's remote seeing and focus simply on its capacity for metaphysical insight. Dharmakīrti had good epistemological reasons for rejecting yogic perception's role in remote seeing, detailed in chapter 3.

Nevertheless, later Buddhists seemed equally wary of Dharmakīrti's rejection of remote seeing and were thus quick to clarify that Dharmakīrti was being rhetorical in this passage. According to them, he meant to emphasize yogic perception's role in gaining *practical* omniscience (*upayuktasarvajña*), the spiritual insight necessary for liberation, in contrast to omniscience in the sense of literally knowing everything (*sarvasarvajña*). While both types of omniscience are said to belong to the Buddha,[64] the former takes developmental priority. For example, Prajñākaragupta (ca. 750–810), one of Dharmakīrti's primary commentators, argues that "being able to see remotely is not tantamount to omniscience, since if that were the case, then even vultures would have it." That is, literally knowing all objects is not sufficient for omniscience. One also needs direct insight into metaphysical truths. Thus, "Those *great* beings with remote seeing have cultivated a *complete* omniscience that was preceded by partial knowledge. That is, beyond that [remote seeing], they cultivated [insight] into reality."[65]

So in place of the seeming antagonism suggested by Dharmakīrti between remote seeing and metaphysical insight, Prajñākaragupta folds both understandings into a progressive framework, wherein those "great" (*mahat*) remote seers—those not content just with clairvoyant acrobatics—first develop insight into reality, practical omniscience, before developing literal knowledge of all things. Prajñākaragupta thus recovers a Buddhist form of unabsorbed yogic perception rejected by Dharmakīrti. Like his non-Buddhist predecessors, he describes it as a type of remote seeing, even invoking *Yogasūtra* 3.25: "yogis sense distant (*dūra*), subtle (*sūkṣma*), etc., objects," including a capacity to read "others' minds."[66] And like Bhāsarvajña (though unlike Bhāsarvajña's predecessors), Prajñākaragupta argues that this remote seeing is a type of mental rather than sensory perception: "Some men can see afar. Some cannot. How are these two something other than mental perception (*samvedanasya pratyakṣa*)?"[67]

Despite Dharmakīrti's efforts to distance yogic perception from remote seeing, it appears that their association was already deeply entrenched in the larger textual context in which he was writing. As such, Prajñākaragupta appears to backtrack Dharmakīrti's rejection of remote seeing to remain in line with standard understandings of yogic perception's unabsorbed capacities toward enumerative knowledge. Buddhists may have felt that if their theory of yogic perception did not account for remote seeing, it would lose its intelligibility. Prajñākaragupta's strategy is thus to make this ability a subsidiary function of yogic perception's spiritual capacity for practical omniscience. Bhāsarvajña in turn may have been influenced by these efforts, since his description of absorbed yogic perception—in contrast to his predecessors'—encapsulates both abilities as well. But like Bhāsarvajña, the Buddhist accommodation of both capacities creates some epistemological hurdles.

The desire to keep Buddhist theories legible to a wider cultural milieu, however, was not the only factor influencing Buddhists to retain remote seeing in their account. I argue that the extramissive connotations embedded in remote seeing are especially intuitive, making them compelling to Buddhist authors, even when they conflict with their theoretical beliefs. In the next section, I explore how extramissive intuitions might have influenced Buddhist theorization in this regard.

Extramission as a Human Intuition

Intuitions

The previous discussion reveals some epistemological ambiguities concerning the connection between yogic perception and *prāpyakārin*. Unabsorbed yogic perception occurs through the senses and ostensibly operates through *prāpyakārin*. But most accounts of *absorbed* yogic perception retain extramissive vestiges even though this is an epistemological incongruity, given that *prāpyakārin* concerns the external senses and absorbed yogic perception is strictly mental. This is typified in Śrīdhara's description of a mind that extends out to perceive another's soul. Buddhaghoṣa's description of the divine eye reveals the same tropes, despite his rejection of *prāpyakārin* altogether. And even Buddhist attempts to distance yogic perception from extramission-latent notions of remote seeing are backtracked by later commentators, like Prajñākaragupta. As such, there appears to be some stubborn resilience to the notion that yogic perception is a type of projective remote seeing.

Vaiśeṣika, Nyāya, Buddhist, and even Jain formulations of yogic perception thus repeatedly run afoul of their own epistemology, since in all these traditions *prāpyakārin* concerns physical contact between a sense organ and an object, and absorbed yogic perception bypasses the senses. And in the Buddhist case, the contradiction is even more egregious, since they claim to reject *prāpyakārin* altogether. The evidence puts us in a bit of an interpretive pickle. If we assume that these authors allowed for no epistemological incongruities, then we must dismiss any seeming similarities between *prāpyakārin* and projective absorbed yogic perception as products of reasoning by analogy. If, on the other hand, we take these similarities seriously, then it appears these thinkers have failed to be epistemologically rigorous, and we fail to be interpretively charitable.

There are some possible methodological solutions to this conundrum. Even if a certain *prāpyakārin* logic may bleed into these authors' analysis of yogic perception, this does not necessarily reveal a lapse of concern for philosophical consistency. *Prāpyakārin* theories can still do work "in the background" and influence philosophical reasoning, despite one's best efforts to remain consistent. In other words, these authors may think extramissively about yogic perception unconsciously, despite their explicit position that *prāpyakārin* does not apply to absorbed yogic perception.[68]

This may explain why Vaiśeṣikas and Naiyāyikas seemingly draw on *prāpyakārin* elements to describe absorbed yogic perception despite its strictly being mental. It may also explain why Buddhist descriptions of yogic perception appear extramissive alongside their rejection of *prāpyakārin*. I focus on Buddhist evidence for extramissive thinking, since it presents the more difficult case: if I can give good evidence that Buddhists are influenced by extramission theory despite rejecting it outright, then this holds for Vaiśeṣika and Nyāya a fortiori.

I propose that the stubborn Buddhist affinity for *prāpyakārin* reveals two levels of conflicting thought processes. Cognitive science commonly explains such conflicting beliefs under "dual process" theories of cognition, in which two different cognitive mechanisms (while most often working in tandem) can sometimes produce conflicting conclusions. Namely, these two processes are our capacity for quick intuitive thinking and slower reflective thinking.

For example, we have a natural intuitive tendency to think of animate objects as alive and inanimate ones as not. This instinct can trip up even the most seasoned botanist when asked if plants are alive. Even entrenched reflective beliefs, informed by years of study, can be hampered by this intuitive association between visible movement and life.[69] This intuition makes evolutionary sense, since it behooves human survival to differentiate quickly what could lunge and bite from what has no capacity to do so. It is better to assume all moving things have agency and are potential threats, even if this means we occasionally mistake some moving things for living things or some unmoving things as nonliving things. Intuitive beliefs are thus especially "sticky," influencing thinking even when they counter our reflective beliefs to the contrary.[70]

This raises a question: *Is extramission intuitive*? Do extramissive intuitions influence optical reasoning in the same way that intuitions about life's mobility work against our reflective understanding that plants are alive? There is strong psychological research that confirms this supposition. The tendency of children to think of perception extramissively was documented by Jean Piaget.[71] More recent research confirms that children commonly harbor an extramissive folk psychology.[72] What is even more compelling, however, is how extramissive beliefs persist among adults, even after educational interventions meant to demonstrate how perception is receptive. Belief in extramission has proven to be "deeply ingrained," with a "resistance to educational efforts" to the contrary.[73] Studies also reveal that extramissive intuitions affect reasoning in other domains, such as estimating at what angle a plank will fall over, even among participants who explicitly reject extramissive beliefs.[74]

Like the intuition that moving things are alive, extramissive intuitions also are evolutionarily adaptive. Humans naturally track others' eyes to glean what is salient in the environment.[75] In other words, others' eyes work like pointing fingers, indicating what is important and what we should pay attention to. We thus naturally think of the eyes as projecting out into the world. If based on this research we assume that extramission is an evolved, pan-human intuition, it is reasonable to assume such intuitions were operative in the minds of our Buddhist authors. Where might we find evidence of their influence on Buddhist formulations of yogic perception?

Metaphors

One possibly is to look at how Buddhists use metaphors. Metaphors, by definition, are uses of language that are intuitively appealing despite our more reflective understanding that they are not literal. Metaphors thus reveal implicit ways of thinking that run counter to our explicit beliefs.[76] For example, extramissive metaphors are deeply embedded in English phraseology. Albeit optically incorrect, we talk of being unable "to see out of a dirty window."[77] English is rife with such fictive motion in its prepositional formulation of perceptual verbs. Looking "into," "toward," "past," or "away" are all perfectly intuitive despite their extramissive connotations.[78]

Is there evidence for similar extramissive phraseology in Buddhist descriptions of yogic perception? I argue that Buddhist descriptions of consciousness as a luminous entity recruits similar projective connotations. Buddhist Sanskrit texts consistently analogize consciousness with light. These analogies marshal two ways to describe light in Sanskrit: (1) qua source, like the sun, and (2) qua extension, the rays that spread out from that source to illuminate objects. *Dīpa* connotes the first, while *prakāśa* or *prabhā*—and their derivatives "*pratibhāsa*" and "*prabhāsvara*"—denote the second.[79]

This distinction maps snugly onto Buddhist uses of light to explain yogic perception if we take extramissive intuitions into account. For example, when Dharmakīrti's *Proof of Other Minds* (**Saṃtānāntarasiddhi*) discusses yogic perception in its capacity as a type of telepathy, he uses Sanskrit terminology denoting light's extension (**pratibhāsa*). This metaphor is apt, since it suggests the telepathic mind's extending beyond itself to reach out and touch another. But Dharmakīrti also argues that, ultimately, there is no true distinction between one's own mind and another's. The appearance of other minds is actually the effulgence (**pratibhāsa*) of one's own mind.[80] Dharmakīrti's claim that there is ultimately no distinction between minds should render the spatial metaphor of extension mute. Nevertheless, his use of *pratibhāsa* preserves this metaphor. His analysis thus recruits a fictive metaphor, in which telepathic yogic perception is likened to light's extension.

Kamalaśīla (740–795 CE) also adheres to Dharmakīrti's ultimate rejection of subject-object duality. Nevertheless, his discussion of yogic perception betrays the same fictive metaphors. In one instance, commenting on Śāntarakṣita's description of yogic perception as "the pure and unwavering light of knowledge (*jñāna-dīpa*)," Kamalaśīla explains that its radiance (*prakāśa*) "illuminates all things and their properties, making them its object."[81] Thus, yogic perception as the cognizing subject is the source of light (*dīpa*), while yogic perception's object is illuminated through that light's extending radiance (*prakāśa*). Like Dharmakīrti, Kamalaśīla employs the spatial metaphors of light's origin and its extension to describe yogic perception, despite his explicit rejection of subject-object duality, which should render such spatial differentiations mute.

Reasoning

Another strategy to reveal traces of extramissive thinking is to examine how Buddhist authors analyze perceptual problems. The influence of extramissive intuitions often manifest when authors are forced to give ad hoc explanations. This is consistent with dual-process theories of cognition. Research shows that our domain-specific reasoning can conflict with our domain-general understanding.[82] In other words, there are cognitive reasons as to why Buddhist analyses about specific perceptual issues might conflict with their general perceptual epistemology.

A prominent example comes from Jñānaśrīmitra (fl. 975–1025), a famed gatekeeper at the great monastic institution of Vikramaśilā. Jñānaśrīmitra wrote *On the Demonstrability of Yogis* (*Yoginirṇayaprakaraṇa*), the only Sanskrit text completely devoted to the Buddhist theory of yogic perception. In this text, Jñānaśrīmitra explicitly denies that yogic perception, of any sort, functions via *prāpyakārin*.[83] Nevertheless, his subsequent analysis suggests a type of extramission. Jñānaśrīmitra argues that it is the mind of yogis, in contrast to their sense organs, that are special, and this allows for remote seeing. The question, then, is how the mind can have a more far-reaching perception than ordinary sense perception.

> Just as you claim that [perception depends on a sense organ because] we invariably observe that a material object's existence as a percept depends on an eye, so too do we observe such a dependence on light, and then it could not be that owls, etc., could see in the dark. . . . That [night] seeing, thanks to the inconceivable power of the mind, transgresses the other case [in which seeing depends on light], and so brings the other [supposition that perception depends on the eyes] into doubt.[84]

The implication is that mental perception is able to directly apprehend objects free of the strictures of a sense organ. Even though, in the case of normal humans, sight depends on light, night vision does not. The existence of night vision, as evidenced by owls, brings the necessity of this dependence into question. So too, Jñānaśrī argues, can we not assume all perception depends on the eye, lending credence to yogic perception as a type of mental sight. This is again consistent with the notion of absorbed yogic perception involving a "twofold contact" between the object and mind.

But even in the case of night vision, Jñānaśrī contends that an "inconceivable power of the mind" is responsible. It is unclear why Jñānaśrīmitra would assume that mental perception should fare better in the dark than the external senses unless we take implicit extramissive intuitions into account. Instead of sensory *prāpyakārin,* it is the mind that spreads its light to illuminate objects at night. This is strikingly similar to the description in the *Bṛhadāraṇyaka Upaniṣad*, where the light of the *ātman* illuminates the dark. And if we recall the longstanding Buddhist tendency to describe the mind, in lieu of the soul, as luminous, then Jñānaśrīmitra's explanation is doubly intuitive.

Furthermore, Jñānaśrīmitra cites owlish night vision as unexplainable by (receptive) sensory perception in the same fashion that Jayanta cites feline night vision.[85] Both author's appeal to night vision as yogic analogues suggest an implicit reliance on extramission to explain yogic perception's superiority. This is, again, suggested by Jñānaśrīmitra's use of fictive motion metaphors. For example, he suggests that, in the case of such supersensory abilities, the consciousness "moves beyond (*atikrama*) the path of the senses,"[86] as if the mind extends farther than their reach. This is also reminiscent of Śrīdhara's claim that in yogic perception "consciousness comes out of the body."[87]

Although Jñānaśrīmitra explicitly states elsewhere that even mental perception is not *prāpyakārin*,[88] his explanations rely on an implicit understanding of consciousness as extramissive. In other words, his reflective rejection of *prāpyakārin* seems to buckle under his ad hoc analysis of night vision. His defaulting to an implicit extramissive analysis of consciousness in this case makes sense given extramission's intuitive appeal.

Implicit extramission is again found in another section of Jñānaśrīmitra's text, where it appears during in his analysis of the vulture's remote seeing. An interlocutor argues that remote seeing is not possible, since visual cognition requires local contact between the eye and its object. Just like how a fire only burns where its fuel is present, vision cannot extend beyond the confines of this immediate contact. Jñānaśrī counters that, while this may be the case for normal vision, remote seeing occurs through mental perception. Thus, the causes for remote seeing are not restricted to one place like a fire that must remain local to its fuel.

> Insofar that those things—e.g., fuel, fire, etc.—that produce smoke and other such effects exist in one place, so too have they no power to produce anything beyond (*atikrama*) that place. But how is it that while our awareness of sense objects occur in one place, vultures' awareness can occur beyond that place? And if it does so occur, it is not limited to one area like the fuel for fire. The totality of conditions for awareness are based on the mental continuum; the intellect is also not limited to one place like smoke is.[89]

Again, Jñānaśrī's language is rife with metaphors of fictive motion. He suggests that the mind can traverse space in a manner not available to the external senses. There is a parallel between his analyses of an owl's night vision and a vulture's remote seeing, the same parallel suggested by Jayanta's reference to cats and Sampāti, the vulture who saw Sītā. In both cases, the mind is purported to be superior to the senses because it has a farther reach, "moving beyond" (*atikrama*) those physical constraints. Jñānaśrīmitra thus implicitly posits the mind as a more powerful extramissive entity. Given the long history of Buddhist analyses of the mind as an extending light, this explanation would be intuitive to Jñānaśrī and his audience.

Conclusion: A Lesson from Hegel

Throughout this chapter, I discuss authors in tension with their own philosophical systems. They universally draw on *Yogasūtra* 3.25 and import its extramissive descriptions of yogic perception, despite its incongruity with their espoused epistemology. Vaiśeṣika thinkers, most notably Śrīdhara, give extramissive descriptions of absorbed yogic perception despite claiming that this mental faculty cannot be *prāpyakārin.* Bhāsarvajña, representing Nyāya, claims that absorbed yogic perception can perceive both metaphysical truths and discrete objects. This marks a notable departure from his predecessors, who argue that the latter only occurs in unabsorbed yogic perception via fourfold contact.

I also examine Buddhist theories. Dharmakīrti attempted to distance yogic perception from the unabsorbed, remote-seeing type. But his commentators, like Prajñākaragupta, appear reticent to exclude this. What is more, Buddhists like Buddhaghoṣa and Jñānaśrīmitra end up importing remote seeing's extramissive connotations despite their rejection of *prāpyakārin.* All of this suggests that there is some powerful intuitive sway to extramission, since it bleeds into discussions of yogic perception even when it runs counter to the discusser's perceptual theories.

As I suggest at the beginning of this chapter, then, the discussion of flawed notions like extramission reveals some compelling facets of human psychology—namely, our high cognitive tolerance for incongruity between global theory and ad hoc reasoning. But how is this relevant to the discipline of philosophy? Identifying a psychological truth is, after all, not the same as demonstrating a philosophical truth.

To this objection, I have two responses. First, philosophy is not *just* about truth with a capital "T." It also requires exegetical nuance. And good exegesis demands we differentiate authorial intention from rational reconstruction. Philosophers, like all humans, are governed by reflective capacities as well as strong intuitive pulls. We forget this when we assume the soundest systematic interpretation is what the author necessarily meant, as if every thought from a good philosopher must be a perfectly cut piece that fits into a larger jigsaw puzzle.

For example, there is ongoing debate as to whether Hegel's notion of the concept was realist or idealist.[90] Many scholars deny that Hegel intended idealism, appealing to the fact that he was a metaphysical realist. But this argument presupposes that Hegel's systematic view determined his reasoning in every instance. Psychology demonstrates that this is just not how thinking works. Likely, Hegel sometimes leaned idealist and sometimes realist when describing the concept.[91] And even though these might not be perfectly compatible, understanding each theory locally, on its own terms, can be philosophically enlightening. I have thus tried to show in this chapter that albeit sophisticated thinkers, theses authors both accept and reject extramission in ways that fail to be explicitly consistent. But by exploring rather than attenuating that inconsistency, we can gain a fuller picture of their thought processes.

Second, exegetical issues aside, the discussion in this chapter is highly relevant to the phenomenology of perception. If we focus squarely on whether extramission is optically accurate, the theory is easy to dismiss outright. But on closer examination, extramission *does* say something truthful about our experience. We experience our visual perception as directive. This is a product of our own embodiment. We move our bodies, our heads, and our eyes to *direct* our gaze toward possible objects of interest. Experientially, seeing is all but passive and receptive. It is active and directed, and even indicative to others.[92]

Perception is thus also intersubjective. We rely on others' eyes to *point* out things of interest to us. It is thus as much distributed as it is personal, since others' eyes are crucial in determining what we take to be salient in the world. Both facets—embodied gaze direction and social gaze detection—belie extramissive intuitions. These intuitions may be optically "wrong." But the experience they undergird is an important arena for phenomenological inquiry, independent of their optical accuracy. At one level, then, extramission *is* right, since it describes how we most naturally experience the gaze. Thus, much like how the appeal of VARK reveals the limit of our accurate self-assessment, the stubborn persistence of extramissive theories unveils a nuanced phenomenology of the gaze. We might miss this with a myopic focus on Truth.

I elaborate on yogic perception's ramifications for phenomenology in chapter 3, concerning omniscience. But chapter 2 continues with epistemology—namely, the epistemic status of report and testimony.

TWO

The Epistemology of Authority and Testimony

Introduction: Hume and Audi

How should we evaluate incredible claims? If a stranger were to approach you on the street and—with slurred speech, glassy eyes, and stumbling a little—told you that they had just seen an alien, you would likely not believe them. If, however, a well-known astrobiologist made a public announcement that, indeed, they had found irrefutable evidence of highly intelligent alien life, would you be justified in believing in aliens?[1] This case is much trickier. On the one hand, we trust their expertise in evaluating cosmic phenomena. On the other hand, the claim's incredulity provokes a higher degree of suspicion and scrutiny. We are reasonably more reticent to accept fantastic claims, and the amount of evidence required to overcome our disbelief is proportional to their abnormality.

Hume

David Hume articulates these intuitions into a general maxim.[2] Although he makes the point with reference to "miracles"—specifically, Jesus's performance of them—we can extrapolate his meaning to any incredible claim. "That no testimony is sufficient to establish a miracle, unless the testimony be of such a kind, that its falsehood would be more miraculous, than the fact, which it endeavors to establish; and even in that case, there is a mutual destruction of arguments, and the superior only gives us an assurance suitable to that degree of force, which remains, after deducting the inferior."[3]

Hume outlines two criteria for justified belief in incredible claims. We are justified if to disbelieve that claim would lead to something even more incredulous. So, what is more likely? That there are aliens, or the astrobiologist is wrong? Statistically, the latter, since even good astrobiologists are wrong far more often than we have discovered aliens. Furthermore, Hume argues that even if the falsity of the claim is more incredible than the claim itself, then at best we must be agnostic. When confronted with two incredible possibilities, it is most prudent to simply withhold judgment until we have more information. In such cases, "there is a mutual destruction of arguments."

"Incredibility" on its own, however, is imprecise. As Karen Jones notes, different communities will find different types of testimony astonishing.[4] Taken psychologically, then, this cannot serve as an epistemic standard. Hume therefore specifies the "ultimate standard" for a claim's credulity is "experience and observation,"[5] specifically, "our observation of the veracity of human testimony, and of the usual conformity of facts to the reports of witnesses."[6] In other words, I rely on my own experience to determine a baseline of truth, and I trust reports to the degree they conform with observable facts.

Many modern scholars identify Hume's view here as reductionist.[7] That is, justified belief in testimony reduces to the listener's sound assessment, based on experience, of its conformity to facts. Hume does not require, however, that the listener *observe* the facts that testimony reduces to in every instance. Rather, he means this conformity generally. We do not have to observe conformity for *every* token of authentic testimony, but we must establish that this testifier is *generally* trustworthy and that this *type* of information conforms to a picture of the world based on observation. Contemporary scholars have called these "local" and "global" reduction respectively. Importantly, the latter is collective, based on our shared assessment of how the world behaves.[8] The problem with testimony about miracles, according to Hume, then, is that they are not the *type* of phenomena we collectively observe. (If they were, we would not need revelatory, prophetic testimony about them.) On the other hand, if someone says ice is in the freezer, then we can be more trusting (assuming they are trustworthy), since ice's being in the freezer is the type of thing we have collectively observed.

Now George Campbell (1719–1796), Hume's contemporary, argued that Hume's global requirement is too strict. Many people have unexpected experiences at one point or another. If miraculous events are equally observable, then reports of those experiences should be believed despite their failure to conform to others' observations.[9] John Stuart Mill (1806–1873) criticized Campbell on this point. He contends that Campbell's position conflates miracles—something categorically contrary to what we observe—with unexpected events, which are rare but still observable.[10] It might be unexpected to see a dog walk on its hind legs. But a levitating person would contradict our shared observations of how the world works.

Still, Campbell's criticism of the requirements for global reduction has some bite. Hume contends that justified belief in testimony requires the listener to have some analogous experience to the attested phenomena. This appears too limiting,[11] since it could potentially toss a large slice of expert testimony out the window.[12] For example, quantum scientists attest that photons can be in superposition, or be both a particle and a wave. And yet our normal, collective observations do not conform with such attestations: that something could be in two places at once or be two things at once. Relative to our observations, this seems, dare I say, miraculous.[13]

Of course, there is not just *one* scientist making such claims; there is a community of scientific consensus. But that collective is a *much* smaller, elite community than the rest of us who must take quantum scientists at their word. And this larger community is unable to fulfill the global requirement, since they have never observed the types of phenomena attested by quantum experimentation. As Karen Jones further demonstrates, *which collective's* observations gain the privilege to represent *the* "global" worldview is often highly contested, political, and directed by power.[14]

Audi

Robert Audi therefore argues that Hume's reductionism has failed to adequately distinguish knowledge from justification. The criterion justifying my belief in testimony is distinct, he argues, from the reductionist criteria that establishes that a testifier has communicated veritable knowledge. In other words, testimony must conform to the facts to be *true;* but I need not observe that conformity—either locally or globally—to justify my trust.[15] Audi thus claims, rather unnervingly, "This case shows, then, that whereas my testimony cannot give you testimonially grounded knowledge that *p* without my knowing that *p*, it can give you testimonially grounded justification for believing *p* without my having that justification—or any kind of justification—for believing *p*."[16]

In other words, I am justified in believing a testifier knows what they are talking about without my having to confirm it. This obtains *even if the testifier is wrong and their claim is unjustified,* since the hearer's justification to believe stands independent of the report's conformity to facts or justification. Such a rationale may seem absurd, but it is the only way we can make sense of expert testimony. Otherwise, we would have to become experimental scientists ourselves to justifiably believe a testifier. This would be the only way to gain the *types* of observations that fulfill the global requirement. Audi thus jettisons this requirement, rejecting that my justified belief in testimony requires my own observation of the "conformity of facts to the reports of witnesses."[17] In place of Hume's reductionism, then, Audi's is highly fallibilist, what he describes as a "credible-unless-otherwise-indicated view of testimony."[18]

While Audi's allowances for *justified* belief in testimony is capacious, his criteria for *true* belief are stricter. He notes that in the case of *credible* testimony, there must be "at least one epistemically sound chain" linking the final report to the source of knowledge, "such as perception."[19] In other words, while justified belief in testimony does not require knowledge of the conformity to facts, such a conformity must prevail if that testimony is to constitute knowledge. Audi's position is thus also foundationalist—perception serves as the foundational warrant for other credible ways of knowing the world. But while true beliefs must always reduce to this perceptual warrant, justified beliefs need not. According to Audi, this marks his departure from Hume.[20]

We can find striking parallels between the debates on yogic perception explored in this chapter and those between Hume, Campbell, and Audi. Opponents to yogic perception, mainly hailing from the Mīmāṃsā tradition,[21] share affinities with Hume. They argue that because no instance of yogic testimony conforms to what is humanly observable, belief in yogic testimony cannot be justified. But they differ from Hume's supposition in a key regard. They argue that *scripture* constitutes a special instance of testimonial veracity in the case of metaphysical truths. Specifically, they contend that the Vedas, the oldest of the Hindu scriptures, are an exclusive record of truth that no human observation can confirm or disconfirm.[22] Thus, although they would agree with Hume that we cannot trust human reports of miraculous events, they argue that the Vedas are an exception, exactly because they do not have human origins.

Defenders of yogic perception find this Mīmāṃṣā position absurd. Their rebuttals mirror the three refutations of Hume adumbrated thus far. First, like Campbell, proponents of yogic perception claim we have clear evidence that miraculous events are observable. Therefore, the credibility of their report prevails even if those events are rare and do not conform to what most people observe. This I dub the argument from *perceptibility.* Second, like Audi's claim about true belief in testimony, these defenders claim that there must be an "epistemological chain" grounding credible testimony to a perceptual event. This claim is thus conditional: insofar as there is true scriptural testimony, there must have been a yogic perceiver that serves as its foundation. This argument only has bite against the Mīmāṃsaka, who takes the existence of authentic scripture as a given. Essentially, this is an argument by *reductio*, since the absence of yogic perceivers would entail there is no credible scripture. As Hume contends concerning the "mutual destruction of arguments," however, such an argument can at best be inconclusive. Some authors will be content with inconclusiveness, while others will try to push the *reductio* toward a definitive proof of yogic perception.

And third, like Audi's claim about justified belief in testimony, proponents of yogic perception adopt a "credible-unless-otherwise-indicated view" of yogic testimony. That is, they will argue that we are justified in believing yogic accounts in the absence of any evidence to the contrary. This is a critique against an argument from ignorance. For the sake of brevity, I dub this "the argument from ignorance." That is, the absence of evidence for yogic perception is insufficient to undermine its existence, as long as there is no evidence for its nonexistence either. When there is insufficient evidence to either end—indeed, as we would expect, since yogic testimony concerns phenomena beyond the normal human pale—then they are credible prima facie.

In this chapter, we also see a continuation of the themes identified in chapter 1 concerning the two roles of yogic perception. The first is yogic perception as enumerative knowledge of discrete and distant objects inaccessible to normal perception. The second is knowledge of metaphysical, or spiritual, truths, like the nature of reality and of the soul. According to Mīmāṃsakas, neither type of perception is possible because only the Vedas are authoritative in such matters. Most other Indian traditions, Buddhist and Hindu alike, will reject this position, arguing that any scripture's authority is merely derivative of what yogis have observed.

The Mīmāṃsā Rejection of Yogic Perception

In chapter 1 we saw an early description of yogic perception hailing from *Yogasūtra* 3.25 as an ability to see subtle, occluded, and distant objects. Verse 3.16 included yogic knowledge about the past and future. Naiyāyika and Vaiśeṣika authors soon expanded on the capacities predicated of yogic perception, including knowledge of the heavens, of the soul, and of others' minds. Barring the soul, Buddhaghoṣa, writing roughly in the same era, locates these same abilities in the divine eye. It is unsurprising, then, that the fifth century CE evinces a Mīmāṃsā reaction to these purported abilities. Mīmāṃsakas argue that only the Vedas, the earliest Hindu sacred texts, can be authoritative about distant places, like heaven, and spiritual truths. If yogis could see these without relying on scripture, then the Vedas would no longer be the only authority on such matters. Mīmāṃsakas were thus highly invested in disproving this purported yogic seeing.

The root text of the Mīmāṃsā school is the *Mīmāṃsāsūtras* of Jaimini (fourth century BCE). His commentators' rejection of yogic perception builds off Jaimini's verses, specifically 1.1.2–4:

> *The meaning of dharma is characterized by the Vedic precepts* (codanā).
> *Now, for the inquiry into dharma's characteristics.*
> *Perception arises from the intellect when human senses make the right contact with objects.*
> *It does not characterize dharma, since it perceives that which is present.*[23]

"Dharma" is highly polysemic. In the texts we consider throughout this book it means both the deepest metaphysical truths about the world as well as what we should do in light of them. It thus has both ontological and ethical dimensions—a type of *normative* truth, both the True and the Good. Jaimini argues that only the Vedas can convey dharma. Perception cannot. Jaimini effectively conflates perception with sense perception, which explains its limited scope.

It is in Śabara's commentary on this verse where we see reference to the *Yogasūtras*. Śabara's dates are uncertain, sometime after Patañjali in the fourth century CE but before Vātsyāyana in the fifth. He comments: "Only the Vedic precepts can bring one to comprehend those types of objects that are past, present, and future, or subtle (*sūkṣma*), occluded (*vyavahita*), and distant (*viprakṛṣṭa*). Nothing else, such as sense perception, can. . . . And because they are preceded by the senses, inference, analogy, and disjunctive reasoning are not causes [for knowledge of dharma]."[24]

Again, we see reference to both *Yogasūtras* 3.16 (knowledge of temporal objects) and 3.25 (knowledge of subtle, occluded, and distant objects). But rather than yogis, only scripture—specifically Vedic precepts (*codanā*)—can provide information on these. Furthermore, no epistemic instrument—be it perception, inference (*anumāna*), analogy (*upamāna*), or disjunction elimination (*arthāpatti*)—can provide knowledge of spiritual matters: dharma. This is because these epistemic instruments rely on perception—they are essentially manipulations of perceptual information.

For example, an inference of fire depends on the perception of smoke. But, because dharma is literally "beyond the senses" (*atīndriya*),[25] there is no perception that could form the basis of an apodictic inference about dharma. Therefore, Śabara argues one must rely on the Vedas for information about both discrete distant objects, the past and future, and dharma. We thus see Śabara deny both of yogic perception's purported abilities—enumerative knowledge of discrete objects and spiritual knowledge of metaphysical truths. According to Śabara, these are the exclusive domain of Vedic testimony.

Śabara's assessment of perception's inability to serve as an epistemic warrant for scriptural testimony parallels Hume's claim that attestations about miracles do not conform to observable facts. Both positions assert that quotidian observations fail to have the requisite epistemic resources to ground such propositions. Unlike Hume, however, Śabara ultimately claims that, even independent of observations, scripture contains veridical testimonies about miraculous phenomena. This is because, according to Śabara, belief in scripture is justifiable prima facie[26]—what would be deemed by later commentators as their "intrinsic validity" (*svataḥ prāmāṇya*).[27] Ironically, this position comes close to Audi's claim that justified belief in testimony is "credible-unless-otherwise-indicated."[28] But they *deny* this prima facie charity to human testimony about spiritual matters, since that testimony relies on human perception. They also deny that testimony must *categorically* be epistemologically chained to perception to be *true*, as evinced by Vedic scripture. Indeed, they conflate justification with truth in the special case of Vedic testimony.[29]

Supersensible Objects

The Vaiśeṣika Rebuttal

One possible point of attack against Śabara's position is his claim that supersensible phenomena are categorically imperceptible. It is a false generalization to assume that just because *most* people cannot see them that therefore they are beyond the purview of what is observable. The earliest Vaiśeṣika response that I have found to Śabara thus makes the argument from perceptibility. It contends that although most people cannot perceive phenomena that transcend the senses, yogis can. This hails from the earliest surviving commentary on the *Vaiśeṣikasūtras* by Praśastapāda. In his text, however, the reference to Mīmāṃsā is not explicit. Nevertheless, his stated position directly opposes Śabara's critique. Again, making use of *Yogasūtra* 3.25, he argues these subtle, occluded, and distant objects are perceptible, as is dharma. Praśastapāda agrees with Śabara that dharma and adharma are supersensible (*atīndriya*), that is, beyond the senses.[30] But their being supersensible does not vitiate their being perceptible. This entails that perception is not restricted to the senses. He mentions certain magical remedies that afford perception of such supersensible objects.

> Those who see these visible objects, empowered by [such remedies], have a perception, which observes subtle (*sūkṣma*), occluded (*vyavahita*), and distant (*viprakṛṣṭa*) objects. But we also accept the observation of how dharma and adharma ripen in living beings—be they in the heavens, atmosphere, or earth—as a mere inference, having the motions of planets and stars, etc., as its sign. And

> we further accept the observation of things like dharma, etc., *without* relying on an inferential sign. This can be either perception or "seer" (*ṛṣi*) cognition.[31]

Magical formulae afford a vision of the subtle, occluded, and distant objects described in *Yogasūtra* 3.25. Dharma can be inferred through perceiving astrological signs. Yogis and adept *ṛṣis*, or "seers," on the other hand, can perceive dharmic truths directly, without having to infer them from some other observable.[32] Praśastapāda's formulation here is thus in line with his earlier distinction between unabsorbed and absorbed yogic perception. While unabsorbed yogic perception depends on the senses, seer cognition does not. Śabara, by contrast, denies both.

It is not impossible that Praśastapāda formulated his position independently of Śabara's critique. But given his pointed use of *Yogasūtra* 3.25, his insistence that dharma is perceptible, and his assertion of a nonsensory (non-fourfold contact) perception—all things that Śabara explicitly denies—it is more likely that he is responding to Śabara's Mīmāṃsā position here.

The Nyāya Rebuttal

If we concede that fantastic events are perceptible, then we must concede that felicitous reports about them are knowledge yielding. This is the essence of Audi's argument about the epistemological chain. Naiyāyikas make a similar point in their own lengthy rebuttal to Mīmāṃsā, arguing that perception provides the warrant for reliable (*āpta*) testimony. In other words, someone's report is reliable to the extent that they have a firsthand experience with the object of their report. Vātsyāyana's commentary on *Nyāyasūtra* 1.1.7 states:

> *Testimony* (śabda) *is the instructions of reliable persons.*[33]
>
> A reliable person is a teacher with direct experience (*sākṣāt*), who is impelled by a desire to make known some object as they see it. Direct experience is the reason for someone's being reliable about some object.[34]

We can anticipate how this definition might apply to yogic perception, even though Vātsyāyana does not use that term explicitly. If yogic perception provides the yogi with privileged knowledge through direct perception, it is based on this privileged access that they become a reliable authority.[35] We can also understand why the Mīmāṃsaka would be threatened by this notion, since it makes something other than the Vedas a source of sound testimony.

Uddyotakara's (sixth century) *Nyāyavārttika* greatly expands on verse 1.1.7 by introducing our familiar Mīmāṃsaka opponent. Ventriloquizing the Mīmāṃsaka, Uddyotakara raises an objection: if things like heaven are perceptible, then just anyone should be able to perceive them, and everyone would become reliable testifiers in such matters. Hume's global requirement, we should note, is simply the converse of this biconditional: any instance of sound testimony must concern an observable. If testifiable phenomena are observable, however, then, according to the opponent, testimony is not a unique epistemic instrument. There would be no need for special teachings about heaven, since this would be something anyone could observe on their own—so argues the Mīmāṃsaka.

Uddyotakara clarifies, however, that he does not mean that just *anyone's* perception is a basis for sound testimony. Only special perceptions afford direct knowledge of things like heaven. Thus, an object's being perceptible does not guarantee that just anyone can perceive it. "We do not say that people like *us* have reliable perceptions concerning heaven, etc. Rather, the person who has such perceptions is the one who gives the teachings. . . . [Objects in heaven are perceptible] because [the heavens are made of a material] substance, and whatever has a substratum is likewise perceptible by someone . . . just like a jar, or whatever."[36]

Uddyotakara's "person" here is a yogi.[37] Like Praśastapāda—who defined yogis as those "different from us"—Uddyotakara discuses those who are not "like us," possessing the supersensory ability to see heaven. Uddyotakara thus makes the argument from perceptibility. His rebuff parallels modern scholars' discussion of expert testimony, which problematizes Hume's global requirement. Scientists, like yogis, are also "not like us," since they have a unique ability to interpret empirical data. And so, our justified belief in their testimony does not require that testimony conform to *our* observables. Nevertheless, scientists and yogis still perceive observables, just of a different sort. The heavens are still made of stuff, and stuff is perceptible. They are just not globally accessible, just like the data of scientific experimentation.

Under a rational reconstruction of his argument, Uddyotakara would fault Hume's global requirement for defining observability *in terms of a community of observers*. Instead, he would argue that it is a quality of *objects*; it is not determined by their perceivers. Likewise, the Mīmāṃsā position is too strict, since perceptibility is not determined by what normal people see. For example, color is not rendered imperceptible per se just because a given community may be collectively blind.

The problem of the global requirement, therefore, is the contingent demarcations of the collective. Try as they might, a lay community will be unable to corroborate whether a given scientific attestation concerns an "observable" phenomenon, since they do not have access to such observations. They could, of course, become scientists themselves. But so too, Uddyotakara would argue, could one become a yogi and confirm the insights of yogic perception! And so, lay epistemic capacities should not serve as a basis of conformity for the whole of testimonial claims.

Still, however, Uddyotakara only provides criteria for when such testimony is *true*—that is, when they concern a perceptible. But if normal people have no ability to judge that perceptibility, then it is unclear under which conditions they would be justified in believing expert testimony.[38] One solution, as suggested by Audi, is that we should believe yogis in the absence of contravening evidence—the argument from ignorance. We will see proponents of yogic perception marshal this argument. But this is the same argument Śabara levels against those who disbelieve the Vedas, maintaining that its injunctions are prima facie justifiable.[39] Those who argue for yogic perception thus have a problem: if the argument from ignorance is sufficient to defend the justifiability of yogic attestations, it would seem equally applicable to a defense of the Vedas' "intrinsically validity," rendering yogic perception superfluous.

This is where the argument from *reductio* will come into play for the pro-yogic perception camp. Although that argument is predicated on the conditions for *true* belief in testimony, we will see it marshalled against the Mīmāṃsaka for why belief in yogic testimony is justified, and why, furthermore, justified belief in testimony simpliciter cannot be intrinsic. In this way, they counter the Mīmāṃsā claim that testimony is a sui generis warrant.

Perception as the Foundation of Scripture

Bhartṛhari's Rebuttal

These pro-yogic perception thinkers repeatedly turn to the argument from *reductio* to lend support for justified belief in testimony: they argue that to reject yogic perception is more problematic than accepting it. We saw Hume argue that this was one necessary criterion for justified belief in miraculous testimony. That is, belief in such testimony would be justified only if its denial would amount to something even stranger, and even then, there would be a "destruction of arguments," rendering the *reductio* inconclusive. Although Hume intended this as a reason to reject miraculous testimony (confident this condition could never be met), the Indian authors I am about to discuss argue that yogic attestations fulfill this criterion. Some even bite the bullet on the inconclusiveness of the *reductio*. But others deny it, arguing the *reductio* proves justified belief in yogic testimony.

In the context of debate against Mīmāṃsakas, the absurdity of the *reductio* concerns their acceptance of scriptural validity. If it can be demonstrated that to reject yogic perception renders reliable scripture incoherent, then Mīmāṃsakas must accept yogic perception rather than relinquish the possibility of authoritative scripture. Proponents of yogic perception argued in a manner that echoes Audi's epistemological chain to construct this *reductio*: there can be no sound scripture without its being grounded in yogic perception.

The first example of this strategy comes from a rough contemporary of Uddyotakara, the grammarian Bhartṛhari (ca. fifth century CE). Bhartṛhari's influence on Dignāga (ca. 480–540)—a seminal figure in Buddhist epistemology, whose work becomes central in following chapters—is well documented.[40] Dignāga was especially taken with Bhartṛhari's *On Sentences and Words* (*Vākyapadīya*), from which he developed much of his theory of conceptual thinking. Like the authors explored so far, Bhartṛhari argues that yogis[41] grasp what cannot be seen by others:

> *The testimony of those beings who see supersensible* (atīndriya) *and un-intelligible* (asaṃvedya) *objects is not overturned by inference.*
>
> *How can someone else undermine that person, who, standing on the side of perception, cannot doubt this observational knowledge as if it were his own?*[42]

Bhartṛhari's argument mirrors those explored in previous sections. He asserts—again, likely contra the Mīmāṃsaka—that supersensible objects (*atīndriya*) can be perceived by spiritual elites, even though they are unintelligible to normal people. Such objects include, just as before, "the past and future."[43] Bhartṛhari also makes clear that perception is the foundation of sound testimony, describing scripture as a type of "uninterrupted" (*avic-cheda*) transmission of an initial perceptual insight.[44] This closely resembles Audi's epistemological chain, especially his contention that testimony is "not generative with respect to knowledge," only "transmissive" of it.[45]

Both Bhartṛhari and Audi thus argue for foundationalism, agreeing perception is foundational to sound testimony. But Bhartṛhari's foundationalism is even stronger than Audi's. Not only does inference depend on perception, but he argues that ipso facto inference has no warrant over sound testimony and the beliefs of those who trust it as if it were their own observation. And so "there is little use in commentaries" for those who have an authoritative understanding of dharma from scripture;[46] and warranted reports of perceptions (in the form of scripture) cannot be undermined by "logicians."[47]

Audi's foundationalism is not this strong. Although he agrees that perception is noninferential,[48] he concedes that inference has some warrant against its report. Again, this turns on his distinction between truth and justification. While true testimony necessarily transmits an unassailable perceptual event, *that* it transmits truth needs justification, and this requires inference.[49] Uddyotakara and Bhartṛhari thus seem to equally eschew the issue of justifiability. The former claims that *true* testimony concerns perceptibles, without providing criteria for when we are justified in believing that something is perceptible. Likewise, Bhartṛhari says that testimony is unassailable because it reports a perception, without providing criteria for when we are justified in believing that testimony is a felicitous report of such a perception.

But Bhartṛhari's argument differs from Uddyotakara's in an important regard. While Uddyotakara's argument concerns the nature of testifiable phenomena—their perceptibility—Bhartṛhari's concerns the nature of testimony—the report of those perceptions. And, while the Mīmāṃsaka opponent can cogently reject that Vedic phenomena are perceptible, they cannot so reject that the Vedas are testimonial. Thus, Bhartṛhari, contra the Mīmāṃsaka, is only tasked with conditionally demonstrating that insofar as scripture is authoritative about supersensible objects that there must be a supersensible perception grounding it. This *reductio* does not require he outline the parameters of justification per se. He only needs to demonstrate that justified belief in scripture is tethered to justified belief in yogic testimony. This *reductio* hinges, of course, on the claim that testimony can only be *true* if it reduces to a perception—the epistemological chain. Forthcoming authors spell out this dependence in more detail.

Jain Rebuttals

Even if we assume this dependency, the *reductio* would at best be inconclusive—Hume's "mutual destruction of arguments." While Bhartṛhari does not directly confront this issue, the Śvetāmbara Jain Haribhadrasūri (fl. sixth or seventh century CE), accepts the *reductio*'s being inconclusive. Though he was incredibly prolific, little is known about Haribhadrasūri's life.[50] The following verses hail from his *Compendium on Commentarial Doctrine* (*Śāstravārtāsamuccaya*), a seven-hundred-verse work examining the doctrines of both Jain and other schools.[51] These first two verses hail from Haribhadrasūri's analysis of his own school.

> *Spiritual recognition* (pratyabhijñā) *is never mistaken, since there is nothing that contradicts its truth. And there is no epistemic warrant for having conviction* (pratyaya) *in yogis.*
>
> *There is no proof* (pramā) *that yogis know objects distinctly and not in an undifferentiated matter. And such a teaching may be disseminated in accordance with the merits of the trainee.*[52]

These first two verses echo Bhartṛhari's argument that yogic perception is impervious to inference or testimony. Yogic insight cannot be overturned by reasoning, since no other epistemic instrument has the probative power to undermine direct insight. But unlike Bhartṛhari, Haribhadrasūri denies that yogic testimony necessarily transmits their realization. Because the provenance of yogic perception is supersensible, *our* epistemic instruments, which are restricted to the senses, have no ability to confirm or disprove their insights, especially given that the yogi may have pragmatic reasons to give a teaching contrary to their knowledge.[53] Thus, we cannot know definitively whether yogic testimony "conforms to facts."

Nevertheless, Haribhadrasūri gives us good reasons, barring this certainty, to trust yogis. He thus offers an inchoate argument for *justified* belief in yogis, albeit *avant la lettre*. This involves Bhartṛhari's *reductio*, Uddyotakara's argument from perceptibility, as well as the argument from ignorance. These occur in two more verses, which concern the ultimate purview of yogic knowledge: omniscience (see chapter 4). The first reiterates Uddyotakara's rejection of the Mīmāṃsā position that supersensible objects are imperceptible. "*And things like dharma and adharma are perceptible because they are knowable objects that exist, like a jar, or whatever.* There is no inference that proves that there is no one for whom all [such objects are perceptible]."[54]

Haribhadrasūri invokes Uddyotakara's familiar example that dharma and adharma are perceptible because they are "like a jar." Because these phenomena are perceptible, there is no reason a priori to assume that no human perceives them—in other words, that no one is omniscient. These constitute the argument from perceptibility and from ignorance respectively. The next verse recapitulates the *reductio*. "*Through disjunction, we know from scripture that those who know about supersensible things* (atīndriya) *exist. Otherwise, there would be no consolation for the common person.*"[55]

Haribhadrasūri essentially argues a version of the epistemological chain. If there exists sound scriptural testimony that correctly attests to dharma and adharma, we can infer that someone must have seen these things directly. That is, if people like us did not author these texts, someone else—namely, the yogi—must have. We therefore have good reason to believe yogis prima facie, since without them we would be without consolation. Insofar there is any guidance for how to pursue dharma, we must take it on yogic authority, which necessitates a yogic perceiver. Although a need for consolation is not a surefire epistemic standard for true belief—again, the truth status of yogic testimony is inconclusive—it appears, at least according to Haribhadra, to provide sufficient justification for such a belief.

The arguments from perceptibility, ignorance, and *reductio* appear to have become a standard line of Jain critique of Mīmāṃsā. A rather late instance comes from another Śvētāmbara Jain, the polymath Hemacandra (1088–1173), who wrote on grammar, philosophy, history, mathematics and became renowned as an accomplished poet. The following excerpt comes from his *Investigation of Epistemology* (*Pramāṇamīmāṃsā*).[56]

> Subtle, hidden, and far-off objects (*sūkṣma-antirita-dūra-arthāḥ*) are perceived by someone, since they are knowable objects (*prameyatva*), like a jar, or whatever. And this is the case since there is no proof to the contrary concerning informative (*avisaṃvāda*) astrological knowledge (*jyotir-jñāna*).[57]

If there is no cognition of a hidden, transcendent object, then whence do people have informative knowledge about astrology?

If you argue that it comes from divinely inspired works, then that requires another source.[58]

This passage encapsulates all three arguments. First, we see Hemacandra's reference to "subtle, hidden, and far-off objects (*sūkṣma-antirita-dūra-arthāḥ*)," again likely cribbing from *Yogasūtra* 3.25. Hemacandra also invokes Uddyotakara's argument from perceptibility that such hidden objects must be perceptible, since they are "just like a jar." Exploiting the argument from ignorance, he claims there is no proof that yogis fail to know such things. Finally, the *reductio* is found in Akalaṅka's verse. The existence of divinely inspired works about celestial objects necessitates yogis who have perceived them as their source.

Later on, Hemacandra extends the *reductio* to the Vedas specifically. The original insight contained in the Vedas "must belong to someone. Otherwise, to whom did the Vedas proclaim the objects of the three times? Such a person," he argues, "must have authority" in the manner. He concludes, "Because there is no proof that establishes otherwise . . . omniscient cognition (*kevala-jñāna*) of supersensible (*atīndriya*) objects is proven."[59] Here, he reiterates the argument from ignorance. Yet unlike Haribhadrasūri, Hemacandra seems to understand this argument to be a definitive proof of yogis' existence, contending that it substantiates supersensible perception, eschewing inconclusiveness. He concludes that omniscience "of supersensible objects is proven."

His reasoning for this conclusiveness belies the most sophisticated argument for the epistemological chain that we have seen so far. He problematizes the Mīmāṃsā claim that justifiable testimony can be untethered from justified belief in yogic perceivers. Even Mīmāṃsakas concede that the Vedas were revealed *to* someone—namely, "seers" (*ṛṣis*). And those seers must have had some authority in determining that that revelation was authentic. Otherwise, the seer would be unable to determine if their revelation was a fiction or the truth, and it would be absurd for others to trust their report. Thus, even justified belief in scripture assumes that its first testifier had some authority in the manner of its authenticity. And since that authority cannot come from testimony *itself* without a regress problem, it must come from a perceptual event (given that even sound inferences depend on perception).

With this stronger argument for the epistemological chain, Hemacandra reverse engineers a proof for the existence of yogis. Knowledge of the soul and astrology (at least, the "divinely inspired" sort) are beyond what we normal folk can deduce from observation. Yet, we have knowledge of them. He therefore concludes there must be yogic seers. Of course, this argument question begs the existence of the very phenomena that yogic perception is supposed to substantiate. Still, the argument has some conditional bite: insofar that we can justifiably believe in phenomena that we cannot glean from our own observation, we must conclude that *someone*, in one form or the other, has observed them.

Buddhist Rebuttals

DHARMAKĪRTI

Buddhists also joined the crusade to defend yogic perception against Mīmāṃsā. Dharmakīrti is perhaps one of the earliest. And like his predecessors, he employs the arguments from perceptibility, by *reductio*, and from ignorance. His repudiation of Mīmāṃsā hails from his auto-commentary on the first chapter of the *Commentary on the Compendium of Epistemology* (*Pramāṇavārttika*). He articulates the *reductio* by appealing to the epistemological chain: the existence of credible scripture entails the existence of individuals with supersensible abilities.

> You may claim that because of some superior intellect, senses, or whatever, he [Jaimini] alone knows and no other. But why is it that only *he* has this superior knowledge of supersensible (*atīndriya*) objects? For example, why should it be impossible to observe someone else [like a Buddhist] who could see objects that were by nature distant in space or time (*deśa-kāla-svabhāva-viprakṛṣṭa*)?[60] There is no evidence repudiating this possibility that fails to amount to that same [ambiguity in your case]. And even if there were such evidence, then that which substantiated any such difference between them for one should hold for the other as well. Thus, only refraining from committing to either (*anabhiniveśa*) is permissible.[61]

Invoking the argument from perceptibility, Dharmakīrti contends that the Mīmāṃsaka cannot claim exclusive knowledge of supersensible objects, since such objects are perceptible to anyone with the requisite acumen. The Mīmāṃsaka thus cannot claim their scriptures have exclusive authority. Dharmakīrti's argument from perceptibility is predicated on the *reductio.* Jaimini must have had some direct insight into the meaning of the Vedas because The words of the Vedas do not say, "This is our meaning and this is not."[62] The Vedas are ambiguous. So, insofar as Jaimini's text is authoritative, he must have marshalled epistemic resources beyond the text itself. This resembles Hemacandra's appeal to authority: if the *Mīmāṃsāsūtras* are reliable, Jaimini must have had some acute perceptual acumen to have composed them.

Next, Dharmakīrti invokes the argument from ignorance. If, according to the Mīmāṃsaka, we ought to doubt that a Buddhist could have such a perceptual ability, then we must extend the same doubt to Jaimini, in which case we would have to remain agnostic (*anabhiniveśa*) about either's authority. Dharmakīrti thus shares Haribhadrasūri's contentment to leave the matter inconclusive, deeming it "permissible." But if the absence of any contradicting evidence gives us amble reason to trust Jaimini, then we must extend the same charity to Buddhist yogic perceivers. Ostensibly, then, Dharmakīrti would argue, like Audi, that yogic testimony is credible prima facie in the absence of contravening evidence.

It is also worth noting that Dharmakīrti's description of the ability to sense distant objects incorporates themes from *Yogasūtras* 3.25 and 3.16, discussing perception of "those objects that distant in space and time." Despite his earlier quips about remote seeing explored in chapter 1—"If you are concerned with the instruments for remote seeing, come, we will seek out the vultures!"[63]—Dharmakīrti here is more in line with traditional argumentation about yogic perception, agreeing that it affords knowledge not just about the reality of things—a spiritual truth—but also about discrete objects in different times and places.

ŚĀNTARAKṢITA AND KAMALAŚĪLA

Śāntarakṣita (725–788) and Kamalaśīla (740–795) are perhaps best known for introducing scholastic Indian Buddhism into Tibet. Both inherit Dharmakīrti's version of the *reductio.* The twenty-fourth chapter of Śāntarakṣita's *Compilation on Reality* (*Tattvasaṅgraha*) on "The Examination of *Śruti*" (Śrutiparīkṣa), including Kamalaśīla's commentary, contains a lengthy recapitulation of the Mīmāṃsaka argument. The commentary quotes Śabara's definition of dharma directly—"Dharma is that which produces welfare."[64] Kamalaśīla's commentary (*pañjikā*) subsequently summarizes the familiar Mīmāṃsaka argument against yogic perception: "Nor does yogic perception have the scope of supersensible objects (*atīndriya*), since it is perception, just like any other perception, [which only involves the senses]."[65] Because the Mīmāṃsaka considers perception coextensive with the senses, they argue yogic perception cannot be supersensory.

Śāntarakṣita retorts that the possibility of accurate scriptural exegesis necessitates yogic perception:

> *Thus Vedic precepts are not sound epistemic warrants for dharma, since their meaning is unascertainable by those whose faculties are dull, whether oneself or others.*
>
> *Seek out a teacher who can instruct on the different meanings of* śruti*: a man whose inner darkness has been dispelled by the light of gnosis.*[66]

In other words, if there is anyone who understands the Vedas, it must be yogis, who have some direct perceptual insight into their meaning. This mirrors Dharmakīrti's claim that the Vedas are ambiguous, and so one must marshal epistemic instruments outside of the text—that is, yogic insight—to decipher them. Only they "can instruct on the different meanings of *śruti*," or heard revelation. This evinces a skepticism toward scripture: while Bhartṛhari, for example, argued that scripture is infallible because of its yogic source, Śāntarakṣita argues that scriptural meaning is underdetermined and requires yogic intervention for its exegesis. They thus interpret the *reductio* differently.

But the *Compilation on Reality* also gives the more standard *reductio*. Kamalaśīla comments on this verse, "Mīmāṃsakas claim that phenomena, etc., are not understood by the meditative power (*samādhi*) of yogic perception. But this . . . is not the case, given the argument for yogis, as will be proven later."[67] The explanation of yogic perception to which he alludes comes in chapter 26, "The Examination of Those who Have a Vision of Supersensible Objects" (Atīndriyārthadarśiparīkṣā).[68] In that same chapter, Śāntarakṣita again argues supersensible perception is presupposed by scripture:

> *The ability of mudras, mandalas, and mantras to free us from demons and* ḍākinīs *and to neutralize poison, etc., is known supersensibly.*
>
> *If the sages, eagles, etc., did not understand these flawlessly through a direct cognition, without having heard of them or inferring them prior, then how could they relay them to others?*[69]

Again, Śāntarakṣita draws on the epistemological chain to make the *reductio*. Insofar as we have effective religious practices—mudras, mandalas, and mantras—there must have been someone with supersensible abilities who first had insight into their efficacy. Otherwise, we would have no knowledge of them. We also see Śāntarakṣita draw on eagles (*tārkṣya*), to whom Sampāti likened himself in the *Rāmāyaṇa* (see chapter 1), as the classical example of remote seeing. Again, despite Dharmakīrti's reluctance to give such abilities attention, subsequent Buddhist authors seemed compelled to give them some account.

JÑĀNAŚRĪMITRA

These arguments were recapitulated in Buddhist literature up until the sunset of Indian Buddhism's golden age in the twelfth century. In the quote below, Jñānaśrīmitra gives a sophisticated rendering of the argument from ignorance. He states, like his predecessors, that yogic perception has a capacity for remote seeing. His Mīmāṃsaka interlocutor disagrees, arguing that perception is limited to the senses, and the senses do not have such long-range abilities. Jñānaśrīmitra counters,

> It is not acceptable to reject such an ability merely because you have never observed it. [Objection:] *But there is no method to develop such an ability.* [Reply:] Even with regard to [substantiating] the nonexistence of such a method, there is no other means besides nonobservation. Thus, that being the case, there is nothing precluding the accomplishment of this ability.[70]

Jñānaśrīmitra reveals the Mīmāṃsā rejection of yogic perception to be inconclusive. The only means to substantiate the absence of any method to develop yogic perception is a failure to observe it. But failure of observation does not constitute a sound denial, and so it cannot preclude its accomplishment.

Although these texts concern magical, yogic abilities, their arguments are relevant to our general understanding of expert testimony. Insofar that there is *any* authentic testimony about difficult-to-perceive phenomena, experts—yogic or otherwise—must be credible prima facie. Cast into the language of Audi, these authors embrace his "credible-unless-otherwise-indicated" view of justification, along with his epistemological chain criterion for true testimony. And like Audi, they would be suspect of the global requirement, arguing it does not give us sufficient epistemic resources to justifiably believe experts. Still, given that we, normal people are ill-equipped to assess when the epistemological chain obtains, prima facie acceptance now seems *too* permissive. Does being trustworthy (the local requirement) really reduce to the *absence* of reasons for distrust? It seems, intuitively, that there are also positive criteria for the local requirement. We trust experts because we have reason to believe that they *are* experts, not just because they have given us no reason to suspect that they are *not* experts.

We saw a potential solution to this problem during the analysis of Uddyotakara, at least in theory: if we could reproduce the perceptions that lead to some instance of testimony, we could confirm its accuracy, essentially becoming experts ourselves. But as the Indian theories thus far stand, they provide no clear avenue to pursue this reproduction. We know that sound testimony entails first-hand perception down the chain retrospectively. But how do we do this in reverse? How do we acquire the "same" perceptions that lead back up the chain and corroborate that testimony?

The problem lies in determining whether the reproduced and original perceptions are the same. If they are not, then the soundness of a given instance of testimony cannot derive from being a felicitous transmission of a perceptual event, since the epistemological chain should be bidirectional, such that testimony is both derived from and leads to the same perceptual content. On the other hand, we have no resource besides testimony itself to guarantee their sameness. For example, if I say to you, "Turn right on Main Street, go one mile, and you will see a large oak tree on your right," we only know that you saw the "same" oak tree on Main Street based on my testimonial instruction. A perceptual event of seeing an oak tree simpliciter *without* this instruction would be powerless to corroborate my report of an oak tree on Main Street. So two perceptual events need to have the same content to corroborate some testimony, but guaranteeing the sameness of that content requires the guidance of the original testimony. This renders the relationship between testimony and perception hopelessly circular.

This seems to be a weakness of foundationalist formulations. If sound testimony is founded on perception, then there is no surefire way to corroborate that testimony without reproducing its instigating perception. But if that testimony serves as a guide toward that reproduction, then there is no longer a unidirectional relationship between perception and testimony, undercutting the foundationalist's fundamental premise.

A Coherentist Interpretation

Although this circularity may call foundationalism into question, it need not necessarily undermine epistemology. According to a coherentist, this circularity is benign. Testimonial accuracy, in practice, just means the mutual coherence between testimony and perception, in *both* directions. In other words, just as much as a perceptual event authenticates testimony, that testimony in turn warrants what perceptual events count as its authenticator. In practice, this warrant functions through the testifier's instruction of how to recreate the perceptual event, which amounts to imparting expertise—either in yogic meditation or the scientific method.[71]

Coherentism, I argue, is especially important for a theory of epistemic development. Trusting experts is one (meager) way of knowing. Developing expertise is another entirely. Any epistemology that explains the acquisition of expertise requires an account of how we move from mere justified belief in report to stronger, first-hand corroboration. And this requires some sort of coherentist explanation of how testimony does not just transmit perceptual information in one direction, but can guide the learner toward the other, such that they can acquire the specific type of perceptual events that corroborate that testimony in the first place. Because these Indian traditions are invested in spiritual practice, and this practice depends on epistemic development, it is unsurprising that we find their adoption of coherentist frameworks.

Veṅkaṭanātha (aka Vedānta Deśika, ca. 1269–1370) adopts a coherentism of this ilk. Veṅkaṭanātha defended the Viśiṣṭādvaita Vedānta, or "Qualified Nondual Vedānta," view. This tradition was founded by Rāmānujā (ca. 1017–1137), but some scholars argue its roots are found in the works of Yāmuna's (967–1038).[72] Philosophically, it could be considered a compromise between the nondualist and dualist approaches of Śaṅkara (ca. 700–750) and Madhva (1238–1317) respectively, though historically Rāmānujā was only in dialogue with Śaṅkara. Rāmānujā agrees with Śaṅkara's monism—the great spirit of

Brahma is all that exists—but qualifies this nondualism, arguing that monism does not necessitate reality's being homogenous. Even though all reality is Brahma, it is not undifferentiated, and so it can accommodate multiplicity and distinctions.

A thorough Viśiṣṭādvaita Vedānta defense of yogic perception against Mīmāṃsā comes from Veṅkaṭanātha's *Purification of Reasons* (*Nyāyapariśuddhi*). Veṅkaṭanātha was incredibly prolific, composing over a hundred works, and is considered seminal in Vaiṣṇavist thought. His is quite late compared to other texts explored thus far, but it succinctly brings together several of their elements.[73]

Veṅkaṭanātha's indebtedness to Praśtastapāda's formulation of yogic perception is obvious. Like Praśtastapāda, he differentiates it from the normal perception of "those like us." He also divides it into absorbed and unabsorbed types. Veṅkaṭanātha further agrees with Praśtastapāda that only absorbed yogic perception occurs exclusively through the mind. Unabsorbed yogic perception, on the other hand, "occurs through the external sense faculties (*bāhyêndriya*)." Veṅkaṭanātha's definition of yogic perception as able to cognize both distant (*prakṛṣṭa*) and hidden (*adṛṣṭa*) objects may be a reference to *Yogasūtra* 3.25, but this is not conclusive.[74]

Veṅkaṭanātha then discusses the relationship between yogic perception and scripture. His analysis is reminiscent of previous arguments concerning yogic perception's role in spiritual authority.

> Yogic perception's object is dictated by what one desires to know, etc. That object must also be attested in [at least] one scripture. That perception, which arises just from the power of meditation, is directed toward the creator of the world, the superintendent of scripture's source. This is because, otherwise, the commentary writers would just be parroting the sounds of [the root text author] who had had a direct yogic perception, and even by developing yogic perception, which is the root of scriptural knowledge of God, one would have no capacity to produce that state outlined in scripture; there would be no point in it.[75]

Here again we see the recapitulation of the *reductio*. Veṅkaṭanātha argues that scripture is only meaningful insofar as it contains the reports of yogis—specifically, their experience of God. But he adds an interesting twist. While previous authors concur that warranted scripture entails the existence of yogis, Veṅkaṭanātha further argues that scripture is instrumental in reproducing yogic insight. It is only through scriptural attestation that the eventual yogi learns about the experience of the Godhead; and only through that learning do they become interested in developing the state recounted in scripture. Without this potential, commentators would just be parroting the root text; they would have no direct experience that could guide their commentary. The text is thus not only a record of yogic perception but is instrumental in its generation. Put another way, the epistemological chain does not just flow from the yogi to scripture, but from scripture back to the yogi. Veṅkaṭanātha thus trades the unidirectional yogic perceptual warrant of scripture for a hermeneutic circle, arguing the contents of scripture are both the beginning and end of yogic insight.

In the place of foundationalism, Veṅkaṭanātha's formulation thus leans coherentist. We can again think about the scientist to make this point. The fact that the scientist needs to learn how to interpret data proves that perception per se cannot unilaterally support scientific testimony. Otherwise, we could all confirm scientific testimony via our own access to the data. The scientist must initially learn these interpretative methods through the testimony of fellow scientists. Likewise, Veṅkaṭanātha argues that the yogi must learn about how to develop yogic perception as "outlined in scripture." In both instances, perception is as indebted to testimony as testimony is a report of perceptions.

But this coherentist, hermeneutic circle is also open to critique. If testimony both entails and produces perception, then its claims become insular, since it produces its own confirmation. The foundationalist does not have this problem, since they claim perception is self-authenticating, and testimonial authenticity is only derivative of perception. Because the coherentist denies either perception or testimony self-authenticates, insisting their mutual corroboration is sufficient, there is a risk of vicious circularity[76]—even relativism.

Challenges to the Epistemological Chain

I will address the coherentist view of yogic perception with greater detail in chapter 3. But whether coherentist or foundationalist, both views are rooted in some version of assent to the epistemological chain—a circular chain in the case of coherentism. And this chain may have some weak links.

I just identified the potential problem for coherentism: if perception and testimony are chained only to each other, and not anchored in anything else, they are epistemologically adrift. On the other hand, the foundationalist views I have explored anchor testimony's truth in perception. But this leaves justified belief in testimony ambiguous. We can never be certain that an instance of yogic testimony is knowledge yielding; we only know that we are not wrong prima facie for believing it.

We might be fine, then, with accepting testimony as fallible and revisable. This may be sufficient for our everyday epistemic needs. But it would seem to fail as a standard for *religious* testimony, which is supposed to be apodictic and unassailable. Yet some Indian thinkers double down on testimony's shortcomings in this regard. They contend that normal people *only* ever have justified beliefs about metaphysical truths—never actual knowledge. This is because testimony can only provide an approximation. And that testimony is constantly revisable as the lay learner gains expertise and increased firsthand experience. (Indeed, Haribhadrasūri made such an argument earlier in this chapter.)

We do not need to appeal to yogic mysticism to explain this mismatch between testimonial and perceptual knowledge. Scientific education involves the same issue. Consider, for example, lay explanations of Albert Einstein's general theory of relativity—that mass curves space-time. Science educators often analogize this to a ball being placed on a rubber sheet, such that it depresses the sheet. When other balls roll on the sheet, their paths curve. So too, the analogy goes, do massive objects curve space-time, affecting the trajectories of other objects. Now, this analogy falls short for several reasons. First, the curvature of space-time does not only occur in one plane like a sheet. It is four-dimensional. Second, space-time is not some membrane that objects move through. Rather, space-time is a geometrical representation of how objects move over time.[77]

So, testimonial accounts given to the nonexpert are often incomplete and fallible. But they are increasingly refined for the lay learner as they approach expertise. This means that testimony and perception are not merely different procedures to acquire the same piece of knowledge, but epistemically distinct. The former may be only partially true, albeit instrumental toward gaining further expertise. Thus, believing it is justified. Only the latter is wholly true, and thus epistemically complete. The authors discussed in this section similarly argue that there is an unbridgeable disconnect between testimonial belief and perceptual knowledge. They therefore problematize the epistemological chain, denying testimony's transparency to perceptual knowledge.

Candrakīrti

This will become clearer from an example. Buddhist texts often analogize yogic perception to another meditative ability: to see the world as if full of bones. The meditator literally *sees* bones everywhere. Meditation on bones or "repulsiveness" (*aśubha*) is an ancient Buddhist practice, extending back to the Pāli Suttas[78] and is discussed in detail by Vasubandhu[79] and Buddhaghoṣa.[80] By making this meditation vivid, the meditator not only develops meditative acumen but disgust with the world, inspiring renunciation and the pursuit of the Buddhist path. Yogic perception is said to work via a similar meditative mechanism and result in the same vividness, so vivid that it is indistinguishable from a perception.[81] The question, then, is whether these vivid appearances refer to actual objects. Are they the apparitions of a powerful imagination, or real?

Candrakīrti (ca. 600–650) is one of the earliest Buddhist philosophers to examine this question in detail in his *Introduction to the Middle Way* (*Madhyamakāvatāra*). His position is revealing about the distinction between subjective and intersubjective truth. He argues that while these bones are real from the perspective of the individual, they are not real communal objects. Though this seems paradoxical, Candrakīrti argues that it must be the case. If the bones were communal, then the yogi's meditation should affect everyone—"the vision of skeletons, etc., would arise to the non-yogi and yogi alike."[82] If, on the other hand, the bones were not real for the meditator, then their appearance to the meditator would have no corresponding external object.

This second consequence does not initially seem problematic—indeed, we normally think of hallucinations as appearances without referent objects. But Candrakīrti recognizes that his opponent, Buddhist Yogācāra idealists (*cittamātra, vijñaptimātra*), argue that if we concede *some* mental events, like hallucinations, with no corresponding object, then it is conceivable that *every* cognition is objectless (see chapter 3). Regardless of whether this is a slippery slope argument, Candrakīrti takes no chances. He counters, therefore, that *all* cognitions must have corresponding external objects. If this were not the case and all phenomena were purely mental events, then the appearances of bones would be just as "real" as any other bones and, therefore, just as communal. Counterintuitively, then, Candrakīrti argues that the only way we can make sense of the private, vivid appearance of bones is to conclude that those appearances have referents for those to whom they appear, but do not for the larger community, to whom they do not.[83]

Candrakīrti thus gives an analogy for the meditated bones, saying they are like eye floaters, what the Indian tradition calls "hairs" (**keśa*). These are understood to be the product of an eye disease (*timira*). Floaters only appear to persons who have the eye disease. People with otherwise healthy eyes do not see hairs tumbling in the world. Therefore, Candrakīrti argues, "Both [the hairs and consciousness of them] are real for a consciousness with an eye disease. For one who sees clearly without an eye disease, both are unreal."[84] Candrakīrti further claims that this is "just like" hungry ghosts (*preta*)—beings who, because of their poor karma, experience pus and blood wherever humans see clean water, such as in a waterfall or river.[85] This example becomes pertinent in chapter 5.

We can appreciate how Candrakīrti's theory of idiosyncratic (yet warranted) perception disrupts the epistemological chain. Suppose I say, "I have floaters." What can Pam, who has never had floaters, do with this testimony? She cannot meet the global requirement—she does not have any analogous observations. We might then invoke the argument from ignorance and contend that she is justified in believing me, there being no evidence to the contrary. But what, exactly, would she have a belief in? Floaters are so foreign to Pam's experience that it is unclear if she could even understand what I was talking about, let alone believe me. Unless she has had floaters herself, my saying "I see hairs everywhere" will not fully communicate the experience.[86]

Candrakīrti's view of yogic perception is much like the state of seeing floaters. When yogis use their meditative prowess to perceive reality as it is (*tattva*), their insight cannot be transmitted through testimony—the audience simply does not have the requisite experience for that communication to mean something. According to Candrakīrti, this is because normal people make sense of the world via conceptual distinctions, while yogis perceive reality without conceptual overlay. He writes in his *Clear Words* (*Prasannapadā*):

"The yogi, who sees reality as it is, cannot make any conceptual designations with forms (*rūpa*) as their basis, such as it its being the opposite of something or not, indicating something or not, being in the past or in the future, or being blue or yellow."[87]

In other words, while testimony and communally shared knowledge depend on linguistic designations, yogic realization transcends these strictures. So, even though yogis "teach others about reality through conceptual distinctions (*samāropa*), the nonyogis (*anārya*) will not understand the nature of that reality through those concepts alone." In an intriguing inversion of the floating hair analogy, Candrakīrti goes on to say that it is as if the greater community has the eye disease and it is only the yogi that sees clearly.[88] In either case, whatever is not communally perceived cannot be transmittable through testimony. Candrakīrti thus appeals to a shared body of conventions (*vyavahāra*) that dictate what types of perceptions testimony can communicate—namely, perception of those things that are commonly observable through linguistic categories.[89]

Hume similarly rejects any testimony that does not conform to (communally) observable facts. Candrakīrti and Hume's reasoning is the same: such events simply do not meet the global requirement. Because those perceptions are idiosyncratic, they cannot serve as a basis of intersubjective knowledge, or warranted testimony. But in place of the foundationalist epistemological chain—according to which perception determines what testimony is knowledge yielding—Candrakīrti's epistemology is thus strongly coherentist, where conventions for sound testimony determine what types of perception may warrant communal knowledge.

But Candrakīrti is distinct from the stereotypical coherentist in one key respect. It is only *conventional* truth (*saṃvṛti-satya*) that is so bound by coherence with conventions. While conventional knowledge must be communal, yogic knowledge is ultimately individual, like the perception of bones and floaters.[90] And this is by design, since yogic perception *transcends* the strictures of conventional knowledge, reaching *ultimate* truth (*paramārtha-satya*). Candrakīrti's accommodation of these two truths (*dvaya-satya*) marks his "Middle Way" (*madhyamaka*) philosophy.

Candrakīrti's argument is thus vastly different than Veṅkaṭanātha's, who sought to show how yogic perception coheres with communal scripture. Candrakīrti, by contrast, argues that whatever can be communally communicated through scripture only represents yogic perception through a glass darkly.[91] This effectively cuts the epistemological chain between scripture and yogic perception. We can only ever understand yogic insights through becoming yogis ourselves, through catching the right eye disease, as it were.

Utpaladeva and Abhinavagupta

Other Indian thinkers beside Candrakīrti also question whether all reports of warranted perceptions are invariably instances of warranted testimony. Interestingly, the following example makes this conclusion from the opposite of Candrakīrti's premise about yogic perception. Candrakīrti argues that appearances in yogic perception are private, but Utpaladeva (900–950) and Abhinavagupta (950–1016) argue that they are shared and observable by others. Utpaladeva and Abhinavagupta are perhaps the most seminal figures of Kashmir Shaivism and incredibly informative for all later codified systems of Tantric practice. They portray yogic perception as an outlier case to the authenticity of inference and testimony. This again effectively breaks the epistemological chain, since reports about veritable yogic perceptions can lead to unsound testimony.

In contrast to Candrakīrti, Utpaladeva describes yogic perception as a type of "emanation" (*nirmāṇa*) that everyone can perceive. In other words, according to Utpaladeva, a powerful yogi meditating on the world as full of bones would create a world full of bones for everyone! But if a yogi can create objects through meditation, this hinders our ability to make reasoned assessments about the world. For example, the classic Indian example of an inference is the deduction of fire from smoke. The ability to make this inference depends on a certain causal regularity. My certainty that fire is present when I see smoke depends on the fact that *only* fire produces smoke. But if the yogi can produce communally observable smoke without fire, just through emanation, then this breaks our inferential capacity.

Abhinavagupta's solution is to treat yogic emanations as an outlier case. Only "if it is determined by some other epistemic instrument according to worldly consensus that an effect is *not* of a yogi's creation" can inferences based on cause and effect or token and type hold, "not otherwise." Furthermore, worldly consensus "is the seed for knowledge had by testimony and inference."[92] Like Candrakīrti, Abhinavagupta thus appeals to communally established conventions to preclude certain types of perceptual events from testimonial consideration. Thus, if I see smoke in the distance and attest to the presence of fire, it is only by convention that we exclude yogic emanations and deem this testimony sound. The possibility of yogic perception renders all inference defeasible, but sufficient for our "quotidian" needs.

Although Abhinavagupta's solution is prompted by the consideration of magical, yogic powers, his point is applicable to our modern epistemological concerns. We can consider, for example, how Newtonian physics is equally defeasible, since general relativity does not always accord with its conclusions. Nevertheless, barring such outlier cases, Newtonian reasoning is incredibly useful at making predictions about the motion of large bodies.[93] This is slightly different than the case of scientific education about general relativity explored in the section on Candrakīrti. There, the issue was testimony's general paucity for communicating the conclusions of first-hand experimentation. There is always a gulf between the scientist's "experience" and the communication of that experience to others. In this section, the issue is not an experiential disconnect. Rather, it is a heuristic concern about which explanatory model we want to use based on the margin of error that we are willing to tolerate.

This difference maps onto a comparison of approaches by Candrakīrti, on the one hand, and Utpaladeva and Abhinavagupta on the other. Because Candrakīrti argues that there can be veritable perceptual events which are completely private, these events can never serve as a testimonial warrant. Utpaladeva and Abhinavagupta, however, do not contend that these events are private. Instead, they develop parameters for the reasonable exclusion of these (communally observable) outlier cases—much like accounting for a margin of error. But all three thinkers agree that conventions are crucial in making these demarcations. Thus, in both theories, warranted testimony cannot reduce to a perceptual event simpliciter, since some such events are excluded from consideration by convention, either because they are private or because they are outliers. These theories thus reject the epistemological chain.

Also like Candrakīrti, Utpaladeva and Abhinavagupta are not concerned *just* with conventional knowledge. Abhinavagupta argues that true insight is to be had outside of communal knowledge.

> Other logicians (*yauktika*) have considered real entities to be the object of normal perception, which accords with yogic perception, toward the apprehension of all objects. But whether there are conventional (*sāmvyavahārika*) authentic epistemic warrants is not our burden. Only our own godly form is the matter at hand, just that self-luminosity, which is unhindered, even given the obstacle of epistemic objects.[94]

Abhinavagupta refers to "logicians" who appear to subscribe to the epistemological chain. According to them, perception conforms with percepts, real objects whose cognition is the basis for sound inference and testimony. But like Candrakīrti, Abhinavagupta claims true insight breaks with the conventional, where one realizes their own "godly" and "self-luminous form." He is thus ultimately unconcerned with whether sound reasoning conforms with observable facts, for what is ultimately real is beyond what we currently observe. He concedes a certain coherentism for our daily needs, where conventions and observations work in tandem. But he agrees with Candrakīrti that true understanding lies outside of this coherentist triad between perception, inference, and testimony. Complete insight is outside these strictures, its link to testifiable phenomena severed.

Conclusion: Scientists and Yogis

Most of the authors I discuss in this chapter, however, understand yogic perception as fundamental to credible scriptural testimony. This point is consistently leveled against those of the Mīmāṃsā tradition, who, by contrast, argue that Vedic scriptural authority exists independent of any foundational perception had by humans. The Mīmāṃsaka makes this point by arguing that perception is limited to the senses, while the Vedas concern supersensible (*atīndriya*) phenomena. Despite the Mīmāṃsā assent to the supernatural, in many ways they are simpatico with Hume's empiricism here, which equally argues that testimony must globally conform to observable facts—namely, those things I can now perceive. Nevertheless, the Mīmāṃsaka takes the existence of the miraculous as axiomatic. Thus, this can only be substantiated by nonhuman, Vedic testimony, which transcends what is observable—the supersensible (*atīndriya*).

Opponents to Mīmāṃsā argue this position is incoherent. Any warranted testimony must transmit *some* perception. Naiyāyikas and Vaiśeṣikas therefore argue that, insofar as there is knowledge of supersensible phenomena, perception cannot be limited to the senses. This is the argument from perceptibility. As supersensory perception par excellence, yogic perception is the foundation of scriptural testimony. But how do we *know* that a given testimony transmits a yogic perception? Because yogis are "not like us," we have no analogous observations that would justify our assent to their claims. This critique resembles criticisms against Hume's global requirement.

Audi thus argues that there is no such global requirement for justified belief in testimony. A conformity to observable facts may be necessary to establish some testimony as *true*. But justified belief is another issue. The authors in this chapter offer two main arguments paralleling Audi here. The first was the argument from ignorance. This is similar to Audi's "credible-unless-otherwise-indicated view of testimony."[95] That is, because the Mīmāṃsaka cannot marshal definitive proof that yogis do not exist, we must provisionally accept yogic testimony. We saw Hemacandra, Haribhadrasūri, and Dharmakīrti all make this point. Hemacandra, in particular, defends it most strongly; in place of agnosticism, he insists that the argument from ignorance entails an outright proof of yogis' existence. Dharmakīrti is more circumspect, arguing that the opponent can only at best say the matter is inconclusive (*anabhiniveśa*). Jñānaśrīmitra used the argument from ignorance toward the same end, arguing that nonobservation of yogis is not conclusive of their nonexistence.

As I have mentioned, however, this argument is not sufficient to make the case. Śabara also argues that belief in scriptural testimony is justifiable prima facie. If such an argument holds for yogis, it should hold for the Vedas, all things being equal. This would render yogic perception superfluous. In addition to the argument from ignorance, defenders of yogic perception therefore also contend that veridical scripture must be epistemologically chained to perception, a point also made by Audi.

This is the second argument, the *reductio*: if we could not believe yogis, there would be no authentic scripture. Bhartṛhari thus states that yogic perception is primary to other epistemic instruments. As a foundationalist, he argues that testimony and inference depend on perception. As such, neither testimony nor inference can bring yogic perception into doubt. Hemacandra and Dharmakīrti further argue that yogic perception is also necessary for accurate scriptural exegesis, since the text's meaning is always underdetermined. Śāntarakṣita and Kamalaśīla corroborate this point. Veṅkaṭanātha even argues that scripture is instrumental in developing yogic perception. Thus, on his account, yogic perception and scripture create a closed, coherentist loop, where neither can function without the other.

Not all authors invoked the epistemological chain, however. We saw Candrakīrti, Utpaladeva, and Abhinavagupta deny that testimony is transmissive of perceptual knowledge. Instead, the conditions for sound testimony preclude certain perceptions by convention. This is necessary for everyday reasoning. If conventions accommodated every perceptual event, they would be impotent to serve our intersubjective needs. Candrakīrti argues that individual perceptions can be warranted even though their reports are not intersubjectively true. Utpaladeva and Abhinavagupta, on the other hand, argue that yogic perception introduces communally shared yet inference-breaking phenomena. These must be excluded conventionally through epistemic instruments. More than this, these authors agree that the content of spiritual insight lays outside of what is conventionally attestable. Thus, yogic perception cannot anchor an epistemological chain that serves as a foundation for testimony, whose warrant is determined by these conventions.

Even though these arguments concern the fanciful world of yogis and magical perceptual abilities, I argue throughout that this discussion has modern-day relevance. How, for example, do we normal folk trust the scientist when we cannot confirm their knowledge? The arguments by *reductio* and from ignorance have some pull here. I, the layperson, have insufficient resources to meet the global requirement for justified belief in scientific testimony. Ostensibly, as we have seen, I could test expert testimony by becoming an expert myself. Still, this cannot serve as a justification a priori, since, as nonexperts, we cannot predict what our future expertise might lead us to conclude. And we cannot be experts in everything.

Yet, if based on this uncertainty I were to distrust the scientist, I could not reasonably follow the advice of scientific institutions. I would not take medicines prescribed by my doctor, get in cars built by engineers, or buy microwave ovens that physicists have told me are safe. This would be an absurd way to live. And so, I must conclude that my prima facie trust in expert testimony is justified. Likewise, concerning the argument from ignorance, it is not a good reason to distrust scientists just because I cannot come to apodictic certainty that they are correct. The absence of definitive proof of their correctness does not warrant my disbelief.

Still, we face a difficult problem: How do we reasonably judge who is an expert? We need some expertise to do so. Yet at which point do we have sufficient expertise to make such judgments, but still insufficient expertise such that relying on testimony remains necessary and retains some epistemic role? Answering these questions would require a more detailed analysis, with wide-ranging social and political implications.

Even if a foundationalist approach does not perfectly resolve these issues, the bulk of the authors in this chapter invoke it to substantiate testimony's epistemic value, relying on the epistemological chain. Veṅkaṭanātha, on the other hand, argued a form of coherentism. On his view, yogic perception does not have a unilateral relationship to testimony. Each is generative of the other. Yogic perception gives rise to authoritative scripture and this scripture helps develop future yogis. This epistemological feedback loop is a central theme of chapter 3.

PART TWO

Indian Buddhism and Phenomenology

THREE

Pragmatism and Coherentism

Introduction: Peirce and Inference

Most of the authors considered in chapter 2 invoke some form of the epistemological chain in their arguments. While perception is self-authenticating, the authenticity of inference and testimony is derivative. Thus, they contend that the authority of authentic scripture reduces to some perceptual event—namely, yogic perception. This view is therefore foundationalist. Put another way, the dependency between perception and the other epistemic instruments is asymmetrical. And so, as Bhartṛhari claimed, even logical inference cannot "overturn" sound perceptual reports. This is why yogic perception is so important in these traditions, since it secures their epistemological bedrock.

I use the term "forward direction" to describe the notion that yogic perception is the foundational warrant for spiritual claims. In this case, the warrant for scriptural authority flows from yogic perception to inference and testimony. But the epistemic flow can also happen in the reverse direction. As Veṅkaṭanātha also claimed, prior to yogic practice, the yogi's meditative object must "be established in scripture." Here, scripture is not just a record of yogic perception. It also instructs the yogi about how to recreate these insights. I dub this "the reverse direction," where scriptural testimony marks the starting point of yogic cultivation. This becomes an important theme in the Buddhist theories I examine in this chapter.

These two directions do not just connect perception and testimony. According to the Buddhists I discuss, it also concerns the connection between perception and *conception*. Testimony and inference are conceptual enterprises. When we hear words or reason about things, we do so via concepts. This is different than seeing something directly. Candrakīrti touched on this distinction in chapter 2, arguing that yogic perceptions cannot be communicated via linguistic conceptions. All Buddhists likewise argue some form of epistemic *disconnect* between perception and conception.[1] Thus, explaining the directional connection between perception and conception despite their epistemic incongruity becomes a challenge for Buddhist authors.[2]

It is also a challenge for Euro-American epistemologists. In the following sections I demonstrate parallels between how thinkers within this and the Indian Buddhist tradition approach this divide. The Euro-American tradition, however, mainly examines this issue from the "forward direction" point of view. And this is an oversight, since a wealth of psychological research demonstrates that conceptualization can *generate* perceptual information as much as it can manipulate such information post facto.[3] Because discourse on yogic perception forces us to consider this generation in the reverse direction, its exploration provides a unique perspective on the nature of perceptual-conceptual epistemic disconnect. As I suggested in chapter 3, the results of this analysis will reveal a coherentist solution, one with affinities to that of Wilfrid Sellars (1912–1989).

On the Indian side, I focus on the thought of Dignāga (ca. 480–540) and his Buddhist lineage, especially Dharmakīrti (fl. sixth or seventh century). These thinkers most commonly distinguish the object of conception from that of perception. The former cognizes universals (*sāmānya*) and the latter, particulars (*svalakṣaṇa*). When I look at something and think that it is a table, I recognize something universal to all tables. According to Buddhists, this recognition does not grasp some essence about the table itself. Rather, it is a mentally concocted concept that my mind applies to objects that seem to me to function as tables. There are thus no tables per se out there in the world. A table is just a projected idea, a concept, a universal. All that is actually there, these Buddhists argue, are atoms buzzing about, individually taking up no space and only lasting for a moment. These momentary, infinitesimal atoms are particulars—all that exist. Although we perceive particulars in the first instant that we look at something, we immediately conceptualize them as universal objects in the next. Thus, this conceptualization is not only responsible for our sense that this is one table among many (a token of a type), but also that it is a singular "thing" with spatial and temporal extension (a mereological whole). Most of our experience, therefore, appears populated with universals. But this is only a result of thinking, not of universals' being in the world.[4]

If this is the case, then we can appreciate how our thinking can quickly get us into epistemological trouble. The space of ideas is much vaster than that of real things. What, then, differentiates fanciful conceptual projections from those that are warranted? Bertrand Russell (1872–1970) gives an intuitive answer. Concepts that can be confirmed by perception are true. Thus, conceptual belief "is true when there is a corresponding fact and is false when there is no corresponding fact."[5] Facts in turn are "given in perception and memory."[6] In other words, it is our perception that determines which of our concepts accurately map onto reality. If I look at a table and think it's a unicorn, I am wrong because the matters of fact given in perception do not suggest a unicorn.

But this still leaves an important question unanswered. Russell notes that perception warrants conceptual universals because within it "matters of fact" are "given." What does it mean for perception to give matters of fact? Sense-data theorists argue that perception gives us only pointillist information about the world. While we perceive patches of blue, amplitudes of sound waves, or instances of roughness or smoothness, knowledge of common-sense objects are conceptually constructed after the fact. Alfred J. Ayer (1910–1989) thus argued that even medium-sized dry goods—tables, chairs, coffee cups, books, and so on—are inferred, not directly perceived.[7] Thus, though the table as a whole is not given in perception, information about certain contours, surfaces, and colors are. This is sufficient to warrant my thought of its being a table over its being a unicorn. Certain combinations of sense data warrant some conceptual projections over others.

Russell and Ayer here describe a type of representative realism, where concepts represent and thus map onto perceived particulars. A similar solution is adopted by some later Tibetan thinkers, particularly those explored in chapter 5. But we might ask if this an accurate description of our experience. When I look at a table, I don't recall seeing contours, surfaces, and colors first and then thinking, "Ah, a table!" I just see a table. If sense data is what is given in perception, and, as Russell states, facts are "given in perception and memory," then shouldn't I *remember* seeing sense data before thinking it is a table? This does not seem to be the case. As Charles Peirce (1839–1914) notes, our perception of objects "comes to us like a flash." Peirce therefore argues that our recognition of objects is not a normal type of inference, like inferring fire from smoke. Rather, it is a kind of abductive inference that is "subconscious." This abductive process spontaneously turns our initial perception into a judgment about what an object is. But we have no conscious awareness of this process, as we do with the process of normal inference.

Furthermore, because the process is abductive—based on heuristics rather than ironclad deduction—it is not apodictic. Abductive judgments are sufficient for navigating our world but do not provide epistemic certainty. Thus, as Peirce notes, they are "extremely fallible."[8] Even cognitions of sense data are abductive. For example, if I really concentrate, I might start to see the table as contours, surfaces, and colors without projecting "table." Indeed, artists seem to suspend certain judgments about what objects are to capture their features more accurately. Such a process, Peirce would argue, does not capture what is "really there." Rather, it evinces training in another type of abductive process, one that renders perceptual input as sense data instead of as medium-sized dry goods. But it is equally fallible and ad hoc. Seeing red is just as conceptual and no more basic than seeing a full table.[9]

The important difference between Ayer and Peirce, then, is whether we have perceptual knowledge. Ayer says yes. We infer objects from our perceptual knowledge of sense data. Peirce says no. We never have perceptual knowledge. Awareness only ever occurs at the end of the abductive process, at which point sensory information has been transmuted into the cognition of a universal, as per Dignāga's definition.[10] According to Peirce, awareness only happens at the level of conceptual thinking.

How does Dignāga, then, understand perception? Some interpretations suggest that he shares affinities with Ayer. For example, Dan Arnold notes that Dignāga and Dharmakīrti advocate "'aspects' or 'images' (*ākāra*) comparable to the 'sense data' of the classical British empiricists" and thus were "represented by doxographers not as direct realists, but as 'proponents of the doctrine that external objects can only be inferred.'"[11] This seems to suggest Ayer's picture, where sense data is perceived and objects are inferred.

But other sections of Dignāga's works suggest Peirce's formulation. For example, he argues that "one apprehends color, or the like, through both the particular, which is ineffable (*avyapadeśya*), and a color, which is a universal."[12] In contrast to Ayer, seeing color is not epistemologically fundamental, but the result of both perceptual and conceptual processes. Also, in line with Peirce, the perceptual component is subconscious, exactly because the perceived particular is ineffable. Just as Peirce says that "abductive inference shades into perceptual judgment without any sharp line of demarcation between them,"[13] Dignāga argues that we cannot have conscious access to the perceptual process that undergirds our recognition,[14] even of colors as colors.

If perception is subconscious, however, then we have now lost any epistemic resource to determine which conceptual projections are felicitous. Russell argued that it was perceptual matters of fact that determine which concepts are applicable to which perceptual cases. But Dignāga and Peirce argue that we have no access to perceptual facts, no perceptual knowledge. Even worse than being fallible, how do we know that our abductive judgments are *ever* sound without access to the perceptual matters of fact that initiate them? This becomes a point of attack by the Nyāya school, particularly Uddyotakara (ca. sixth century), against Dignāga.[15] If the particular is completely ineffable, how can it warrant our conceptual knowledge? Dharmakīrti answers pragmatically. Conceptual thinking simply seems to work. Although universals are mental concoctions that do not inhere in the world, thinking with them is effective. The idea of a chair is good enough to help me find something to sit on. Dharmakīrti's pragmatism thus reflects Peirce's theory of fallibilist abduction, noting that our conceptual judgments are the product of habits of thought,[16] which are effective even if they are not accurate.

Peirce, Dignāga, and Dharmakīrti thus seem largely kindred spirits. Peirce argues that because perceptual information eventually arrives in consciousness via abductive processes, the culminating judgments are always fallible. Nevertheless, that abduction remains effective because it is always revisable. Likewise, Dignāga and Dharmakīrti argue the cognition of conceptual universals is mistaken (*bhrānti*), since conceptual processes occlude particulars, the only things that truly exist.[17] Like Pierce's abductive processes, conceptualization manipulates perceptual information about reality, such that by the time it enters our awareness, it is always-already construed into universals. Nevertheless, cognition via universals is still informative (*avi/saṃvāda*), since that conceptualization is by and large effective at achieving desired ends (*arthakriyā*).[18] Dharmakīrti thus cautions that as soon as we use thinking to make claims about reality per se, we have overstepped its utility.

This solution is thus largely an appeal to a black box. We can talk about the outputs of conceptual judgments but can say nothing about the reality that undergirds them.[19] Although perhaps unnerving, this perfectly serves our quotidian epistemic needs. Pragmatically, we don't need access to these inputs as long as the outputs behave as expected. It is like ordering at a restaurant. I just need to know which words on the menu will bring me which foods. I don't need to know how the chef—like the abductive manipulations of perception—converts the ingredients out there in the world into the food I experience.

But Dharmkīrti does not only discuss the forward direction—from ingredient to plate, as it were—the pragmatic conceptualization of perceptual input. Yogic perception is supposed to work in the reverse direction. This is because Buddhists understand yogic perception as the result of repeated meditation on a concept until that cognition flips over into a perception. In other words, through intense, meditative focus on the conceptual end-product, it is possible to reverse engineer that concept back to its perceptual basis, resulting in yogic perception. In other words, we should be able to trace back the epistemological chain and perceive the perceptual inputs that make up the concept upon which we are meditating. This would be akin to the ability to decipher the ingredients from the name of the dish on the menu.

But this possibility would seem to break Dharmakīrti's black box solution. If perception is ineffable, then what benefit could there be in such a reversal? How could yogic perception be knowledge producing if there is no perceptual knowledge? Furthermore, Buddhists claim that conceptual universals, the end product of the abductive process, grossly mispresent the world, erasing the perception of momentary and infinitesimal atoms for what appear to be objects that take up time and space with abstract properties that appear repeatable over several instances. How, then, could a mistaken concept be a starting point for a warranted perception? There is thus both an epistemological and ontological component to the conundrum. Concerning the first, the question is how yogic perception can be knowledge producing if perception occurs below the level of awareness. Concerning the second, the question is to what degree reality conforms to conceptualization, such that whatever appears to the yogi after having meditated on a universal represents a real object.

Yogic perception therefore becomes an intriguing test case for Dharmakīrti's pragmatism. While this pragmatism is predicated on the forward direction, where conceptual universals are the end products of ineffable processes, yogic perception forces the reverse, with universals being the starting point for the development of perceptual knowledge. The reverse direction threatens to weaken Buddhist epistemology and ontology: that perception is ineffable and that universals are fictitious constructions both seem at odds with the notion of yogic perceptual knowledge. This issue informs a central point of debate between Buddhists and their opponents. It also has larger ramifications for how we should understand the relationship between perception and conception generally.

Before beginning this in-depth analysis, I provide some necessary background and a brief discussion of the development of yogic perceptual theory within the Buddhist tradition.

The Buddhist Theory of Yogic Perception

Pāli Precursors

Although different Buddhist traditions have different theories about the content of liberative insight, there is ubiquitous agreement that direct insight is soteriologically necessary. It is often described as a type of "seeing" (*darśana*) that transcends mere intellectual understanding. Indeed, direct seeing becomes the defining feature of yogic perception when it is first defined by Dignāga in the sixth century. But even before the moniker "yogic perception" was used to describe this state, the necessity of direct insight was longstanding in Buddhism—an idea as old as the tradition itself, traceable back to the earliest Pāli *suttas*.

The *suttas* contained in the Pāli canon were undoubtedly instrumental in yogic perception's intellectual development. The *suttas* are rife with conversion narratives that extol direct insight as a superior feature of the Buddhist religion. One such story concerns the Brahman Kūṭadanta. Knowing the Buddha to be learned, Kūṭadanta requests Gautama to instruct him on the proper way to perform a sacrifice. Kūṭadanta's plan is to perform a sacrifice according to well-known Vedic customs, including the slaughter of several livestock. Instead, the Buddha suggests examples of increasingly more profitable forms of sacrifice, starting with replacing live sacrifices with vegetarian offerings and continuing with making these offerings to Buddhist arhats[20] directly.

The highest form of "sacrifice," however is to become an arhat oneself, such that "having realized the clairvoyant forms of knowledge oneself, one teaches" (Pāli *sayaṃ abhiññā sacchikatvā pavedeti*). This stock phrase occurs some thirty-six times in the *sutta* canon. Interestingly, it is usually used as an epithet for the Buddha—"the one who teaches having realized the clairvoyant forms of knowledge himself."[21] Here, however, it is used prescriptively. Thus, in lieu of following Vedic injunctions for sacrifices that will ensure a higher rebirth, the Buddha implores the Brahman Kūṭadanta to realize the truth for himself and be liberated from rebirth altogether.

Kūṭadanta's response is predictably zealous. He promises not only to abstain from sacrificing the animals, but to build them safe refuge and to strive for liberation. After this conversion, the Buddha gives him a teaching on the Four Noble Truths,[22] leading to his subsequent realization.

> Just like a clean cloth free of stain may take to dye perfectly, so too did the stainless and clear dharma eye arise to the Brahman Kūṭadanta in his seat thereby, as he realized, "Whatever arises also ceases." Then, the Brahman Kūṭadanta became someone who saw the dharma, who attained the dharma, who found the dharma, who penetrated the dharma, whose doubt was deflated, whose uncertainty disappeared, who gained confidence, and who need not rely on others to understand the Master's teaching.[23]

Kūṭadanta's conversion narrative suggests he transitions from an intellectual understanding of the Four Noble Truths to their direct understanding. The way this direct realization is described employs several tropes that are repeated throughout Pāli literature. The last line describes those "who need not rely on others to understand the Master's teaching" (Pāli *aparappaccayo satthusāsane*). This is part of another stock phrase that occurs ten times in the *sutta* canon and is usually reserved for those disciples who gain a direct realization of the Buddha's teaching. It is also most often associated (as it is here) with the "dharma eye" (Pāli *dhamma-cakkhu*), suggesting a direct perception of the dharma over and above mere intellectual comprehension.

This insight became codified in the *suttas* as attaining "Stream Entry" (Pāli *sotāpanna*), because entering the stream will inevitably lead to liberation. Stream Entry is described as a "path" (Pāli *sotāpatti-magga*) attained through "seeing" (Pāli *dassana*).[24] Visionary analogies for Stream Entry are myriad in Pāli texts. It is also achieved through the dharma eye and involves direct insight into the Four Noble Truths.[25] Attaining stream entry earns one the title "Noble One" (Pāli *ariya*). Like Kūṭadanta's insight, Stream Entry also entails no longer doubting the teachings or having to rely on the Buddha's spiritual instructions, having directly understood their truth for oneself.[26]

Later explanations of yogic perception employ many of these same tropes subsumed under the dharma eye: direct realization, no longer relying on a teacher, becoming a Noble One, and gaining a type of vision that graduates one to a new path. We saw in chapter 1 that the supersensory abilities attributed to yogic perception, such as remote seeing, derived from descriptions of the *divine* eye (*dibba-cakkhu*). It seems in later Buddhist literature that yogic perception came to encompass *both* of these functions: the remote seeing of the divine eye as well as the spiritual insight of the dharma eye.[27] This will become clear as we proceed.

Vasubandhu and Asaṅga

The notion of stream entry undoubtedly informed what came to be known in later texts as the "Path of Seeing" (*darśana-mārga*). Asaṅga (fl. fourth century) and his brother, Vasubandhu (fl. fourth to fifth centuries), were largely responsible for systemizing a theory of spiritual progression that centered the Path of Seeing as an important milestone. The founders of the Yogācāra tradition, Asaṅga and Vasubandhu, were likely influenced by the sutras recorded in the Pāli canon, either directly or indirectly, perhaps in the form of their Sanskrit recension, the *Āgamas*. The Path of Seeing is, like Stream Entry, an equally pivotal point in the adherent's progression.

Vasubandhu's *Treasury of Higher Knowledge* (*Abhidharmakośa*) gives perhaps the most detailed exposition of both how to achieve the Path of Seeing and what its realization entails. It is his formulation that is most influential for the texts I cover in this book.[28] He argues that one directly realizes the Four Noble Truths on the Path of Seeing. This appears similar to the path of Stream Entry, where one also realizes the Four Noble Truths. Also like the path of Stream Entry, the Path of Seeing culminates in becoming a Noble One (Pāli *ariya*, Skt. *ārya*).[29] Upon becoming a Noble One, eventual success in gaining nirvana is assured.

Asaṅga makes clear that it is through yogic meditation that one achieves the Path of Seeing. He further stipulates that this meditative feat occurs through the cultivation of both concentration (*śamatha*) and insight (*vipaśyanā*). These are two facets of meditative ability in the Buddhist tradition. The first is the ability to fix the mind on a meditative object with clarity, stability, and duration. The second is to analyze that object with acute discernment. Asaṅga describes a meditative method with these two in tandem that occurs in three steps: (1) questioning the reality of external objects, such that one concludes only the mind exists (*vijñaptimātra*); (2) questioning the reality of the mind itself, such that the reality of the mind comes into doubt; and (3) using this discursive analysis to transcend subject-object duality. What is the culminating realization? There is no fundamental building block to phenomena, neither subjectively nor objectively.[30]

Asaṅga discusses these three steps in his *Collection of Mahāyāna* (*Mahāyānasaṃgraha*).[31] Addressing step 1, he explains that through its meditative contemplation, one gains the first stage on the Path of Seeing. "The bodhisattva[32] engages with the characteristics of these knowable objects as if they were mind only." The meditator realizes that everything that appears to them—sights, sounds, tastes, and so on—are always-already mental. They contemplate the fact that one never has any access to nonmental objects outside awareness. Perhaps, then, *nothing* exists outside awareness.

When the meditator directly realizes this possibility—when they "see" it rather than just understand it—"they arrive on the [first stage the on the Path of Seeing called] 'Superior Joy.'" Asaṅga reiterates the necessity of meditative acumen for reaching this stage, claiming that it occurs "through a consciousness honed by transcendent concentration and insight . . . focused on the various teachings."[33] Thus, concentration and insight are necessary to attain the Path of Seeing. This attainment also resembles Kūṭadanta's realization of Stream Entry: both involve direct insight into the teachings. But the content of this realization differs. In place of the Four Noble Truths, Asaṅga argues that the aspirant first realizes that all appearances are mind only.

But within the three-part model, this realization is only provisional. Asaṅga further describes steps 2 and 3: "Turning away from the notion of mind only, the bodhisattva destroys the notion of there being perception of objects. . . . Then, there is not an appearance of mind only." As the meditator reflects further, they realize their skepticism about objects is equally applicable to perception itself. Without an object, how can one speak of perception at all? In what sense is there a mind if it is not cognizant *of* something? This line of inquiry brings the conviction that only the mind exists into doubt, at which point, "when the bodhisattva resides in what is called 'nonconceptual cognition toward all phenomena' . . . they have a nonconceptual gnosis that equalizes both subject and object."[34] In the absence of any subject-object structure to consciousness, conceptual distinctions dissolve, leaving the meditator in a nonconceptual state.

But Asaṅga does not argue that step 3 involves *just* the quieting of conceptual distinction making. In the final step, the meditator's phenomenal content also changes drastically. By jettisoning concepts, the meditator also puts a stop to appearances. Nothing appears at all! Thus, conceptualization and phenomenal appearances are vitiated together. Indeed, according to Asaṅga, the latter depends on the former. The ultimate goal, then, he argues, is to reach this nonconceptual, appearance-less state. Describing this final goal as the pinnacle within a hierarchy of meditative abilities, he writes:

> To understand reality (**tattva*), their understanding must become error free in accord with three types of awareness. Objects appear to those bodhisattvas and meditators, who have gained control over their own mind, according to their inclination. Then, those yogis who have an aptitude for concentration apply their insight to phenomena, and to them objects appear in the manner that they understand them—[namely, as unreal]. But for those who have gained nonconceptual wisdom, it is said that no objects appear. . . .
>
> *In nonconceptual wisdom, none of those objects appears at all.*
>
> *So, take to heart that there are no objects. And since there are no objects, there is no consciousness.*[35]

Asaṅga thus describes three levels of meditative acumen that roughly accord with the three steps of developing meditative realization (figure 3.1).

At level 1, meditators first are able to generate appearances meditatively. This may refer to the *kasiṇa* method explored in chapter 1, where one

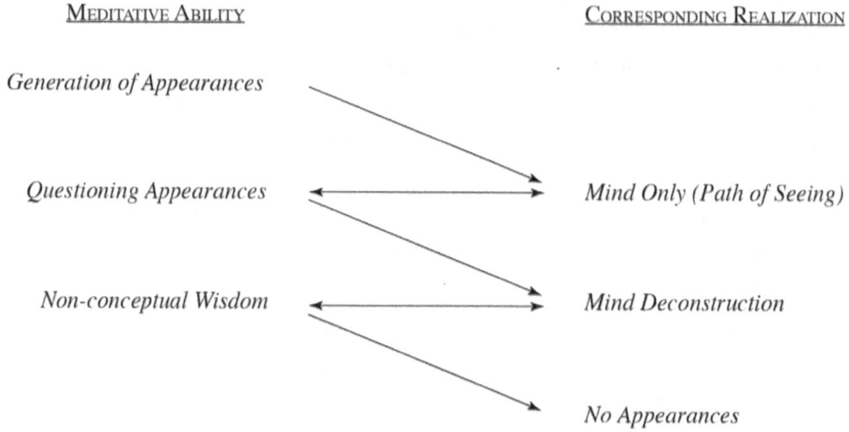

Figure 3.1 Asaṅga on Meditative Ability Versus Meditative Realization.

meditates on an element to control it. Meditation on bones, explored in chapter 2, is another possible example of the yogi's ability to generate appearances.

This meditative ability sets up the conditions for the realization of mind only. Discovering they can generate appearances just by meditating, the meditator begins to question the reality of external objects. Eventually, this understanding becomes so entrenched in level 2 that the yogi sees these appearances as *just* appearances—that is, as not referring to any external objects. Level 2 is thus analogous to the realization of the Four Noble Truths upon Stream Entry, but in this case, it is the realization of mind only on the Path of Seeing.

It is thus telling that Candrakīrti in chapter 2 argues that the meditative appearance of bones was *not* indicative of mind only. He was targeting Asaṅga's Yogācāra methodology specifically, which uses this meditation to gain an insight into mind only. But Candrakīrti is guilty of strawmanning here, since Asaṅga describes mind only as a heuristic, meditative step, not as an ontological conclusion. The spiritual path is only complete at level 3, *where nothing appears at all*—the eradication of all appearances. This corresponds with the "nonconceptual wisdom" mentioned in the above list of three levels—similar to Candrakīrti's notion that yogic insight is beyond what can be articulated.

The relationship between conceptualization and appearances is incredibly important going forward. Not all Buddhist authors agree with Asaṅga's assessment of the third level, which came to be known as a False Aspectarian position (*alīkākāra/nirākāravāda*). Instead, they argue that appearances remain in the absence of conceptualization, asserting a True Aspectarian position (*sākāravāda*).[36] This debate resurfaces as we continue. But it is also important to note Asaṅga's description of the second level, which not only continues themes from the Pāli stratum—direct insight into the teachings—but introduces several others that will be recuring in this book's analysis: that yogic mediation (1) affords one the Path of Seeing; (2) is predicated on concentration and insight; and (3) is precipitated by generative meditation methods, likely the *kasiṇa* method and mediation on bones.

Dignāga and Dharmakīrti

It is not until Dignāga and Dharmakīrti that these precursors become explicitly codified under the appellation of "yogic perception" in Buddhist sources. Fifth- and sixth-century India saw an explosion of intellectual exchange among religious factions. With several religious enclaves well established and all vying for influence, the Indian intellectual milieu developed a sophisticated shared language with which to compete, including a system of formal logic, discussions of epistemic instruments, and a copious list of agreed-upon logical fallacies. It is within this milieu that Dignāga and Dharmakīrti developed their theory of yogic perception.

Participating in this efflorescent age of Indian epistemology, Dignāga was the first Buddhist figure to create a clear taxonomy of epistemic instruments, the means by which we gain knowledge of the world. His formulation parallels that of his Nyāya and Vaiśeṣika predecessors. But unlike those who came before him, Dignāga only accepts two main epistemic instruments: perception (*pratyakṣa*) and inference (*anumāna*). Perception is the instrument that affords our direct experience of the world. It only perceives particulars (*svalakṣaṇa*), which, if we recall, are the fundamental building blocks of reality according Dignāga. Inference is responsible for our knowledge about the world beyond what can be gleaned by direct experience. Yet these inferences are still *based* on direct experience. The classic example is inferring fire from smoke. Even if we cannot directly see a fire on the other side of a mountain, we can infer its presence if we see smoke. Because we know smoke is only produced by fire, the presence of smoke entails the presence of fire. Because inference involves reasoning about conceptual objects, all inferences cognize universals (*sāmānya*).

Dignāga further divides perception into four categories.[37] These are sense perception (*indriya-pratyakṣa*)—seeing, hearing, touching, and so on—mental perception (*mānasa-pratyakṣa*), yogic perception (*yogi-pratyakṣa*), and reflexive awareness (*svasaṃvedanā*). It is here that we find the earliest Buddhist definition of yogic perception, which resonates with Pāli descriptions of the dharma eye. For example, his *Compendium of Epistemology* (*Pramāṇasamuccaya*) states that "yogis see just the object, *independently from the guru's instructions* [emphasis added]."[38] Dignāga thus concurs with the *suttas* that true realization is marked by independent authority and not having to rely on others, even the teacher.

Dignāga's notion that yogic realization involves seeing "just the object" (*artha-mātra-dṛk*) is also reflected in the Pāli *suttas*, where there are hundreds of references to "seeing things as they really are with wisdom" (Pāli *yathābhūtaṃ sammappaññāya* √*pass* or √*dis*). Both phrases denote a perception with the veil of ignorance lifted, such that the object itself appears as it really is (Skt. *artha-mātra*, Pāli *yathā-bhūta*). But Dignāga also elaborates on what this means epistemologically. He explains that the ignorance hindering our ability to see reality "as it is" concerns conceptual proliferations via universals, which one superimposes on reality. Thus, the "guru's instructions" does not simply denote one's intellectual understanding of the dharma as learned from one's teacher but is also a synecdoche for all conceptualization. Dignāga therefore explains in his autocommentary that "those yogis have a perceptual vision (*darśana*) of just the object, independent of any conceptual understanding (*vikalpa*) of scripture."[39] His formulation thus also appears to echo Asaṅga, who notes that yogic meditation is meant to discover directly "the intention of the various teachings."

In this way, Dignāga elevates the mark of self-possessed authority—direct understanding without the need of the teacher—to an epistemological principle: the ability to see reality perceptually without the confusion of conceptual overlay. Although the teacher and the teachings may impart some necessary instructions, "seeing without the teacher" describes the ultimate goal of spiritual practice. This goal again echoes the themes of chapter 2, where Buddhists claim their tradition's authority is based first and foremost on direct experience.

Buddhists still must explain how this nonconceptual, perceptual, and direct realization of reality can be cultivated. Without a clear delineation of praxeology, the epistemology means little. The tradition quickly identified a particular type of meditation as the sine qua non for gaining this direct insight. Dharmakīrti, who greatly elaborated Dignāga's system, understood it as repeated and sustained focus on a conceptual teaching through mediation. The goal of this practice is for that meditative object to eventually appear vividly and clearly before the meditator, as if it were "right in front of them." Dharmakīrti argues that "yogic awareness constituted by meditation has a clear appearance with the web of conceptions dispelled."[40]

Dharmakīrti gives several analogies for this sustained practice, such as when "one is driven crazy by desire, sorrow, and fear."[41] He understands these intense emotions as instances of obsessive rumination that lead to hallucinations. For example, extreme grief over a deceased loved one or desire for an absent lover can create vivid apparitions of those people. Importantly, Dharmakīrti also notes that purely concocted meditative objects can become vivid apparitions. This includes meditative objects already explored, such as repulsiveness (*aśubha*), or bones, and the earth *kasiṇa*. Dharmakīrti elaborates in his commentary on Dignāga's text, the *Commentary on the Compendium of Epistemology*:

> *Although considered unreal, meditative objects,*
> *Like repulsiveness (*aśubha*), the earth* kasiṇa*, etc.,*
> *Are constructed as nonconceptual clear appearances*
> *Through the power of meditation.*
>
> *Therefore, whether existing or nonexisting,*
> *Whatever one meditates upon intently*
> *Will end up forming a clear, nonconceptual cognition*
> *Once that meditation is perfected.*[42]

Dharmakīrti argues that anything meditated upon, whether real or not, will eventually appear clearly with enough practice. But if anything can become clear and perceptual through habituation, what distinguishes yogic perception from hallucinatory delusion? Dharmakīrti, however, does not assent that just *any* instance of meditative clarity constitutes yogic perception. Vivid and nonconceptual appearances are necessary but not sufficient. Vivid meditative hallucinations lack the epistemic efficacy required to be considered informative. Thus, only informative meditative representations—specifically, that of the Four Noble Truths[43]—constitute yogic perception.[44] Although inference is also informative, Dharmakīrti further clarifies that yogic perception, unlike inference, is furthermore unmistaken (**abhrānti*).[45] This grants it its superior epistemic capacity.

Dharmakīrti's theory of yogic perception thus has four primary characteristics: (1) it is nonconceptual, (2) it is unmistaken, (3) it is vivid, and (4) it is informative. At this point, we notice a seeming redundancy in Dharmakīrti's formulation. Recall from the introduction that Dharmakīrti understands informativity to be a lower epistemic bar than being unmistaken. He argues that conceptual thinking is informative *despite* being mistaken. Although it is epistemically effective at achieving certain ends, it misrepresents reality. Perceptions, on the other hand, are unmistaken. This is because, according to Dharmakīrti, mistakenness (*bhrānti*) is caused by ignorance. And ignorance only arises under conceptual influence,[46] while perceptions are categorically concept free.[47] So, why does Dharmakīrti import criteria for conceptual soundness—informativity—to account for the accuracy of yogic perception?

Now, Dharmakīrti also discusses perceptual errors (*pratyakṣa-ābha*) caused by distortions (*upaplava*).[48] Despite being nonconceptual, these are considered a mistaken cognition (*bhrānti-jñāna*), like seeing a mirage. Furthermore, perceptual errors are a source of uninformative (*visaṃvādin*) inferences, such as incorrectly inferring the presence of water based on seeing a mirage.[49] Dharmakīrti also makes clear that meditation on anything *other* than the Four Noble Truths, like bones and the earth *kasiṇa*, will culminate in a perceptual distortion (*upaplava*).[50] So, yogic perception is a unique instance of meditative clarity that, by virtue of its informativity, is not distortive and therefore constitutes an epistemic warrant. But this appears to belie an incongruity. If informativity is defined pragmatically, then why should meditation on bones or the earth *kasiṇa* be so excluded? The former inspires renunciation while the latter affords supernormal powers. This should bespeak their efficacy.

There thus seems to be an incongruity in Dharmakīrti's theory. In some places, he argues cognitive mistake is a function of false conceptualizations of perceptual data, what I have dubbed the "forward direction." This position is foundationalist, since it assumes that perception is self-authenticating, and any error is the result of conceptual processes. But this leaves little recourse to differentiate veritable yogic perception from meditative hallucination, since both are perceptual. He thus also argues for a nonconceptual form of error caused by perceptual distortion.[51] In the case of yogic perception, this perceptual distortion is defined by that perception's failure to conform to the Four Noble Truths. This latter position thus leans coherentist, since it invokes conceptual criteria to determine perceptual warrant. In other words, as much as perception warrants correct conceptual usage, concepts in turn determine a perception's warrant—what I have dubbed the "reverse direction."

Even if we grant the coherentist solution, the use of conceptual informativity to warrant yogic perception's authenticity raises a problem. Even though the Four Noble Truths are informative about reality, they still distort reality by virtue of being conceptual. If yogic perception takes this concept as its starting point, then what prevents yogic perception from inheriting those same mistakes? This leads to a dilemma. Option (1), conceptual thinking is not inherently distorting, and so neither is yogic perception based thereupon. But in that case, there would be no need to cultivate yogic perception, since conceptual thinking already accurately represents the world. Or, option (2), conceptual thinking is mistake-laden but has pragmatic efficacy. In this case, yogic perception based on conceptual thinking would inherit the same mistake. Again, this would render it epistemically redundant, since it does not escape the mistakes of conceptual thinking. So, either both are mistake-free or distorting. In either case, yogic perception appears redundant.

Dharmakīrti's supporters thus must explain how yogic perception is superior to conceptual thinking even though it takes conceptual universals as its founding meditative object. As we see, they vacillate between a pragmatic form of coherentism and a representationalist form of foundationalism in making their case.[52] Again, these issues are prompted by yogic perception's unique operation in the reverse direction. Because meditative clarity can be generated by imagining anything, Dharmakīrti is forced to rethink perception as self-warranting. He must ground its warrant in something other than its being vivid and nonconceptual. This creates a tension between his explanations of the forward direction and the reverse direction. In the former, it is perception's foundationalist self-authentication that grounds conception and testimony. Sound concepts are informative *about* infallible perceptual experience. In the latter, conception's epistemic efficacy grounds perception's warrant. Nevertheless, perception in turn provides the empirical basis for that efficacy's verification. This forms a coherentist circle. Subsequent authors discussed in this chapter grapple with how to square both directions.

Jñānaśrīmitra's Solution

To reiterate, the difficulty for Dharmakīrti's theory of yogic perception is that conceptual thinking via universals is mistaken (albeit informative). If the cultivation of yogic perception takes conceptual universals—those gleaned from Buddhist teachings—as a starting point, then it would seem any perception based thereupon would *also* be mistaken, thus undermining its status as perception. Jñānaśrīmitra counters that this only appears to be a problem because of a category mistake. The question of yogic veracity only exists from within our conceptual purview. But ultimately, yogic perception transcends quotidian epistemic procedures. And so, to evaluate it using those epistemic considerations mistakes its scope. Jñānaśrīmitra explains in *On the Demonstrability of Yogis* (*Yoginirṇayaprakaraṇa*):

> If until another [nonyogi] cognizes an epistemically warranted object, there can be no epistemic warrant, and as long as there is no epistemic warrant, that other cannot be aware of an epistemically warranted object correctly (*abhranta*), then there could be no epistemic instrument at all. Committing onself to focused attention would amount to nothing.[53] And therefore, since that object has yet to appear clearly . . . there is some uncertainty about the establishment of such an object. But when it is established [in yogic perception], no calamity can befall it, such as its failing to have a percept, or whatever.[54]

If yogic perception had to conform with other, mistaken epistemic procedures, then it could never reveal those procedures' mistake. The nonyogi would then have nothing to meditate upon. So, from the point of view of those procedures, some doubt persists until that meditation is perfected.

Jñānaśrīmitra thus argues that it is only from our nonyogic, conceptual standpoint that doubts about its epistemic warrant arise. But when one fully develops yogic perception and transcends that conceptual framework, such concerns become irrelevant. Jñānaśrīmitra, at least here, thus rejects a coherentist framework. Yogic perception is foundational for its own set of metaphysical conclusions, even if they cannot be fully corroborated by our current epistemic means.

The Critique of Concepts

Vācaspatimiśra's Criticism

Still, Jñānaśrīmitra's solution is not entirely satisfying. It appears incongruous with Dharmakīrti's theory of yogic perception. As Dharmakīrti clearly states, not just *any* clear meditative perception constitutes yogic perception. It must be the clear appearance of an epistemically warranted object. But here, Jñānaśrīmitra argues that yogic perception cannot be verified through an epistemically warranted object, since it escapes the strictures of normal epistemic procedures. What prevents this concession for *any* meditative clear appearance? On this view, any private perceptual event would seem to warrant its own, sequestered set of conclusions. (Indeed, we saw Candrakīrti make such a concession, at least partially, arguing that private percepts exist *for* their perceiver.)

Vācaspatimiśra (fl. ninth or tenth century) attacks this very weakness. Vācaspatimiśra was an eclectic figure, writing influential commentaries in support of both Mīmāṃsā and Nyāya traditions. In this section, I explore his Mīmāṃsā critique of Dharmakīrti's position. He argues that if yogic perception is knowledge yielding, then concepts cannot be mistaken. Vācaspatimiśra gives a sophisticated analysis of the problem in his *Grain of Reasoning* (*Nyāyakaṇikā*),[55] a commentary on Maṇḍanamiśra's (ca. eight century) *Investigation of Injunctions* (*Vidhiviveka*). The *Grain* first presents a possible argument in support of Dharmakīrti's position, only to deconstruct it and demonstrate how it is untenable.

Vācaspatimiśra first ventriloquizes a hypothetical Buddhist interlocutor that argues in favor of Dharmakīrti's theory. Specifically, they argue meditation on a concept yields a knowledge-yielding yogic perception. As we explored earlier, the pertinent conceptual object here is the Four Noble Truths—namely, that all phenomena are impermanent and without a self.[56] Even though the Four Noble Truths qua concept are mistaken, they are not mistaken when perceived via yogic perception. This is because the meditative conceptual object that is the basis for yogic perception—impermanence and selflessness—arises "in an uninterrupted succession" (*pārampaya*) from a cognition of the real particulars that they conceptualize.

The interlocutor uses the analogy of inference of fire from smoke to illustrate this uninterrupted succession. Inferences of fire from smoke are apodictic because smoke is necessarily caused by fire. If there is smoke, there is no interruption or intervention between it and its cause, fire. The relationship between fire and smoke also holds, the interlocutor argues, between selfless, impermanent entities and a conceptual understanding of the Four Noble Truths. That is, just as smoke is invariably created by fire, so too does the concept of the Four Noble Truths arise from observing reality. In both cases, there is an "invariable concomitance" (*avyabhicāra*) between the cause and the result. This is what guarantees that meditation on the Four Noble Truths corresponds with real particulars.[57] By reverse engineering the causal connection between perception and conception, meditation on the Four Noble Truths arrives back at a perception of reality.

The criterion of "uninterrupted succession," however, seems insufficient to guarantee epistemic warrant. Drunkenness is invariably created by alcohol. Even though alcohol is a real substance, the cognitions it produces are not warranted. By Dharamkīrti's own lights, inferences thus need not only to arise from real things but also to be helpful at "achieving desired ends" (*arthakriyā*). Pragmatics are the primary concern. If I say my inference of fire from smoke is epistemically warranted, it means that I could use that inference to find an actual fire. Otherwise, it is impotent.

An inference's soundness thus *means* its instrumentality in obtaining desired particulars. What does a sound inference of the Four Noble Truths provide? If, according to the interlocutor, the inference of fire is efficacious in the same way that inference of and subsequent meditation on the Four Noble Truths is—since the former is meant to exemplify the latter—then they should be equally instrumental in obtaining desired particulars. But this is not the case. Inferring smoke from fire, we can walk toward that smoke and find actual fire. But how odd would it be if by *meditating* on inferred fire, so that it appeared clearly, we would fulfill the same desires as if we had actually reached that fire? Vācaspatimiśra explains:

> But even given that the presence of a fire is established through inference, why should that clear cognition, the meditative object of fire, be authentic, since it arises from mediation? [If you agree that meditation on fire is as authentic as actually encountering it], you would have to say that when someone muttering "Om"[58] was ascending a hill, the knowledge of that fire born from connection with a sense organ would necessarily accord with its clear appearance afforded by meditation, and this is absurd.[59]

Vācaspatimiśra gives an excellent retort. The perception of an object cannot possibly be epistemically equivalent to vivid imagination. If that were the case, our most vivid imagination of fire would appear no different from that fire when we actually saw it, with all its attendant nuance of shape and color. If we recognize that the appearance of fire in meditation cannot afford us all the particularities of an actual fire, then there is no good reason to think that the clear, meditative appearance of the Four Noble Truths constitutes an encounter with real, momentary particulars themselves. After all, if the meditative appearance of fire cannot cook anything, why should we expect that the meditative appearance of impermanence would be salutary?

Jñānaśrīmitra's Rebuttal

Jñānaśrīmitra was well versed in the *Grain* and directly quotes it at several points in his *On the Demonstrability of Yogis*. He understands Vācaspatimiśra's critique as a charge of violated parsimony. Summarizing Vācaspatimiśra's argument, he says, "If meditation on fire is not yogic awareness just because it is does not take the ultimate object [of the Four Noble Truths], then absurdly there must be different types of perception."[60] That is, we cannot assert by fiat that the clear meditative appearance of the Four Noble Truths is authentic yogic awareness while the clear meditative appearance of fire is not. The criteria for what constitutes veritable perception must be consistent and not ad hoc. The challenge, then, is to differentiate yogic perception from the meditative appearance of fire under consistent criteria. Jñānaśrīmitra builds off Dharmakīrti's pragmatism to do so. He argues that the cases are different because the efficacy of each inference is realized in different ways.

> [The goal] achieved by a fire that is only inferred to merely burn and cook [is gained] through approaching the place where that fire is. In that case, meditation on fire is useless if that place remains out of reach. When that meditated fire appears clearly before oneself, indeed it is mistaken with respect to the object of the actual fire. Even though this is the case for meditation intent on alleviating anguish, how is there the absurdity of its constituting a different type of perception?[61]

Jñānaśrīmitra argues that it is impossible to evaluate the pragmatic value of meditation in a vacuum. Its warrant is relative to a goal. In the case of fire, the goal cannot be fulfilled by meditation. Fire's clear meditative appearance is useless, since it cannot cook or burn. But in the case of the Four Noble Truths, its meditative clarity *does* succeed in alleviating anguish and reaching liberation. This is true *even if,* like meditation on fire, meditation on the Four Noble Truths misrepresents its object. So, the clear mediative appearance of the Four Noble Truths fulfills desired aims in a manner that the same appearance of fire could not fulfill what we expect actual fire to accomplish. (Why the appearance of the Four Noble Truths has this soteriological power, however, is an open question.[62])

But even pragmatism is insufficient to preclude all those meditative appearances that Dharmakīrti wants to exclude from yogic perception. The clear appearance of bones and the *kasiṇas*, for example, fulfill intended goals—such as developing renunciation and meditative acumen—but are *not* considered yogic perception. Jñānaśrīmitra is thus forced to give additional criteria for yogic perception's epistemic warrant. He opts for a type of representationalism, arguing that yogic appearances are uniquely warranted in how they represent their object. This uniqueness is predicated on a distinction that becomes a trope throughout his text—the distinction between objects themselves (*vastu*) and their properties (*vastu-dharma*). Yogic perception is unique because it represents the *properties* of objects rather than objects themselves. Because reality is in constant flux, the conceptualization of enduring objects is mistaken. Thus, the Four Noble Truths are the *only* conceptual framework that captures this flux, since they describe real properties—namely, impermanence and selflessness—rather than unreal objects.

> All of those things [like the *kasiṇa* or bones] that have no basis (*nirālambana*) appear within meditation on an object, but not within meditation on the *properties* of that object. And those properties of objects—their momentariness, etc.—which are undertaken for meditation out of indifference toward samsara, take on a clear appearance.... Objects are unstable, in the clutches of annihilation and change, and so meditation on them is not informative. But the *properties* of objects—their momentariness, etc.—never cease. Thus, a clear appearance of *that* object—[i.e., properties]—always has a basis.[63]

Jñānaśrīmitra argues that meditations on the *kasiṇas,* bones, and fire equally fail to be accurate for the same reason. Their clear appearance is mistaken—not because they are imagined—but because they represent, enduring "stable" objects. But meditation on momentariness—the very transitoriness of the world—produces vivid appearances which *do* accurately represent the world, exactly because all things are truly momentary. Thus, meditation on this property is uniquely unmistaken.

Jñānaśrīmitra's solution, however, vacillates along the lines of the same tension we observed in Dharmakīrti's epistemology. He first differentiated yogic perception from meditation on fire pragmatically—meditation on the Four Noble Truths *affects* liberation via their clear appearance. This imports Dharmakīrti's criteria for sound concept formation in the forward direction, according to which such concepts, albeit mistaken, are instrumental in accomplishing desired ends. But when forced to explain how yogic perception is distinct from other *pragmatic* meditative appearances, both end-products of the reverse direction, Jñānaśrīmitra seems forced to readopt a representationalist view. He argues that yogic perception is not *just* effective but represents reality in a manner unlike other meditative appearances—that is, by representing its properties.

This brings his original pragmatism into question. If the meditative appearance of the Four Noble Truths is an epistemic warrant because it accurately represents objective properties, then why isn't the meditative appearance of fire as well, since it represents an object? Jñānaśrīmitra would respond that any clear appearance of an object is *not* an accurate representation by virtue of its appearing static. But then his reasoning hopelessly begs the question: the appearance of properties is accurate because it is efficacious, while that efficaciousness is predicated on its being accurate.

Eschewing the issue of circularity, even the representationalist prong of Jñānaśrīmitra's argument is not without its problems. If the Four Noble Truths and yogic perception represent the same properties—impermanence and selflessness—then this would appear to render one of them redundant. And considering that yogic perception necessarily follows a sound inference of the Four Noble Truths, then it would seem superfluous, since it only recapitulates what was previously garnered by an inference. This is the exact critique brought by the next Buddhist critic.

The Critique from Redundancy

Sucaritamiśra's Criticism

The previous debate concerned whether yogic perception is appropriately unmistaken given that it takes a mistaken concept as its starting point. Another seminal Mīmāṃsā text, Sucaritamiśra's (ca. 930–980) *Kāśikā*, grants its being unmistaken but questions its usefulness, since it does not appear to afford any new information. Dharmakīrti himself argues that any cognition of "that which has already been apprehended" is not epistemically warranted "since the means of avoiding objects to be avoided and gaining those to be acquired is the principal criterion of an authentic cognition."[64] In line with his pragmatist paradigm, Dharmakīrti stipulates that an epistemic instrument must afford novel insight about how to stay away from what we do not want or obtain what we do. If it does not give any new information to this end, it is redundant and not an epistemic instrument.

Here arises a problem for his theory of yogic perception. Dharmakīrti has already affirmed that developing yogic perception presupposes having a sound inference, namely of the Four Noble Truths. What new information does a *perception* of the Four Noble Truths thus afford? If yogic perception offers no new insight, then it cannot be an epistemic instrument. It is this potential weakness that Sucaritamiśra exploits. He asks:

> What one meditates upon has been understood by another authentic epistemic instrument. So what is the point of meditation, since that has been established? And what even is that epistemic instrument? It cannot be inference, given that dharma and adharma are not grasped beforehand, since there is no perception of a sign that entails either. . . . Only an object that is something to avoid or acquire is the thing that is desired to be known. And those two are established from scripture alone. So meditation is useless. Even the compassionate one, the Buddha, should be able to explain his scriptural teachings to his students with effort. One need not exhaust themself with meditation.[65]

Sucaritamiśra argues the Buddhist is in a dilemma. Yogic perception depends on a sound inference. The yogi thus must already have a sound understanding of dharma, the Four Noble Truths. But dharma is exactly *what is to be realized* in yogic perception. If one already had access to some inferential sign, the perceptual basis by which one makes an inference, then yogic perception would be redundant. But if there is no such sign, since dharma is supersensible, then meditation has no object by which to develop yogic perception in the first place. Sucaritamiśra also uses Dharmakīrti's own definitions against him. Informative knowledge is defined pragmatically as knowing what "to avoid or acquire." If this is known prior to meditation, then "meditation is useless," since one already has the necessary guidance. The pragmatic efficacy of that knowledge is not enhanced by its clear meditative appearance.

Ratnakīrti's Rebuttal

On this point, Jñānaśrīmitra's student, Ratnakīrti (ca. eleventh century), provides the most thorough Buddhist response. Again, his rebuttal hinges on a pragmatist interpretation. The "new knowledge" that yogic perception provides is the salutary nature of its clear appearances. Because these effects are unique to yogic perception, it is not epistemically redundant. Referencing Sucaritamiśra's argument, he writes,

> That other instrument *is* inference. But when one conceptually determines the reality of objects in the form of the Four Noble Truths, without a direct perception, the obscurations (the mental afflictions and the obstructions to knowledge)

> are not destroyed. So, to that extent, the argument for meditation is sound, also for one's own sake. And when that mindstream does have a direct perception of reality, given that that direct perception is possible, others will be impelled toward that direct perception following their own determination.[66]

Ratnakīrti insists the pertinent question is what perception can *do* that concepts cannot. Yogic perception, he argues, has the capacity to destroy mental obscurations in a manner that conceptual understanding lacks. This holds not only for oneself but affords that perceiver the ability to help others gain the same capacity. Because perception is uniquely instrumental at bringing about these results, it cannot be epistemically redundant. Ratnakīrti thus refuses to take the bait from Sucaritamiśra and engage in a discussion about perception's representational capacities. Whether yogic perception and inference of the Four Noble Truths represent the same fact is irrelevant.

But like Jñānaśrīmitra, Ratnakīrti quickly reappropriates a representationalist framework. It seems that he finds the rebuttal against yogic perception's redundancy on pragmatic grounds incomplete. And so, he feels called to thwart any charge that yogic perception is *representationally* redundant as well. Like his teacher, he argues yogic perception involves the cognition of a property (*vastu-dharma*) not an object (*vastu*).

> Indeed, momentariness must be apprehended either by perception or inference, since there is no other type of epistemic instrument. As long as one is focused on momentariness, etc., they have no perception of it. But the direct encounter with the reality of objects (*vastu-tattva*), which appears with complete clarity, is a perception, even considering that that determined reality had been individuated by an exclusion[67] through inference. Thus, it does not apprehend something that has already been apprehended, since inference does not come into contact (*asparśana*) with the reality of objects.[68]

Ratnakīrti concedes that the reality of objects is determined prior to yogic perception through inference, as captured by the Four Noble Truths. On the other hand, yogic perception, he argues, comes into closer "contact" with that reality than its inference.[69] But these considerations, such as a cognition's proximity to a state of affairs, should be irrelevant in a pragmatist framework. Nevertheless, Ratnakīrti argues that yogic perception gains its epistemic preeminence through its clear representation of a property—reality (*tattva*). And so, the same question begging reemerges. He invokes pragmatism to eschew considerations of yogic perception's representational capacity—in which case it would be equivalent to inference—only to invoke representationalism again to substantiate its pragmatic superiority.

Again, it is only within the context of Jñānaśrīmitra and Ratnakīrti's discussion of yogic perception that this tension between pragmatism and representationalism come to the fore. When explaining how yogic perception is superior to inference, both appeal to its pragmatic capacity to engender liberation. But in explaining how yogic perception is unique as an *unmistaken*, clear, meditative appearance, they appeal to a type of representationalism. These two currents are in conflict, since the very reason Dharmakīrti proposes pragmatism is to explain how concepts are epistemically warranted even though they are representationally mistaken. If yogic perception is *unmistaken* (compared to other meditative appearances) because of its representational capacity, then conceptual thinking becomes warranted in a manner that threatens the need for yogic perception in the first place.

Conclusion: Sellars and Coherentism

This chapter explores an incongruity in Dharmakīrti's epistemology. In the forward direction, he is a strict pragmatist. Yet in the reverse, he argues representationalism. This distinction also entails another epistemological incongruity. In the forward direction, Dharmakīrti advocates a type of foundationalism. Even though the process is a black box, perception causally dictates which concepts are epistemically warranted. But in the reverse direction, Dharmakīrti relies on conceptual criteria to differentiate warranted from unwarranted perceptions based on what they represent. As elucidated by his commentators, the main criterion concerns whether the perception was instigated by a concept that felicitously represents the properties of objects, namely their impermanence and selflessness, as dictated by the Four Noble Truths. This is *not* a foundationalist view, since it rejects that perceptions are self-authenticating. Some instances of mediative clarity, like of bones or the earth *kasiṇa*, are not self-warranting even though they are perceptual.

Dharmakīrti thus has certain affinities with Wilfrid Sellars's coherentism on this point. Sellars famously critiqued "the myth of the given." He argues that nothing is given to us naked and indubitably in perception. Epistemic warrant is constructed in the symmetrical interaction between perception and inferential thinking.[70] So, what we deem "perceptual" is based on our reasoning about the "standard conditions" under which perception obtains. For example, we may say that a tie "looks" green under artificial light. But we know that its looking green differs from its "actual" color in standard conditions—that is, in broad daylight—where the tie "looks" like the color that it is.[71] Perception thus cannot be self-authenticating, since we must use inferential processes and our knowledge of standard conditions to determine what sensory events constitute veritable instances of perception.

This parallels Dharmakīrti's analysis of yogic perception. Just as Sellars discusses "looking" as distinct from perception, Dharmakīriti differentiates clear meditative appearance from yogic perception. Both thinkers appeal to conceptual criteria for standard conditions to differentiate how things look—whether produced by meditation or artificial lights—from how they are correctly perceived. According to Dharmakīrti and his commentators, these standard conditions derive from the Four Noble Truths. This discussion thus reveals the importance of considering Dharmakīrti's theory of yogic perception in the reverse direction when accounting for his epistemology in general, since current scholarly debate on whether Dharmakīrti is a foundationalist largely ignores it.[72]

But Dharmakīrti is not a full-blown coherentist of Sellars's ilk either. This is because his explanation of yogic perception appears to be an outlier case. It is in this limited instance that conceptual thinking and perception are mutually constitutive—a unique feature of the reverse direction. But in the forward direction—indicative of quotidian, nonmeditative perceptual states—perception disproportionately determines epistemic warrant. According to Dharmakīrti, therefore, all things being equal, conceptualization is epistemically secondary to perception.

In this regard, Dharmakīrit is similar to Peirce, agreeing that concepts abductively translate perceptual data into fodder for pragmatically effective inferences. Like Sellars, Peirce has his own analysis of color misrecognition. "I may think a thing is black, and on close examination it may turn out to be bottle-green. But I cannot think a thing is black if there is no such thing to be seen as black."[73] So, according to Peirce, pragmatic concepts, like color, are necessarily born out of direct experience. He argues that the only reason something "looks" black is because there is such a thing to *see* black. Therefore, even if we grant that conceptual thinking has some role in determining *when* perception occurs, the *what* of our conceptual toolkit is beholden to perception. Peirce thus appears to attack Sellars' position avant la lettre.

Dharmakīrti explains conceptual formation (in the forward direction) similarly. For example, I may see a shimmering light and think that that is a jewel. That light may be from a lamp or the reflection of a jewel. In either case, my cognition is mistaken, because reflecting light is not itself a jewel. But if I end up finding a jewel, this conceptual projection would have been informative. And if I do not, it was a conceptual misapplication.[74] Nevertheless, the fact that I can mistake a "lamp" for a "jewel" means that both concepts must be informative in some context, since even conceptual misapplication evinces an entrenched, cognitive habit where that concept has withstood pragmatic culling.[75] Unlike the reverse direction, this habit is not the product of concerted meditative effort, but a natural product of some concepts' being epistemically effective and others not.

We can thus anticipate how Dharmakīrti's concession that meditation can alter these habits would throw his pragmatic picture into question. In the forward direction, concept application is pragmatically constrained by perception. But in the reverse, it is not, since Dharmakīrti concedes that unreal perceptual events may be born from unwarranted conception in meditation. This requires inferential criteria to determine perceptual accuracy. There are thus two conflicting currents in Dharmakīrti's thought, the first Peircean and the second Sellarsian. This tension is inherited by Dharmakīrti's commentators and manifests as a vacillation between pragmatist and coherentist frameworks.

We saw this vacillation play out in two instances. Against Vācaspatimiśra's charge that meditation on fire is no different than yogic perception, Jñānaśrīmitra appealed to pragmatism. The appearance of the Four Noble Truths in yogic perception achieves their goal in a manner that the clear meditative appearance of fire could not. But when it came time to differentiate yogic perception from other pragmatic, meditative appearances—bones and the earth *kasiṇa*—Jñānaśrīmitra was compelled to invoke a coherentist framework tempered by representationalism. He argued that the conceptual object of yogic meditation represents objects' properties, granting the resultant yogic perception its epistemic warrant.

Ratnakīrti, Jñānaśrīmitra's student, demonstrated the same vacillation. Against Sucaritamiśra's charge that yogic perception is redundant, Ratnakīrti appealed to pragmatism. Appearances in yogic perception have an effect that an inference of the same object lacks. But when faced with explaining this efficacy, Ratnakīrti appeals to a concept's representationalist capacity. Yogic perception is salutary because it more closely "touches" reality than inference. The superior accuracy of this representation guarantees that yogic appearances have special soteriological characteristics. Both Ratnakīrti and Jñānaśrīmitra's therefore root yogic perceptual warrant in some type of perceptual-conceptual coherence, mediated by representation.

At first blush, these incongruities seem to be the result of Buddhist attempts to accommodate a fanciful notion of perception into an otherwise consistent epistemological framework. Had Buddhists just stuck with the forward direction, their pragmatism would at least be consistent. I argue, however, that they belie a more fundamental philosophical issue.

Specifically, these debates are a microcosm of how to handle outliers generally—a requirement for any comprehensive epistemology. And Dharmakīrit's theory of yogic perception negotiates psychologically confirmed outliers of this sort.[76] For example, as Dharmakīrti identifies,[77] conceptual rumination motivated by sorrow and grief can generate vivid hallucinations of the deceased.[78] Furthermore, these hallucinations can be therapeutic in the bereavement process.[79] And there are other instances of beneficial, complex hallucinations. Synesthesia is a condition where sensory data becomes crisscrossed, such that one sees sounds or hears colors. This condition is shown to provide cognitive benefits in several domains.[80]

So, how would a pragmatist explain these outliers? Are these hallucinations epistemic because they afford benefits? Traditionally, pragmaticism doubles down in such cases. Peirce even argues that belief in God is nondelusional solely based on its psychological benefit. This is sufficient for its being a "direct experience" of God.[81] And this follows from Peirce's analysis of color. I might misidentify an experience of God, but insofar as that I can have an experience of God at all, that experience is functionally veritable.

But again, Peirce's analysis only deals with a limited case of misrecognition. As suggested by Dharmakīrti and confirmed by psychological data, conceptual thinking also generates perceptual content; it does not just influence how that content is abductively interpreted. So, if through conceptual habit I come to see a unicorn where there is none, would we have to conclude that there is such thing as a unicorn? Assuredly not. The analysis of yogic perception and its analogues in modern, psychological literature thus reveal the limits of Peircean pragmatism. Concepts are not just pragmatic heuristics that arise in response to perceptual data. They can create that data, even in ways that are beneficial. And so, we need more strict criteria to determine which concepts are epistemically sound.

Representationalist criteria is an intuitive solution. As we saw, Dharmakīrti tempers this with a Sellars-sympathetic type of coherentism. That is, standard conditions stipulate that things look as they *exist* when they appear momentary. And so, concepts that represent this fact are epistemically complete. But this has its own limits as well. Like Sellars's analysis of the tie in daylight, what guarantees that the Four Noble Truths provide definitive standard conditions? Why not claim that static objects are the standard, or how things look in *artificial* light? (Indeed, we spend as little time meditating as we do outdoors.) As Lorraine Code further demonstrates, such standard conditions exist relative to epistemic communities, each of which may be engaged in incommensurable epistemic projects.[82] But here then rears the specter of relativism, jettisoning any hope for a universal epistemology. To absolve this, we may be tempted to revert to pragmatic criteria for standard conditions. And so round and round we go.

Even though I have not arrived at a definitive solution to these problems, in this chapter I demonstrate how discourse on yogic perception—despite its superstitious accretions concerning supernormal powers—holds important epistemological considerations. I show how pragmatism can blur the lines between hallucination and perception in a way that seems untenable. And yet coherentist solutions differentiate them in ways that seem arbitrary. These are challenges not just for theological explanations of yogic perception, but for an account of perception and conception's relationship in general.

In this chapter, I mainly focus on the conceptual side of yogic perception, exploring how concepts inform yogic perception and what that means for its epistemic warrant. But Dharmakīrti makes clear that yogic perception itself transcends conceptually circumscribed knowledge. Regardless of its conceptual impetus, or post facto conceptual interpretation, then, what is *this* perceptual experience supposed to be like, where one *sees* reality without concepts? What can even be said about a nonconceptual experience? This forms the subject of chapter 4.

FOUR

Omniphenomenology

Introduction: Husserl and Heidegger

Chapter 3 focused on the tension between perception and conception in Buddhist theories of yogic perception. On the one hand, Dignāga and Dharmakīrti argue a black-box theory of perception. Although perception provides the fodder for our conceptual judgments, we have no perceptual awareness. By the time the world comes to us, it is always-already encumbered in conceptual categories.[1] Conceptualization thus misrepresents our preconceptual encounter with the world. This flow from perception to conceptual I dubbed "the forward direction." On the other hand, Dignāga's and Dharmakīrti's theories of yogic perception demand that at least some concepts accurately signify percepts, since yogic perception is warranted through the accuracy of its meditative concept. If only the clear appearances of accurate concepts constitute yogic perception, then those concepts must describe the content of yogic perception to some degree. Suddenly, perception appears less of a black box than their theory initially suggests. This epistemic flow from the meditative conceptual object to its direct yogic perception I dubbed "the reverse direction."

This chapter focuses more squarely on the question of perceptual content in yogic perception, the result of the reverse direction. I have already explored *what* yogis see in some depth in previous chapters. Yogis purportedly see discrete objects *and* their nature—their knowledge is both enumerative and metaphysical. But what is the quality of such a perception? And what does it mean to see these objects nonconceptually? I take these to be phenomenological questions more so than strictly epistemological ones. In place of *what* yogis see, this chapter asks *what is it like* to see it? This question is prompted by the Buddhist soteriological promise of the ability to perceive the world without concepts. On the one hand, the black box suggests there is no such experience at all, since it precedes awareness. On the other, Buddhists describe nonconceptual yogic perception as the most direct encounter with the world. Bracketing the epistemological pitfalls of this seeming incongruity, here we approach it phenomenologically.

I rely on a particular data set to explore the question of yogic phenomenology, focusing on those sources that describe yogic perception as a type of omniscience. Omniscient yogic perception encapsulates both of its purported abilities. To be omniscient is both to have enumerative knowledge of all objects and to perceive their reality. According to most Buddhists, such an ability can only be had by perception, since conceptualization obscures how objects exist. Yet what we call "objects" in our everyday experience is also strictly the product of conceptual categories. There is no chair independent of my idea of a chair. An omniscient yogi thus must nonconceptually perceive reality while (somehow) maintaining access to conceptual objects, lest their omniscience be incomplete. What could such an experience be like?

We might also ask why a phenomenology of yogic omniscience is worthwhile. If we do not believe in omniscient buddhas, and thus, if there is nothing that it is to be like a buddha, this exploration will be no more fruitful than pondering what it is like to be a rock. Regardless of whether buddhahood is possible, I argue that looking at Buddhist theories of yogic omniscience offers important interventions into phenomenological reduction. All branches of phenomenology assert that, one way or the other, the way we conceptualize our experience is removed from our most immediate experience. Martin Heidegger (1889–1976), for example, argues that our "ordinary" sense of time differs from its "primordial" understanding. In everyday experience, we think of time as a series of moments, one strewn after the other. The future is simply another moment at which we will eventually arrive. But this conception of time is an overlay upon a more fundamental experience. Namely, our sense of the future is our "being-toward," meaning our anticipation about the potentiality of being.[2] The future is fundamentally, then, not some future moment out there waiting in the distance, but a product of one's own anticipatory capacity—a horizon more so than a destination.[3]

Taking a phenomenological interpretation of yogic perception, I suggest that conception is the equivalent of Heidegger's "ordinary," while yogic perception is the equivalent of his "primordial." The yogi comes to a direct, unmitigated experience of being, unencumbered by the conceptual overlay that normal people—through learned habit and innate ignorance—project onto that experience. By constructing this parallel, I argue that exploring yogic perception prompts us to reevaluate the primordial, which the German and French phenomenological tradition (by and large) understands as inextricably first-person. That is, they claim that our most immediate experience is structured by a fundamental dichotomy between the individual and the world they inhabit.[4]

This is where a Buddhist phenomenology of yogic perception offers an intervention. It argues that even our sense of being a first-person subject inhabiting a world is a conceptual overlay upon a more immediate experience. Instead, our primary encounter with the world is aperspectival and coextensive with the world itself. This is why seeing the world without concepts leads to omniscience, since nonomniscience is predicated on some separation between one's experience and the world, which is itself only a conceptual overlay. In place of a first-person account of the primordial, Buddhists, I argue, offer a no-person phenomenology with the illusion of subjectivity dissolved.

Western phenomenological traditions, on the other hand, are besotted with a type of first-person solipsism. For example, Edmund Husserl (1859–1938) proposes a transcendental idealism, which he marshals to deconstruct subject-object duality. But it is still circumscribed within the first-person perspective. This is most evident in his eidetic reduction, where he attempts to describe "the pure thing seen," our most direct experience. Here, "pure seeing" is actually an amalgam of first-person perspectives, which are "retained" and "taken together" in order to "get to know the object."[5] Even though Husserl uses this method to bracket subject-object dichotomy, his phenomenology makes the first-person fundamental, reasserting the basicness of subjectivity. And because his phenomenology is constructed from what is given to the first person, it amounts to a type of solipsism.

Heidegger's critique of Husserl on this point is well known. He argues that Husserl's eidetic reduction is not felicitous to our actual experience, which instead is always-already encumbered in subject-object dichotomies. Thus, while Husserl brackets this dichotomy based on his conclusion that it is post facto to experience, Heidegger understands this dichotomy as phenomenologically primary—our sense of existence is fundamentally "being there" (Dasein), that is, being in a world with which we are in relation but is distinct from us in a sort of irreconcilable antinomy. Thus, any attempt to reduce away the experience of being in the world misrepresents our fundamental mode of being.[6]

Although Heidegger's intervention absolves phenomenology of solipsism, it retains a primacy for first-person subjectivity.[7] Being there is predicated on the assumption that a distinction between oneself and the world is phenomenologically basic.[8] This distinction is inscribed in Heidegger's analysis of Dasein as fundamentally structured by its anticipation of death. Death is "that possibility which is one's ownmost, which is nonrelational, and which is not to be outstripped."[9] Thus, death circumscribes one's own potential for being—it reveals its ultimate impossibility. This is distinct from death as "publicly interpreted," where it is not understood as the limit of being but as an actual, repeatable occurrence that befalls other people.[10] In the same way we conceptualize primordial time into ordinary time, so too our most intimate encounter with death becomes banalized into a public event. In place of a structure of being, it is fancied to be a mere event.

Despite Heidegger's efforts to the contrary, then, his ontology resonates some solipsistic overtones. This is evinced by his assertion that death qua what happens to others is derivative of the nonrelational recognition of our own impossibility.[11] As Heidegger notes, the public "idle talk of the 'they'" must "comport itself" to "that ownmost possibility of Dasein," which "lurks" in our everyday talk about death.[12] In other words, our quotidian discourse about death as a happening is a distorted form of our more primordial and ownmost Being-toward-death. Public discourse about death occurs as a bastardization of what is most authentically true for me.

But it is unclear why *my* "ownmost possibility of Dasein" should be more ontologically basic than Being publicly construed. From a non-first-person point of view, death is just one occurrence in a world that persists afterward. Why, then, must the limit of my Dasein be considered primordially coextensive with Being itself? This appears to beg the question. And how could my ability to contemplate the possibility of my impossibility even be "nonrelational" such that it retains priority? How else can I come to think about my death if not for first seeing the event of death in the world? Thus, rather than construe "publicly interpretable" death as phenomenologically secondary to Dasein's ultimate impossibility to be, we might also conclude this "ownmost" impossibility of being is phenomenologically post facto to a more primordial, public form of death.[13]

I argue that, taken phenomenologically, the Buddhist texts we consider argue this public form of being as our most fundamental. On this view, omniscience is our most primordial state. In a type of Heideggerian inversion, they argue that conceptualizations create the fancy of our being individual and distinct from the world. In place of a first-person analysis of experience, Buddhists offer a no-person view, where being is not Dasein juxtaposed against the world—"being there," as localized to some perspective—but posited as being simpliciter, just *sein,* a nonlocalized being coextensive with the world itself—or perhaps an *Überallsein,* "being everywhere."

If such a phenomenology is unique, it must be distinct from the first-person prioritizations found in Western phenomenology. We have already seen this prioritization in Husserl and Heidegger. It also informs many of the phenomenological lineages that they inspired. Jean-Paul Sartre (1905–1980), for example, argues that even Heidegger has strayed too far from the fundamentality of personal consciousness. He says that "the *cogito* must be our point of departure," which is "the first condition of all reflection."[14] Maurice Merleau-Ponty (1908–1961) disagrees slightly. He argues that "being-in-the-world can be distinguished from every third person process . . . as from every *cogitatio*, from every first person form of knowledge."[15] Nevertheless, "the body is the vehicle of being in the world."[16] Although being-in-the-world is not strictly first person, it is embodied, individualized in the body. From a Buddhist point of view, the conflation of experience with localized embodiment is another form of conceptual ignorance.[17]

I argue that in contrast to these traditions, a phenomenology of yogic perception—especially as it relates to omniscience—pushes phenomenology beyond the first-person and thus away from the solipsistic primacy of subjectivity. This project is not just negative, but it proposes a type of non-first-person experience. Omniscience is just this nonperspectival experience, coextensive with reality itself. It should be stressed, however, that this is a highly metaphorical interpretation of omniscience. In place of an epistemological claim about literal knowledge of all things, I take omniscience here phenomenologically as describing a nonperspectival way of being in the world. Throughout this chapter, I dub this phenomenological read of omniscience "omniphenomenology."[18] And I say a bit in the conclusion about why we should take such an experience seriously.

Knowing All Through One

The Scope Problem

To reiterate, my omniphenomenological read of the proceeding texts suggests our first-person perspective is not basic to experience but a conceptual interpretation of something more fundamental. To reinvoke the Heideggerian inversion I proposed, while the first-person perspective is our "ordinary" way of being in the world, the elision of perspective is "primordial." In this section, I parallel this distinction to the Buddhist differentiation between conception and yogic perception. While we conceptualize our experience as perspectival, perspective is elided in yogic perception. This will become clear in the following pages.

As we saw in chapter 3, Buddhists largely theorize conceptual thinking as the construction of universals. Universals in turn are sets containing all of those things that instantiate the property designated by that concept. Thus, my thought of "red" references all those things that are red. Similarly, my thought of "impermanent" would reference all impermanent things. Universals thus must be instantiated in all their instances, since this is what guarantees their membership in the class that the universal defines. But this raises an epistemological problem. Colors, for example, exist on a gradient. If I slowly mix red with another color, eventually I will conclude that it is no longer red. But how do I know where that line is? Unless I have already seen *all* of those colors included in the spectrum of red—unless I know where that color is supposed to start and stop—how do I judge whether any one instance of "red" truly falls within the boundaries of that universal?

We might say this is only a problem for boundary cases, and that members more toward the "center" of the universal are easily identifiable. But this would be a circular argument. How can we even be clear where the "center" of the universal is or what the most typical instance looks like unless we have already accounted for all instances? Calculating an average, for example, assumes we already know all the data points in our set. We could, then, say that universals are pure superimpositions and their "centers" are predefined. But then we have no guarantee that these universals cut at natural joints. In sum, it seems we need to know all the instances of a universal to define it, and yet we need to define a universal first to decide which instances fall within its scope.

It appears, then, that complete knowledge of a universal and of all its instances rise and fall together. Aristotle (384–322 BCE) discusses this conundrum in the context of triangles. For example, Mary knows that all triangles have interior angles whose sum is 180°. This seems to suggest that Mary is aware of all triangles. If *t* is a triangle and Mary is not aware of it, then how can she be aware that *all* triangles have interior angles whose sum is 180°? Aristotle solves this issue by revealing that it plays on a scope ambiguity in the universal quantifier "all." It is thus not the case that for all *t*, Mary knows *t*'s interior angles sum to 180°. That is, Mary does not have knowledge of each and every *t*; there are plenty of triangles of which she is simply not aware. Rather, Mary knows that for all *t*, *t*'s interior angles sum to 180°. That is, her knowledge is *about* all *t*. Put succinctly, knowledge of a universal rule is not the same as enumerative knowledge of all instantiations of that universal.[19]

I contend that Aristotle is essentially arguing a form of the forward direction here. In the forward direction, I have perceptual encounters with discrete particulars that I conceptualize post facto as a given universal. With repeated exposure to each triangle *t*, I eventually develop a general understanding of "triangle" with certain properties that hold for all *t*.[20] This describes an inductive process by which we come to know universals, moving from specific perceptual events to general conceptual understanding.

But let's assume for the moment (per the Buddhist) that cultivating the *reverse* direction harbors some epistemological advantage. This process cannot be inductive, since it *begins* with a generality. Nor can it be induction in reverse, since its end product is not specific. If it were, then meditation on a concept would culminate in the perception of one instantiation. For example, by meditating on "red" I would come to see a singular red balloon. Yogic perception, however, is purported to afford a deeper understanding of that universal. The question for Buddhist exegetes, then, was to determine how yogic perception grants this greater understanding if perception only apprehends individuated particulars.

Based on these assumptions, the only consistent response is that yogic perception eventuates *a perception of all that universal's instances.* In the forward direction, many perceptions of particulars can be generalizable into a universal. But in the reverse direction, a concept cannot be respecified into an isolated particular, since this would be no different than normal perception. On the other hand, yogic perception cannot be a "perception" of a universal, since this would be conceptual. The only possible object of fully developed yogic perception is all the referent particulars of a given universal. Thus, although I conceptually know all triangles have interior angles that sum to 180°, to *perceive* this fact is to see all triangles with interior angles of 180°—that is, to have enumerative knowledge of all triangles.

The Buddhists I explore in the next section make just such an argument. Yogic perception leads to omniscience because it perceives the referent particulars of its instigating concept. If the initiating concept in sufficiently broad, it can cover all phenomena, and thus lead to total omniscience of all discrete objects. My analysis here should not be confused with support for such a position. Rather, I am simply illustrating that the seeming bizarre conclusion that one becomes omniscient by meditating on an abstract concept is perfectly consistent with Buddhist epistemology, especially their understanding of yogic perception as a reversal of the normal flow from perception to conception.

Even if this theory is epistemologically suspect, it provides useful fodder for an omniphenomenological project. It suggests that conceptual processes create our experience of objects as instances of universals, and thus as belonging to a larger category of objects to which I have no direct access. This, in many ways, is the definition of a first-person perspective, such that what I see is just one instance of a whole array of similar but inaccessible objects. When I see something and think "red," my recognition of redness is inextricable from an awareness of a plethora of red things outside my purview. In fact, this sense of my experience of a red thing's being part of a class of red things to which I have no access may be the phenomenological basis of my first-person perspective. Put another way, conceptual attributions construe my own experience as a piece of some greater whole—that mine is only one perspective of a greater reality.

This chapter explores the possibility of a deeper, nonconceptual omniphenomenology. In a nonconceptual space, where objects are not seen as one token among an inaccessible many, perception becomes coextensive with the world. This may seem to veer toward solipsism, and indeed, we will see some Buddhists go this route. But it is not the only interpretation. On another read, solipsism is still conceptual. "What I see is everything that exists" denotes a universal "existence" exhausted by that the totality of my experience. But in a nonconceptual state, we cannot meaningfully differentiate personal experience from some greater reality, either as its totality or its partiality. This deconstructs perspectivalism without tipping over into solipsism. It is this deconstruction that I argue is phenomenologically captured in Buddhist theories of yogic omniscience. In the upcoming sections I explore how Buddhists discussing omniscience thus flirt with the line between solipsism (where the world is my experience) and literal knowledge of everything (where I experience the whole world).

Śāntarakṣita and Kamalaśīla

This theory that meditation on a universal gives way to a yogic perception of all its instances was first proposed by Śāntarakṣita and Kamalaśīla. I first consider Śāntarakṣita's *Compilation on Reality* and Kamalaśīla's commentary. Here, Śāntarakṣita gives a detailed account of the relationship between yogic perception, omniscience, and mental cognition.[21] He argues that omniscience must be a type of direct, mental cognition that does not rely on the senses. Omniscience, however, does not occur in the first instance that one achieves yogic perception on the Path of Seeing, but after long cultivation.[22] Eventually, the yogi mentally perceives all those things that are currently, for us, only the object of the senses: "*What is seen now by normal people, those various objects observed by various epistemic warrants, we will likewise observe at another time [in the future but with the mind].*" Like previous authors, Śāntarakṣita counts the objects in *Yogasūtra* 3.25 among these. He argues that this mental perception explains "vision of objects which are distant, subtle, etc., (*dūra-sūkṣma-ādi*)."[23]

By including "various types of epistemic instruments," Śāntarakṣita alludes to objects normally known through concepts as part of a yogi's mental purview. He appears, then, to be in line with Jñānaśrīmitra's representationalist description of yogic perception. Both agree that yogic perception's epistemic warrant is a product of its ability to perceive directly what concepts capture only indirectly, through a glass darkly. But while Jñānaśrīmitra restricts yogic perception to the "properties of objects" (*vastu-dharma*), Śāntarakṣita argues yogic perception perceives objects (*artha*) more generally, including medium-sized dry goods, at least when that yogic perception is refined to the point of omniscience. In addition to these abilities, Śāntarakṣita also includes the apprehension of object properties, arguing that yogic perception perceives the "reality inherent in all objects" (*samasta-vastu-sambaddha-tattva*).[24] Thus, Śāntarakṣita argues that yogic perception (eventually) affords both enumerative knowledge of discrete objects and metaphysical knowledge about how they exist.[25]

In fact, on Śāntarakṣita and Kamalaśīla's account, these two abilities are closely related. Because it is nonconceptual, omniscient yogic perception does not see "reality" as an abstract property, disembodied form its instantiations. Rather, by perceiving reality, it perceives everything that is real. Kamalaśīla explains:

> As soon as one reaches the culmination of intense meditative practice[26] on the reality of all objects, characterized by their impermanence, etc.—which is contained in all objects themselves—there is a mental cognition with the scope of real objects. That mental cognition constitutes a perception insofar that it is both a clear appearance and is informative. Omniscience is accepted as this mental cognition, since it grasps all objects simultaneously.[27]

Kamalaśīla argues that by meditating on the nature of all objects, all objects themselves appear. Śāntarakṣita himself states this explicitly elsewhere. He writes, "*The reality* (bhāvikatva) *of emptiness,*[28] *selflessness, etc., is established. Thus is the yogi's knowledge resulting from meditation on these real objects an epistemic warrant. It is a perception because it appears clearly and it is an epistemic instrument because it accords with real things. . . . It [eventually] becomes a simultaneous clear appearance in a singular consciousness. And therefore let there be just such a recognition of all phenomena.*"[29] In other words, by meditating on the emptiness or selflessness of an object, one also gains epistemically warranted knowledge of empty or selfless objects themselves. Śāntarakṣita next argues that it is through this meditative process that one eventually gains omniscience: "*It is the omniscient one, that crown jewel of men and gods, that has accomplished [this meditation], encircling the entirety of knowable objects in a single moment by a single mind.*"[30] Sara McClintock thus dubs this purported ability "knowing all through one"—that is, by yogically apprehending a singular concept, one sees everything.[31]

Vācaspatimiśra's Objection

Although it may appear fanciful, Kamalaśīla's theory of omniscient yogic perception was taken seriously enough by non-Buddhist opponents to warrant critique. Vācaspatimiśra felt it worth his while to deconstruct it in detail in his *Grain*. Showing his deep grasp of the debate, Vācaspatimiśra first gives an accurate and detailed description of his opponent's theory of yogic perception. Following Kamalaśīla,[32] he notes the Buddhist argument that "there is a direct perception of all objects as selfless. This being the case, insofar that that awareness functions in a mindstream furnished by meditation on real entities, which are all objects, it has a perceptual basis in [all] objects."[33]

Vācapastimiśra then offers a well-constructed critique without strawmanning his Buddhist opponent. His response is intuitive: Why would it be the case that just because all objects are selfless that meditation on selflessness would afford knowledge of all objects? This seems to be an odd conflation. "True, meditation on testimonial and inferential objects, [like selflessness], can be a cause for consciousness of a clear appearance. We have no qualms about that. But even though that [clear appearance] might come from that object, the culmination of a meditation on that form whose scope had reached clarity would never furnish the distinctiveness of a gustatory object."[34]

Knowledge about the selflessness of all objects does not carry with it knowledge of all objects that are selfless. For example, a clear understanding of a mango's selflessness should not furnish the meditator with a vivid experience of its sweetness. To think otherwise fails to keep track of the universal quantifier, as Aristotle identified: knowledge of a universal is not the same as universal knowledge. Meditation on the selflessness of all objects will, indeed, grant a perception of *all objects' shared selflessness,* but not a perception of *all selfless objects* along with their bundled properties.

The Buddhist may question, however, what exactly is the distinction between the selflessness of all objects and all selfless objects. As we saw earlier, a property like selflessness is defined as the set of all things that are selfless. For this reason, Dharmakīrti argues that the very distinction between universal and particular is itself a conceptual differentiation.[35] If properties and the set of objects that instantiate them are ultimately indistinguishable, how, then, could it even be possible to perceive "selflessness" *without* seeing all selfless things? To argue this is possible would be to abstract selflessness away from its instantiations in the exact fashion that Buddhist ontology disallows.[36]

But Vācaspatimiśra is careful to note that he is *not* suggesting that selflessness and selfless objects are thus, somehow, disconnected. He is aware of the Buddhist argument that the separation between selflessness and selfless objects is a false reification. But even this, he argues, will not help their account. "Ultimately real entities that are selfless and essentially distinct are not within the scope of scripture or inference. Furthermore, your meditation is absorbed on the mere other-exclusion of those things—[e.g., their selflessness]. That meditation cannot constitute a scope including ultimately real particulars."[37]

According to Vācaspatimiśra, the Buddhist confuses an ontological fact for an epistemological possibility. Śāntarakṣita and Kamalaśīla only demonstrate that all phenomena cannot be disentangled from their selflessness *ontologically*. But this fact does not transfer into an epistemological claim that to know selflessness is to know all selfless objects. Vācaspatimiśra's move here is thus the same as Aristotle's. Knowing a universal rule, as gleaned from inference or scripture, is not the same as having universal epistemological access to all the objects about which that rule applies.

But on the other hand, Vācaspatimiśra's charge of epistemic-ontological conflation also indicates that he has failed to evaluate the Buddhist on their own terms. On the Buddhist position, it is only in conception that one can cognize a property independent of its instantiation. But perceptually, this is impossible, since perception affords no such distinction. Thus, if meditative absorption on that property leads to its yogic perception, it cannot apprehend selflessness at the expense of selfless things. The ontological fact of their indistinguishability must obtain at the level of yogic perception, which only perceives things as they are.

Still, Vācaspatimiśra may retort, even if properties and their property bearers are perceptually indistinguishable, this is no guarantee that by meditating on "red" I would see *all* red things. Maybe I would just see *one* red thing. Nevertheless, the Buddhist account of the reverse direction precludes this possibility. While the forward direction moves from specific to general, the reverse cannot move from general back to specific if it is to be at least epistemologically equivalent to the cognition of a universal. Thus, even if Śāntarakṣita and Kamalaśīla's position appears far-fetched, it is internally consistent given that he accepts three premises. If (1) perception perceives particulars, (2) a universal is ultimately indistinguishable from its particular instantiations, and (3) yogic perception apprehends a universal perceptually, then, QED, perfected yogic perception *of* a universal must perceive all particular members of its set. On the other hand, this conclusion could justifiably be considered absurd and evince a flaw in one of these three premises via *reductio*.

Jñānaśrīmitra's Rebuttal

The success of the Buddhist theory of omniscient yogic perception thus hinges on the ultimate entanglement between universals to particulars. Buddhists argue that yogic omniscience is simply the epistemological realization of their ontological identity. But this argument raises obvious objections. There are two hurdles to giving such an account. (1) How is it that yogis perceive objects *at all* without universals? Buddhists claim that even the particulars belonging to a given set can only themselves be individuated into *members of* that set via conceptual construction. If yogic perception vitiates conceptualization entirely, then how can it be cognizant of discrete, selfless objects? (2) Even if yogis can perceive such objects, what guarantees that the scope of that perception encompasses *all* objects? What cognitive mechanism guarantees this?

In this section I confront question 1, turning to Jñānaśrīmitra to do so. Jñānaśrīmitra was well acquainted with Vācapaspatimiśra's criticism of omniscient yogic perception in the *Grain*. But his rebuttal demonstrates an equivocation. In one instance, he rebukes Vācaspatimiśra's introduction of Kamalaśīla's theory of omniscience as out of bounds. After describing Kamalaśīla's position in detail, he claims, "But this argument is to be disregarded, since it is outside of the discourse of Dharmakīrti's *Commentary* and its commentary by Prajñākaragupta, among others."[38] This is because the framework from which the *Commentary* is written, the Sutrist (*sautrāntika*) view, does not recognize Buddhahood and omniscience as the goal of Buddhist practice and focuses, instead, on arhatship. (Sutrists are also representational, external realists, as will become pertinent forthcoming.)[39] In the Sutrist context, then, yogic perception simply perceives the Four Noble Truths qua the properties of objects—it does not perceive those objects themselves. Put another way, it brings metaphysical knowledge but not enumerative knowledge.[40]

Immediately after this section, however, Jñānaśrīmitra makes a sudden, roundabout turn. Despite Kamalaśīla's theory's being off topic, Jñānaśrīmitra appears compelled to support it.

> Still, if one were to gain such a meditative state [where they directly perceive the Four Noble Truths],[41] that person, whose mind would be clear of obstructions, would make effort sustained over a long time toward a mind whose operating scope is all objects, with the highest aspiration to attain the aims of others in all their forms due to their excessive compassion. That person will gain a special method of this sort. From practicing this method, the most vivid knowledge—which represents the state of each atom and all objects in their diverse positions in space and time—should arise.[42]

Jñānaśrīmitra gestures to the bodhisattva path, where the development of compassion leads to buddhahood, replete with total omniscience. How, then, according to Jñānaśrīmitra, do we explain yogic perception of such objects? On the one hand, they are mere conceptual constructions. On the other, they are supposedly perceptible by yogis, even though perception vitiates conception. This is the critique leveled by Vācaspatimiśra, which Jñānaśrīmitra has yet to confront.

On this point, Jñānaśrīmitra cites Dharmakīrti and his commentator, Prajñākaragupta. These predecessors claim that the way yogis perceive discrete objects "cannot be known by us."[43] Even though Jñānaśrīmitra only cites Prajñākaragupta directly, he identifies this view as belonging both to Prajñākaragupta and Dharmakīrti in the lineage of the *Commentary*. In the next section we will see Dharmakīrti, outside the Sutrist strictures of that text, explain total omniscience through the language of inconceivability. But even in the *Commentary*, Dharmakīrti does allude to this notion in verse 3.532cd, below with Prajñākaragupta's commentary for clarity:

> *The state of a yogi's comprehension is inconceivable* (acintya)
> *Relative to the impure mind, which comprehends objective characteristics.*[44]

> Thus, how yogis sense distant (*dūra*), subtle (*sūkṣma*), etc., objects and others' minds is inconceivable now [for us normal people].[45]

Prajñākaragupta tellingly invokes *Yogasūtra* 3.25. But the key addition here is that yogic perception's ability to grasps these objects is "inconceivable" (*acintya*). We also saw Śrīdhara claim that yogic perception is the result of an "inconceivable power." But in Dharmakīrti's and Prajñākaragupta's case, "inconceivability" describes an epistemological paradox more so than an incredible power. Namely, the appeal to inconceivability solves the problem of how yogic perception can perceive discrete, conceptual objects. Recall that for non-Buddhist realists, like Vācaspatimiśra and Praśastapāda, this is unproblematic. They consider universals to be real and thus perceptible. Dharmakīrti, Prajñākaragupta, and Jñānaśrīmitra, by contrast, must appeal to inconceivability. We simply cannot explain, from our point of view, how yogis perceive those objects that for us are conceptually constructed. But they must, or they could not be omniscient. And despite Jñānaśrīmitra's initial reticence to discuss omniscient yogic perception, he concludes his entire text with an assent to this point: "The yogi, whose necessary mediation on Four Noble Truths has reached its completion, will meet the source of the inference of all objects as they desire, and then they will have a direct perception of all objects."[46] Here, he displays obvious affinities with Kamalaśīla's theory.

Despite this seeming equivocation, a charitable read of Jñānaśrīmitra reveals what Sara McClintock has dubbed a "sliding scale of analysis."[47] This denotes a particular Buddhist hermeneutic where the exegete modifies their explanation based on the level of sophistication at which they are conducting their analysis. So, despite Jñānaśrīmitra's initial rejection of omniscient yogic perception in a Sutrist context, his final assent signals a deeper level of analysis—specifically, a Yogācāra framework (see chapter 3). And unlike Sutrists, Yogācārins accept omniscience, reject external objects, and are phenomenalists.[48] Still, this appears to exacerbate rather than relieve the incongruity, since in the Yogācāra context, external objects do not exist. Hence the paradox: What does it mean to be omniscient of nonexistent objects? The appeal to inconceivability may be consistent with paradox. But it fails to give a satisfying answer to the conundrum.[49]

However, despite its epistemological shortcomings, an omniphenomenological read may cast Jñānaśrīmitra in a more positive light. If we bracket nonconceptual *knowledge,* we might ask what a nonconceptual *experience* might be like. Dharmakīrti's writings suggest that even the distinction between concepts and particulars, properties and their bearers, is itself only a convention.[50] So, it would make sense that nonconceptual awareness would be inconceivable from our point of view, encumbered as it is by conceptual categories. If there is something that it is like to be a yogi, then, it is fitting that it should escape our linguistic capacity. Jñānaśrīmitra's appeal to inconceivability may thus be more than just a lackluster polemical defense. It suggests the impossibility of describing a nonconceptual encounter with the world.

Furthermore, as I suggested earlier, conceptual distinctions are intimately connected to perspective. As Dharmakīrti suggests, the distinction between concept and percept is not fundamental. If we take the concept as the most basic unit of perspective, then perspective is equally nonfundamental. Nevertheless, there is little we can say about an experience with these divisions elided, since language is rooted in the same structures that make experience seem perspectival. This, again, all suggests a nonperspectival but indescribable omniphenomenology, something expanded upon in the next session.

Reflexive Awareness and Omniscience

Dharmakīrti and Prajñākaragupta

In the previous section, we addressed question 1—that is, how is it that yogis perceive objects at all? We saw Jñānaśrīmitra appeal to yogic perception's inconceivability. I demonstrated that this argument relies on an equivocation on the nature of perception. It cannot be conceptual, or else yogic perception would be redundant. Nor can it vitiate conceptual objects either, or else yogis could not become omniscient. Jñānaśrīmitra insists this is a false dilemma. Though inconceivable by us, yogic perception neither accommodates nor vitiates conceptual objects. This seems to be a cop opt, but it also appears consistent with a nonconceptual omniphenomenology.

What then of question 2—that is, what guarantees that yogic omniscience has the sufficient scope? There are two possible solutions. One is literal, hinging on representationalism. On this view, yogic perception really represents all discrete objects. The second interpretation hinges on phenomenalism.

This is the view that mental representations do not refer to external objects. If this is the case, then we are all, in some sense, always-already omniscient, since nothing exists outside of our awareness. This view is thus solipsistic. But it makes omniscience appear less mysterious. Omniscience would just be the mind's knowing itself completely.

But just like Jñānaśrīmitra's appeal to inconceivability to reject that yogic omniscience must be either perceptual or enumerative exclusively, Buddhists in this section reject the dichotomy between representationalism and phenomenalism as a false dilemma. Both interpretations are conceptual interpolations of a nonconceptual state. Neither can accurately capture what yogis see. Therefore, they refuse to assent to either lemma.

At certain points, Buddhist seem to suggest a solipsistic approach. This is most poignant in Buddhist descriptions of yogic perception as an instance of reflexive awareness (*svasaṃvedanā*). "Reflexive awareness" denotes the mind's ability to be aware of itself. This awareness is approximate to Kant's notion of apperception, though not identical. According to the Yogācārin, it is responsible for (though does not necessitate) our first-person, subjective experience. Only insofar as we are aware of ourselves do we experience ourselves as a subject.[51]

Furthermore, the Yogācārin contends that *all* phenomena are simply an instance of the mind's cognizing itself. This would seem tantamount to solipsism. But according to Yogācāra, the *fact* that subjectivity is a result of reflexive awareness, and not (as it seems) the result of an ontological distinction between oneself and the world, belies that subjectivity is illusory.[52] Counterintuitively, the appeal to reflexive awareness to explain the illusion of subject-object duality *elides* the subject, which cannot exist if there is nothing distinct from mind. This, according to Yogācārins, is the ultimate realization, which I interpret as a non-first-person omniphenomenology.

Dharmakīrti explains the function of reflexive awareness in reference to yogic telepathy, something we identified as a key element of yogic perception in chapter 1. The following comes from his *Proof of Other Minds* (**Saṃtānāntarasiddhi*). As its title suggests, Dharmakīrti's goal in this work is to establish the existence of other minds. Here, Dharmakīrti is in full Yogācārin form, no longer restricting himself to the framework of the realist Sutrist. Dharmakīrti argues that even though we conventionally call telepathy a perception of "other" minds, ultimately there is no such distinction between one's own mind and another's, exactly because all cognition is fundamentally reflexive.

> Because their mind has yet to be purified (**āśraya-aparāvṛtti*),[53] the yogi has yet to destroy the subject-object distinction. Their knowledge of other minds is thus an epistemic warrant conventionally, since it is informative, just like seeing forms, or whatever. Through the power of yoga, knowledge mimicking the particular mental images of other minds arise as a clear appearance to them.[54]

Conventionally we may say there is cognition of other minds, but ultimately this distinction is itself merely conceptual. Although it seems to the not-as-of-yet-enlightened yogi that they are reading another person's mind, all they are actually doing is "cognizing the effulgence (**pratibhāsa*) of their own mind, which *resembles* mental images of that [other mind]." Despite yogic perception's being ultimately reflexive, "there is a conventional determination of 'knowledge of other minds.'"[55]

Dharmakīrti's phenomenalist analysis appears solipsistic—telepathy is *really* just one's own mind cognizing itself. But like Buddhists explored in previous sections, Dharmakīrti refuses to come down squarely on solipsism either. Immediately following the passage quoted above, he, like Jñānaśrīmitra, appeals to inconceivability: "Because this [telepathy] has a clear appearance that mimics the mental image of another mind, it is perception; and because it is informative (**avisaṃvāditva*), it is considered as an epistemic warrant (**pramāṇa*). The Bhagavan's comprehension of all objects is inconceivable because it is completely beyond objects of knowledge or linguistic designations, [able to know all objects through reflexive awareness]."[56]

These are the concluding words of the *Proof.* Both Jñānaśrīmitra and Dharmakīrti conclude their texts with a nod toward inconceivable, total omniscience. And like Jñānaśrīmitra does in his text, Dharmakīrti seems to be hedging against a possible misinterpretation that the enlightened state retreats into idealist isolation. Even though a buddha's cognition is only reflexive, they still have warranted and informative perceptual knowledge about the world and others' minds.[57] How this is possible, given that Yogācārins argue that our cognitions never escape reflexivity, is again "inconceivable."

Prajñākaragupta's commentary makes Dharmakīrti's intention to hedge more explicit. Prajñākaragupta's remarks follow Dharmakīrti's claim that "The state of the yogi is inconceivable" in the *Commentary.*[58] He interprets Dharmakīrti within the framework of omniscient yogic perception *cum* reflexive awareness.

> What is the use in pondering how the completely pure mental continua of the yogic *lords*, [the buddhas], cognize these objects? Let it be. Thinking it to be like this or that is only ever partial. [Objection:] *How could it be that by apprehending one's own intellect one apprehends everything? It is understood that it is not apprehended, since that would lead to another object [besides the intellect].* [Reply:] This is unreasonable. Hence,
>
> *In that case, those objects that exist as subtle objects, etc., no longer have the status of objects [for the yogi].*
>
> *Whatever arises to an awareness of form, etc., after the fact was not there before [in yogic perception].*[59]

How can one know the entire external world by knowing the mind? Prajñākaragupta could have appealed to solipsism, arguing that there is no outside world to know. If solipsism holds, omniscience obtains de facto. Indeed, he concedes that external objects do not appear qua object (*grāhyatā*) to yogis in meditation. But outside of that context, within post-facto conventional discourse, knowledge stemming from those perceptions evinces omniscience of such objects. As far as what this perception is like for meditating yogis, however, Prajñākaragupta tells us to let the question go. Any possible answer offers only a poor facsimile. Prajñākaragupta thus marshals inconceivability in a manner resembling the previous section.

It may be easy to dismiss Dharmakīrti and Prajñākaragupta as espousing mystical nonsense. But we can give them a more charitable omniphenomenological read. Both authors theorize what an experience not structured by subject-object duality would look like. In such a state, neither representationalist realism nor phenomenalist solipsism applies. The former reifies the object while the latter reifies the subject, both making a cut between oneself and the world; realism as world qua presence and solipsism as world qua absence. Omniphenomenology refuses to make this cut. Furthermore, the primacy of reflexive awareness does not amount to solipsism on this omniphenomenological interpretation. Rather, it suggests that our initial encounter with the world is an experiential whole, which is only post facto construed under subject-object dichotomies. To experience the world *as* reflexive awareness, rather than be fooled by that reflexive awareness into reification, vitiates any first-person perspective, such that dualisms between oneself and a greater world do not arrive.

Bhāsarvajña's Criticism

The problem with this line of thinking, however, is that it only qualitatively distinguishes omniscience from our ordinary experience. On this view, omniscience is simply a direct encounter with the world without a subject-object overlay. Yet, according to Buddhists, omniscience also has *content* that our normal cognition does not. Omniscient yogis *know* things about the world that we do not, such as all that has come to pass and all that will. How could precognition and retrocognition come from seeing the world without subject and object? This question initiates Bhāsarvajña's attack. His *Ornament for Logic* contains one of the few instances of a Nyāya critique of the Buddhist theory of yogic perception.

He does not disagree, however, that yogic perception can be omniscient, else he would be at odds with his own Nyāya orthodoxy. Rather, he takes issue with the assertion that omniscience is achieved through reflexive awareness. Namely, "If omniscience has no percept (*nirālambana*) and is merely reflexive awareness, then what distinguishes yogic perception from other perceptions?"[60] If Dharmakīrti means to make sense of cognition without appeal to external objects, then Dharmakīrti has eviscerated any way to differentiate correct cognitions from incorrect ones. The distinction between a vivid hallucination and the appearance of a warranted object only obtains relative to the external objects they purportedly represent. If all cognition is reflexive, this distinction becomes meaningless, as well as any distinction between omniscient and normal cognition a fortiori.

Bhāsarvajña notes, however, that maybe Dharmakīrti is not speaking from a Yogācārin theory of reflexive awareness. Perhaps he is still speaking from the Sutrist acceptance of external objects. If so, the authenticity of yogic perception derives from its ability to represent external objects. But Bhāsarvajña explains that even in this case, Dharmakīrti has a problem. "Do you agree with the position of the Sutrists? If you do, then how is it that yogic perception can have knowledge of past and future objects, [since according to Sutrists, the past and future do not exist]? There can be no mental image of something that does not exist."[61]

As Bhāsarvajña identifies, the Sutrists are strict presentists, arguing only the present moment exists. How, then, could yogic perception be omniscient about the past and future, since the past and future do not exist? Bhāsarvajña thus offers a two-pronged attack against both Buddhist representationalist and phenomenalist interpretations of yogic omniscience. The phenomenalist view cannot hold, since it fails provide criteria to differentiate correct from incorrect perceptions. The representationalist view cannot hold either, since, given their presentism, the Buddhists must agree that any representation of the past or future would be fallacious. Buddhist therefore have no viable theory of yogic omniscience.

Jñānaśrīmitra's Rebuttal

The Buddhist has a potential, straightforward response to Bhāsarvajña here. They could simply bite the bullet on either prong. Accepting phenomenalism, they could concur that reflexive awareness renders distinctions between correct and incorrect perceptions irrelevant. If nothing exists outside of the mind, all perceptions qua perceptions are authentic. Or, accepting representationalism, they could counter that a failure to know about nonexistent things is not an epistemic failing. If everything is momentary, then there is no past and future to cognize—knowledge of the present would be sufficient for omniscience.

It is revealing that Buddhists do *not* opt for either alternative. Again, this is indicative of their refusal to abide by the terms of the phenomenalist-representationalist dilemma. Jñānaśrīmitra and his student Ratnakīrti both tackle Bhāsarvajña's critique on this point. As in the previous section, both of their analyses belie a certain equivocation. They first eschew the issue, arguing omniscient yogic perception is out of bounds. But both eventually appear compelled to defend it. We start with Jñānaśrīmitra's reply.

Initially, he argues that Bhāsarvajña misses the mark. Dharmakīrti discusses yogic perception from a Sutrist point of view, according to which it is neither reflexive *nor* omniscient. Thus, Bhāsarvajña's charge that the Sutrist cannot make sense of omniscient yogic perception is a red herring. "The objection from Bhāsarvajña's *Ornament* from the perspective of Yogācāra is off topic, since we proceed to make our point already assuming the existence of external objects. In that case, his objections leveled against complete omniscience are dismissable, since we don't assume that [complete omniscience exists in this context]."[62]

We saw Jñānaśrīmitra appeal to doxography similarly in the previous section. But like that section, Jñānaśrīmitra again seems unable to resist the bait and defend omniscient yogic perception. He continues: "But we have also shown that another possibility cannot be ruled out, that it is like a dream that comes true. So, it is not the case that just because there is no mental image of the past or future *in* the present that there is no mental image of the past or future *as* a time other than the present. If that were so, no object [would be temporally indexed as] past or future at all."[63]

In dreams, we seem able to return to the past, reliving childhood memories, for example. Or we may dream about the future, imagining where we will be in ten years. What separates such dreams from *actual* instances of seeing the past and the future? A representationalist would say that a veritable instance of precognition should represent some future existing object. But a phenomenalist would counter that this would be a nonstarter, since we have no access to objects beyond representation. Instead, according to Jñānaśrīmitra, veritable precognitions are like dreams that "come true." Here, he offers a verificationist solution. Although all phenomenal appearances per se are authentic, later "waking" experience can confirm or disconfirm their status as prescient. It is only when the dream comes to pass, via other appearances always already in the present, that I can verify that the dream was a precognition. This is a sufficient epistemological criterion for precognition. In fact, it is the *only* way to substantiate precognition.

In the next section we see how Ratnakīrti expands on this argument. Most compelling at this juncture, however, is Jñānaśrīmitra's pivot away from representationalism. He at first insists that the debate must stick to a Sutrist framework, only to propose a phenomenalist appeal to dreams. But this shift evinces a Buddhist reluctance toward both representationalism *and* phenomenalism. Ultimately, as clarified by Ratnakīrti, their oneiric appeal suggests an omniphenomenology eliding the very distinction between representationalism and phenomenalism. This will become clear in Ratnakīrti's more detailed analysis.

Ratnakīrti's Rebuttal

Ratnakīrti proceeds in the same manner as his teacher, Jñānaśrīmitra. He argues that Bhāsarvajña's critique "from the perspective of Yogācāra in the *Ornament* is irrelevant, since we have laid out our argument assuming external objects." Ratnakīrti also concurs that yogic omniscience is out of bounds: "We are talking about meditation on all objects as momentary and selfless only in relation to practical omniscience, not from the perspective of complete omniscience. Thus, that there is no cognition of past and future objects is no refutation."[64] Again, in a Sutrist context, the concern is the metaphysical knowledge needed to free oneself from suffering (that is, the Four Noble Truths), not enumerative knowledge of all things.

Nevertheless, like Jñānasrīmitra, Ratnakīrti is reticent to abandon yogic perception's role in total omniscience. He proceeds, "But this does not mean that we relinquish total omniscience." Quoting the same passage from Jñānaśrīmitra about complete omniscience that we read before,[65] Ratnakīrti adds, "It is like how, even in the absence of a causal connection, a dream can come true through divine intervention."[66] His elision of causality in this example anticipates a sophisticated epistemological explanation of how total omniscience occurs.

> Normal people know a thing through identity (*sārūpya*) or through a causal connection (*utpatti*). But yogis grasp things merely through identity. This is the reason. And it is said in the *Commentary* [3.532bcd]:
>
> *In contrast to impure minds, which conceives subjects and objects*
> *The state of a yogi is inconceivable.*[67]
>
> Thus, even if there is nothing which produces a cognition of the future and the past, their clear appearance within yogic knowledge are not falsified.[68]

Ratnakīrti gives a sophisticated analysis of what it means to be informative. When we say that a cognition is informative about reality, we could mean two things. First, we could mean that we infer the presence of objects based on their causal connections, like between fire and smoke. This renders reality inextricably temporal. But there is a second possibility: Being informative describes a relationship between appearances and assessments about their shared identity. In other words, when we say that a cognition is informative, we mean that it coheres with other appearances. Warrant becomes a function of how phenomenal appearances imbricate, without the need to posit a temporal ontology.

Jñānasrīmitra made this same point—if veiled—through his analogy to dreams. If we claim that a dream has come true, and thus that that dream was prescient, we need not appeal to some metaphysically real, future object with which that dream corresponds. We verify the truth of that dream by its coherence with other appearances, by its "coming true," and the ongoing failure to falsify it. While conventionally we may construe this as the appearance *of* a future object, its warrant is only ever verified through its coherence with other appearances as they arise.[69]

Although normal people think of informativity as occurring in both modes, both through causal and token-type relationships, Ratnakīrti argues that the yogi can infer the temporal content of their visions through identity only, having jettisoned any temporal metaphysics. He elaborates further in response to an interlocutor who argues that perception by definition necessitates a percept, and thus an external object which is its cause and with which it corresponds. "Therefore, even if there is no proximate object, through meditation, the awareness mimics that object's spatiotemporal aspects. So how is there no percept, given that, by determining it as such, there is a recognition of its being distinguished by that determined time, just like a dream that comes true?"[70]

Ratnakīrti's assessment is again indicative of a verificationist framework. When we say that a cognition has a veritable percept, we just mean that it is verified by a later experience, not that it corresponds with some "real" object that caused its perception. Similarly, any correspondence with the "past" or "future" is determined post facto, based on a conceptual comparison of appearances that dictates their accuracy. But yogic perception per se has no referents. Indeed, any purported percept is a post hoc construction.[71]

We may intuitively think that, surely, there is a difference between hallucinating a past or future event and *actually* peering through time to see some past or future object. But Ratnakīrti suggests that such instincts are mired in ignorance; all we really have are appearances. No noumenal objects in the present, past, or future can adjudicate the veracity of those appearances. If they lead to desired ends—for example, if a precognition allows one to effectively predict a future event or a retrocognition reliably recalls a past one—then they are informative.

Even though both Ratnakīrti and Jñānasrīmitra initially claim they are arguing from a Sutrist, representationalist framework, they quickly pivot toward its rejection, arguing that appearances alone can account for yogic omniscience. They both use the analogy of a dream that comes true to make this point. But does this amount to phenomenalism? It might seem so at first. But ultimately, their position is closer to a verificationism, bracketing questions of appearances' metaphysical status—whether they represent (realism) or alone exist (phenomenalism). Ratnakīrti and Jñānasrīmitra thus refuse to construe warrant in terms of the relationship between mind and world, either through theorizing their connection or equating them.

As I have been arguing throughout, Ratnakīrti's and Jñānasrīmitra's rejection of representationalism and phenomenalism is indicative of a nonperspectival omniphenomenology. Conventionally, we do indeed speak of warrant qua correspondence. This correspondence is endemic to a subject-object framework, as is its attendant first-person perspectivalism. Yogic perception elides these strictures. But this does not devolve into phenomenalist solipsism either. Yogic appearances precipitate effective judgments about the objects that populate our world. Still, how yogis themselves perceive those objects in the absence of subject-object dichotomies is inconceivable. Buddhists further argue that the culmination of this dualistic collapse leads to yogic cognitions that never fail to be verified by future appearances—effectively, omniscience.

Conclusion: The Oceanic Feeling

Throughout this chapter, I argue that Buddhist descriptions of yogic perception can be read omniphenomenologically as a non-first-person experience of the world. I argue that these Buddhists understand the subject-object dichotomy to be a post-facto conceptualization upon our more fundamental, nondual experience. Thus, within yogic perception, which perceives reality at its most fundamental, experience and the world are coextensive. Furthermore, this coextensivity is not a form of a solipsism. It is neither the case that the world is just my experience nor that I experience the whole world. Both statements abide by subject-object dichotomies, which Buddhist theories of omniscience problematize. From the standpoint of our "ordinary," conceptual framework, we can only say that such states are "inconceivable."

We saw different Buddhists articulate this point in different ways. But all of them suggested some collapse of dichotomies. Śāntarakṣita and Kamalaśīla, for example, collapsed the distinction between universals and their instantiations. In yogic perception, the distinction between the conceptual cognition of a universal and perception of its referent instantiations breaks down. This is why yogic perception affords omniscience. Dharmakīrti's appeal to reflexive awareness presents a similar collapse, but between subject and object. Omniscience is reflexive exactly because in that state the distinction between subject and object no longer abides.

In the context of Jñānaśrīmitra and Ratnakīrti, this collapse is most prominent in their vacillation between Sutrist and Yogācārin frameworks, avoiding both representationalism and phenomenalism. Initially, they reject that yogic perception affords omniscience, since that assertion is not made within the representationalist, Sutrist framework that constitutes their analysis. But they ultimately do not adopt this position, feeling compelled to defend the Yogācārin account of yogic omniscient. Still, despite Yogācārin idealism, this concession is not an assent to phenomenalism. Instead, they appeal to a verificationist schema. This allows them make sense of yogic perception's warrant without resorting to realist representationalism or trivialist idealism. When yogic perception makes correct predictions, it is like a dream that comes true. Its warrant comprises internal consistency, the mere imbrication of appearances, not a mind's ability to correctly assess an external world.

We may wonder, however, the value of this supposed omniphenomenology. Even if we admit that subject-object structures are the product of conceptualization, that does not guarantee some experience where this framework is suspended. Indeed, in the previous chapter I argue that nonconceptual states are below the level of awareness. It would thus be folly to give them an omniphenomenological analysis, since without awareness, no such experience is possible. Still, Buddhists insist that unlike normal sense perception—which, indeed, does not reach the level of awareness—yogic perception *is* an experiential state. In fact, it is the *summum bonum* of awareness, the enlightened state of omniscient buddhas. Nevertheless, even if we grant that such an experience is possible, it is still an outlier. It would seem to have little import for normal life, or how normal folk go about their day and experience the world. Buddhists reserve their account of this "inconceivable" state for highly adept yogis, not humdrum being in the world.

Such extraordinary experiences, however, might be more common than we think. In addition, they might also have drastic ramifications for our understanding of everyday being. Take for example the fascinating case of Jill Bolte Taylor. Dr. Taylor is a neuroscientist who at the height of her career had a major hemorrhagic stroke in the left hemisphere of her brain. She was able to remain lucid, arguing that what she experienced was the shutdown of her left hemisphere, ushering in "a deep inner peace" and her "journey into my right hemisphere's consciousness."[72] Her account of that morning is compelling:

> By this point I had lost touch with much of the physical three-dimensional reality that surrounded me. My body was propped up against the shower wall and I found it odd that I was aware that I could no longer clearly discern the physical boundaries of where I began and where I ended. I sensed the composition of my being as that of a fluid rather than that of a solid. I no longer perceived myself as a whole object separate from everything. Instead, I now blended in with the space and flow around me.[73]

Taylor describes exactly the type of subject-object elision that has been a theme of our Buddhist authors. More than this, she suggests the same coextensivity between the self and the world. "By the end of that morning, my consciousness shifted into a perception that I was at *one* with the universe."[74] Taylor's stroke thus seems to be a prime example of the non-first-person state described throughout this chapter. In place of Heideggerian thrownness, where one feels thrust into a world beyond oneself,[75] Taylor describes a world indistinguishable from herself. In such a space, the very distinction between self and the world has "melted" into each other.[76]

Taylor's account is phenomenologically rich on its own, independent of her assessment of its neurological cause. Nevertheless, her conclusion that it was precipitated by the disfunction of her left hemisphere is revealing. She argues that this hemisphere houses areas of the brain that define the boundary between oneself and the outside world.[77] If her feeling of being one with the universe was precipitated by her brain's temporary inability to make that distinction, then Buddhists may be on to something when they argue that nonconceptual yogic perception culminates in omniscience. This, of course, presupposes we read omniscience phenomenologically as the loss of the first-person perspective, the elision of mind-and-world structures.

Such experiences are not merely the domain of cognitive malfunction. Alan Lightman recounts having a similar omniscient experience as a result of starring into the night sky: "My body disappeared. And I found myself falling into infinity. A feeling came over me I'd not experienced before. . . . I felt an overwhelming connection to the stars, as if I were part of them. And the vast expanse of time—extending from the far distant past long before I was born and then into the far distant future long after I will die—seemed compressed to a dot."[78]

Lightman describes both a spatial and temporal connection to all things that, taken omniphenomenologically, resembles the descriptions of omniscience found in this chapter—especially a connection to the past and the future.[79] Indeed, Romain Rolland famously described this "oceanic feeling" of the eternal as the essence of "religious sentiment."[80]

But these experiences are not merely confined to the height of spiritual fervor. In fact, it may describe our most basic way of being in the world. Psychological research demonstrates that our sense of a distinction between ourselves and the world is learned, not innate. For example, children have difficulty understanding the distinction between knowledge of the world and the world itself.[81] Some theorists thus argue that omniscience, or the conflation of perspective and the world, is our most intuitive view.[82] In other words, the conceptual differentiation between the world as it is and the fact that each individual carries limited perspectives on that world is a post facto, learned, reflective form of thinking. Young children, by contrast, conflate the world with perspective and assume that everyone knows the world in whole, having yet to form an epistemic-ontological differentiation. This further suggests that omniphenomenology describes our most fundamental experience, where, free of perspectival structures, we feel merged with time and space.

The ramifications of omniphenomenology go beyond the phenomenological reduction, however. The way we conceive of our most fundamental experience, either as fundamentally coextensive with the world or separate from it, affects our relationship to that world—especially as populated by others. For example, as I note in the introduction to this chapter, Heidegger subscribes to a phenomenology of separateness. He defines Dasein vis-à-vis its being-toward its own impossibility, its death. Being is thus a carved-out positive—literally "being there" (Dasein)—contrasted against its negative space, its nothingness. In this way, Dasein stands apart from the world that serves as its negative, that which will no longer be there for Dasein once it no longer has its being to be.

Calvin Warren's poignant book *Ontological Terror: Blackness, Nihilism, and Emancipation* gives a lucid analysis of how this construal of Dasein, however, does not concern human Being as a whole. Rather, it is inscribed in whiteness and its attendant social dichotomies. It is only in contrast to a black nothingness that whiteness can take its place. Whiteness thus draws its being against the "ontological terror" of black nothingness. It both needs and hates the black other, since—just as death structures Dasein—blackness structures whiteness, both its being and as its threat.[83] Warren thus argues that Heidegger, "because of his Eurocentric perspective," does not consider how black being is denied Dasein and is, instead, mere equipment for Dasein.[84] Whiteness is given place in the negative space created by black erasure through physical and political violence.[85]

Heidegger thus conflates a *particular* bourgeoise ennui, one characterized by the lone individual who must come to terms with their place in the world, with the whole of human Being.[86] The result is normative: collective identity[87] is reduced to a palliative balm against innate isolation—an inauthentic public, "they self"[88]—while Dasein, in its authentic individuality—the "Self"—is realized in a "moment of vision."[89] As Warren demonstrates, this is both predicated upon and continuative of whiteness as the positive corollary to a black negative space that threatens it.

If, as Warren suggests, subjectivized phenomenologies are both the product and perpetuator of racism, then omniphenomenological interventions, by problematizing Eurocentric individualism, should provide a remedy. This is because in place of a subjectively structured phenomenology, omniphenomenology proposes an *unstructured* phenomenological reduction.[90] Omniphenomenology is thus accommodative rather than normative. Since Being does not necessitate any particular structure, all structures become equally authentic. This frees us to structure the person-world complex in more equitable ways by ameliorating the antagonistic structure inherent in Heidegger's Dasein as Being against the world.[91] This might include a more capacious and inclusive sense of group identity as well as deeper empathy for others.[92]

I should reiterate, however, that my phenomenological interpretation of Buddhist arguments for omniscient yogic perception would likely be foreign to the Buddhist authors that I cite. Their belief in omniscience was likely literal and not figurative; they would resist reading omniscience as a metaphor for a phenomenology. There are assuredly points I make with which they would agree. In particular, the Yogācārin authors that we reviewed saw themselves as trying to deconstruct the metaphysical baggage of realism *without* positing a metaphysical idealism in its place. In this sense, Yogācārins are indeed engaged in a phenomenological project that attempts to bracket unhelpful metaphysical dichotomies.[93]

But even on this point, it seemed difficult for subsequent Buddhist traditions to remain metaphysically agnostic. Especially in the context of highly scholastic Tibetan traditions, the pressure to present a clear metaphysical position seemed to win out with time. This is the theme of chapters 5 and 6. Specifically, I demonstrate how some traditions sided with representationalism, along with its attendant realism, while others argued antirepresentationalism and antirealism.

PART THREE

Tibetan Buddhism and Language

FIVE

Gelug Representationalism

Introduction: Russell and Representationalism

I discussed in chapter 4 how Buddhist authors avoid both representationalism and phenomenalism: appearances in omniscient yogic perception do not represent external objects, but this does not amount to a privatized phenomenalism, where yogic omniscience is nothing more than glorified solipsism. Jñānaśrīmitra was a pivotal figure in this discussion, and his arguments are consistent with his larger philosophical view. He argues a type of phenomenological reduction where appearances are fundamental, identified in chapter 3 as the True Aspectarian view (*sākāravāda*). Within this reduction, dualistic metaphysical distinctions do not obtain. Thus, appearances are neither representations distinct from something real, nor exhaustive of reality itself. Such ontological distinctions are merely superimposed on appearances post facto.

But as I explained in chapter 3, Asaṅga ultimately rejects appearances. He holds a False Aspectarian view (*alīkākāra/nirākāravāda*). According to him, while yogis are still befuddled by appearances, buddhas escape befuddlement exactly because nothing appears to them. We should note, however, that nothing appearing is not the same as *the appearance of nothing*, for this would still be an appearance. It is not clear, on this view, that enlightened cognition has no phenomenal content whatsoever. Rather, whatever that content is, it is not the type of thing that appears to us now, or that could be described as an "appearance." The False Aspectarian thus rejects phenomenological reductionism, since, according to them, there is nothing of our current experience that remains once our befuddlement is elided.

Without phenomenological reduction, however, the debate between representationalists and phenomenalists reasserts itself. If appearances cease when one sees reality as it is,[1] then appearances are distinct from a perception of the real, and we are back to the metaphysical problem of their relationship. Even if appearances cease eventually, might they still represent the real, albeit poorly? Or, are appearances completely sequestered, constituting a phenomenal world detached from reality, like a dream that we will eventually wake up from?

These are not easy questions to answer, and responses to either one raise issues. On the latter, which constitutes a phenomenalist interpretation of this issue, appearances do not represent anything. But then what differentiates false from accurate appearances, even within the dream? All epistemic distinctions would seem to collapse. But the former, representationalist solution seems self-subverting. If appearances represent reality perfectly, then they are transparent. But then, they would be superfluous—we might as well accept naive realism. But if they are opaque, how could we ever know with certainty that they represent accurately, having no access to what they represent? Thus, if we are to accept any notion of appearances as distinct from reality, then we are hard-pressed to construe their relationship.

As I foreshadowed in chapter 3, these ruminations about representationalism versus phenomenalism were at the core of Bertrand Russell's philosophy, and how he resolved it remains an issue of debate. Some argue that Russell flirted with both phenomenalism and representative realism.[2] Russell himself, on the other hand, rejects he ever subscribed to the former. He concedes that it is impossible to find empirical evidence for anything beyond appearances. But Russell claims this fact just describes our "egocentric predicament," not some metaphysical truth.[3] Nevertheless, although our egocentric predicament does not necessitate phenomenalism, it does not preclude it either. Neither is it clear, given such a predicament, what empowers us to argue for realism in its stead. That accurate appearances represent real objects becomes nothing more than fiat on the concession of our egocentric predicament, since that predicament precludes empirical evidence of real objects.

A similar tension is reflected in the Tibetan commentarial tradition on the Indian sources we have explored so far. Chapters 5 and 6 focus squarely on how Tibetan exegetes navigate the issue of appearances and their relationship to reality. A corollary to this issue is conceptual correspondence, explored in previous chapters. Just as we can question whether appearances, the phenomenal content of our experience, represent real objects, we can further wonder whether our concepts have corresponding referents. These two issues are related, since we build our concepts from what appears. Therefore, if appearances do not represent objects, transitively, concepts cannot have real referents.[4] The degree to which appearances represent and concepts correspond is a major dividing line between the Tibetan schools explored in this chapter, especially as it pertains to yogic perception.

Representationalism in the Tibetan Milieu

For reasons that are not entirely clear, scholastic Buddhism became almost entirely extinct in India within two centuries of Jñānaśrīmitra's death in the eleventh century. Without Tibetan support, including massive translation projects and funding for Indian Buddhist experts to educate a new generation of Tibetan Buddhists, many more texts and teachings from the Indian Buddhist tradition would have disappeared completely. But with renewed resources, Buddhist discourse on these issues continued to flourish, transplanted in foreign Tibetan soil.

Inheriting a wealth of Buddhist thought from their Indian predecessors en masse, Tibetan thinkers were especially invested in developing a comprehensive doxographic structure to account for the various Buddhist views they encountered. Their reasons may have been practical as much as philosophical. Receiving more than a millennium's worth of tradition in Buddhist scholastic learning over the course of a couple hundred years, Tibetans were likely searching for systematic ways to make sense of its breadth. But their doxographies were not just taxonomic. Tibetan Buddhists used doxography to develop a hierarchy of views, each progressively more accurate than the next.

Not all Tibetan doxographies agree, however. Some exegetes place phenomenalism and others representationalism as the highest view. In the

Buddhist context, however, these terms must be nuanced from how they were understood by Russell and his conversation partners. The Buddhist phenomenalist view, like the phenomenalism addressed by Russell, argues that appearances do not represent any underlying reality. Appearances may be construed post facto as constituting a shared life-world, and this may be sufficient for intersubjective experience. But this world is not undergirded by something that is truly, ontologically communal.

But unlike Russell's sense of phenomenalism, Buddhist phenomenalists generally assert that there is some ultimate reality behind appearances. Whatever that reality is, however, it is not the foundation for appearances. It is thus completely beyond the ken of what normal, unenlightened folk know now. We cannot even call it "real," since our very notion of real is derived from appearances. This view thus amounts to a type of phenomenalist antirealism—or perhaps better stated as antirepresentationalism. Normal people only have access to appearances, and what appears is not real at all. The goal of yogic perception, then, is to get beyond appearances by eradicating them, so that the real reveals itself. I come back to this viewpoint in chapter 6.

Here, however, I tackle another doxographic strategy in which appearances *do* represent reality. But as appearances, they slightly distort real objects. Namely, appearances distort *how* objects exist, such that they appear to have all those qualities that Buddhist analysis reveals to be impossible: being permanent, endowed with a self, and not empty. Even though appearances distort how things exist, they still accurately represent *what* things are. Thus, this is a representationalist realist view, but also with a caveat. Appearances are accurate save how they represent objects' mode of existence, and this failure is what causes all our problems and suffering. The goal of yogic perception is to correct this distortion so that objects appear in conformity *both* with how they exist *and* what they are. In contrast to phenomenalist antirealism, I dub this a type of quasirepresentationalist realism.

To give a succinct analogy, the Buddhist phenomenalist antirealist says appearances are like a blindfold, blocking our view of the real, while the quasirepresentationalist realist argues that appearances are like poorly prescribed glasses, creating blurs that represent the world in part but distort it in others. The debate between these views is thus whether yogic perception is like removing a blindfold (vitiating appearances) or fixing the prescription (correcting appearances). In this chapter I explore the "glasses" theory of yogic perception, mainly focusing on thinkers from the Gelug (*Dge lugs*) school. For political reasons perhaps more so than any inherent philosophical superiority, the Gelug school became the dominant intellectual power in Tibet from the seventeenth century onward. But it was founded several centuries earlier by Tsongkhapa Losang Drakpa (Tsong kha pa Blo bzang Grags pa, 1357–1419), whose work comprises the bulk of my analysis. But first I turn to a pre-Gelug thinker who would prove to be incredibly influential to Tsongkhapa and subsequent Gelug thinkers.

Chapa on Yogic Perception

Chapa Chökyi Senge (Phywa pa Chos kyi Seng ge, 1109–1169) was a founding figure for the study of epistemology (*pramāṇa, tshad ma*) in Tibet. As abbot of the famed Sangpu Neutok (*Gsang phu ne'u thog*) monastery in Central Tibet for eighteen years, Chapa solidified his monastery's reputation as the mecca for Tibetan epistemological studies in its heyday. He was a strong proponent of the power of reason and highly resistant to Buddhist theories arguing that the goal of Buddhist praxis was to reach some mystical state that escaped reason's purview.

Chapa was thus confident that we can make reasonable assessments about the world based on what appears to us. Nevertheless, he recognizes that those reasonable assessments may contradict how the world appears prima facie. For example, even if observations of the world are distorted, it is based on our observations that we can come to conclude that reality is impermanent. We see things break, and even the most stable things eventually undergo change. Nothing ever lasts. Still, when things appear, they appear to be permanent from moment to moment. Thus, we rely on appearances to conclude that things are impermanent even though things still appear to be permanent. The same holds true for an optical illusion. The optical illusion appears even though we rely on other observations to realize it is an illusion.

According to Chapa, one primary goal of logic is to identify which appearances are distortions and which have epistemic value. Distortions are called "elaborations" (*spros*), since they are the result of the mind elaborating upon what actually exists. As we saw in chapter 4, however, Buddhists believe that all conceptual thinking is a type of elaboration. How, then, can conceptual thinking undermine false conceptual elaborations? Chapa argues this is not a major hurdle. For example, the conceptual claim that reality is free from elaborations is a concept that (when understood fully) uproots elaborations themselves. Furthermore, "freedom from elaborations" (*spros bral*) accurately corresponds with reality, even though it distorts that truth by virtue of being conceptual. This is indicative of quasirepresentationalist realism.

Chapa's opponents argue this is nonsense. Concepts cannot both distort and represent reality accurately, they argue. On the phenomenalist, antirealist read, then, concepts have no referent whatsoever. They cannot even capture their own failure to correspond accurately. Thus, even the concept "freedom from elaborations" so fails. Nevertheless, the antirealist must agree that such a concept, at least at first, is instrumental toward realization. Indeed, before realization, conceptual reasoning is the only instrument at one's disposal. So even though the goal is to eradicate concepts, concepts must be employed to do so—to fight fire with fire, as it were.

Chapa identifies, however, that this antirealist position has a bootstrapping problem. If even the concept "freedom from elaborations" has no referent object, then it could not even be instrumental toward realizing reality, since it is as disconnected from the real as the concept "unicorn." Chapa thus argues in his *Essential Teachings of the Three Mādhyamikas from the East* (*Dbu ma shar gsum gyi stong thun*)[5] that this antirealist position is untenable.

> If you assent that freedom from elaborations is not actually a knowable object, then you implicitly must agree that the inference which negates elaborations is not an epistemic warrant since it has no epistemic object (*gzhal bya*). And thus, it would have to be a type of mind other than an inference or perception, [which is absurd].[6]

If, as the opponent claims, we only know objects through elaborations, then "freedom from elaborations" would denote the *absence* of any knowable objects. The inference of "freedom from elaborations" would thus equally produce no object of knowledge. But this would be self-subverting, since no epistemic process could then substantiate "freedom from elaborations." This is because inferences categorically posit some object of knowledge—they are probative—while perception apprehends positive particulars, not absences.

In response, Chapa's interlocutor argues that they can substantiate "freedom from elaborations" indirectly. The probandum of such an inference is still an absence. But instead of elaborations as the negatum, the opponent proposes an "ultimate entity" (*don dam pa'i dngos po*), that is, some *thing* that really existed as elaborated. The inference proves that no such object exists, since *nothing* ultimately exists as elaborated. So, in place of establishing the absence of elaborations, which would be self-subverting, the interlocutor proposes an inference that denies an impossibilium, an ultimate entity. It is in the void of this denial that the realization of freedom from elaborations can rush in.

> [Objection:] *Indeed, inference never analyzes freedom from elaborations. Nevertheless, it analyzes an ultimate entity* (don dam pa'i dgnos po) *as a negatum. Thus, it is not the case that this inferential reason is bereft of an epistemic object.* [Reply:] Is this epistemic object commensurate with emptiness or not? If not, then it is just an incomplete version of emptiness. If it is, the epistemic object should only be emptiness itself. And so, that contradicts an ultimate entity's being the epistemic object.[7]

The opponent argues that they can arrive at the necessary negation through Modus Tollens. This might be of the form, "If elaborations are accurate, things exist ultimately." Through an inference that rejects ultimately existing things, one arrives at freedom from elaborations. Such an inference takes "ultimate things" as its object. So, the opponent argues, it escapes the fault of making freedom from elaborations an epistemic object, which would render it an elaboration paradoxically. But Chapa demonstrates that the opponent merely kicks the can down the road. There are two options: either the subject of that inference, "an ultimate entity," is the same as emptiness, true freedom from elaborations, or not. It cannot be the same, since that would render emptiness an elaboration in the very manner the opponent wants to avoid. But if it is different than emptiness, then it is not the true target of the inference, even *via negativa*. On the opponent's view, even the negation of an ultimate entity is antithetical to the target probandum, since emptiness is purportedly beyond any elaboration. Thus, the opponent cannot give a cogent account of how the subject of the inference is an epistemic thing and yet the probandum is not.

Chapa thus argues that his opponent's position suffers from a general self-contradictory view of inference. The opponent argues that inferences can negate without positing anything. According to Chapa, this is incoherent. They must, at the very least, posit negations. But Chapa goes even further than this. He argues that negations must be predicated on some positive entity. For example, my question, "Where are my keys?" implies my perception of a table where they are not found. Even categorical denials imply existence. "There are no unicorns" implies a world without them—a world that serves as the warrant for their absence. The contrary would be absurd. There are no unpredicated absences, applicable to nothing. Chapa thus argues that absences cannot be free-floating. There can be an absence of certain qualities in an object, but any absence must instantiate of some object. Thus, no negation of ultimate entities can vitiate entities entirely.[8]

This is all indicative of quasirepresentationalist realism. "Freedom from elaborations" must represent some object; it cannot be a statement of objects' total vitiation. Yet as a concept, "freedom from elaborations" is itself an elaboration, and so, yogic perception is required to grasp true freedom from elaborations without the medium of elaborations. Nevertheless, like many of the authors in chapter 3, Chapa insists that the inference of this concept correspondences with that true freedom, and further warrants meditation based thereupon. Chapa makes this point explicit in the next section. He notes that some opponents argue that inferences provisionally posit "freedom from elaborations" as an epistemic object, while yogic perception of "freedom from elaborations" has no epistemic object at all. But Chapa again argues that moving from this provisional inference to yogic realization would be impossible. If yogic perception had no epistemic object, then, "Yogic perception would entertain freedom from elaborations, which is not an epistemic object, as an epistemic object. It would thus be in error. But if it does not entertain such an object, then it would have no epistemic object at all, [and there would be nothing to meditate upon]."[9]

Recall that yogic perception is developed through meditation on a salutary concept—in this case, "freedom from elaborations." But if "freedom from elaborations" has no referent—since, according to the opponent, it vitiates all objects—then any inference with "freedom from elaborations" as its probandum would be false. Any yogic perception based thereupon would likewise be erroneous. On the other hand, it is impossible to cultivate yogic perception without any such an object, since then one would have nothing to meditate upon. According to Chapa, then, we must conclude that this initiating, inferential concept corresponds with reality.

In many ways, Chapa here is agreement with his predecessors, like Jñānaśrīmitra. We saw how the latter took great pains to demonstrate that meditation on a conceptual property like momentariness corresponds with actual momentary entities. But we also saw Jñānaśrīmitra vacillate between representationalist and pragmatist theories. According to the latter, appearances in yogic perception can be soteriologically effective even if they do not refer. Chapa positions himself more squarely on the side of representationalism: because probative inferences necessarily substantiate epistemic objects, yogic perception based thereupon must warrant those same objects. Mutatis mutandis, if accurate inferences about reality are possible, appearances in turn must also represent reality, at least sufficiently enough to serve as fodder for these inferences. Hence, Chapa's quasirepresentationlist realist view.

Tsongkhapa on Yogic Perception

Tsongkhapa Losang Drakpa's (1357–1419) interpretation of these issues held near total hegemony within monastic curricula across different Tibetan schools. As I suggested, the primacy of Tsongkhapa's views may have more to do with political fortune rather than any innate philosophical superiority. The Gelug school, of which Tsongkhapa was the founder, eventually came to political supremacy in the seventeenth century. With increased political power came increased religious influence. For example, Nyingma (Rnying ma) monasteries (another Tibetan Buddhist school) were forced to use Gelug textbooks in their curricula up until at least the beginning of the twentieth century.[10] Given that Tsongkhapa's view represents a minority position within a much more diverse Tibetan philosophical landscape, the dominance of his interpretation in Tibetan monastic curricula is all the more notable.

Although Tsongkhapa disagreed with Chapa on many points, he undoubtedly shared Chapa's belief in the referential capacity of reason.[11] Like Chapa, Tsongkhapa was invested in showing that yogic perception perceives an object substantiated by inference. Also, like Chapa, he appears to eschew pragmatic arguments. Even when restricting himself to the viewpoint of

Dharmakīrti's position, Tsongkhapa did not feel comfortable abandoning the epistemological framework of correspondence in favor of pure pragmatism. He thus argues that yogic perception represents properties that inhere in objects; yogic perception is not *merely* efficacious toward liberation. Indeed, according to Tsongkhapa, this efficacy *depends* on yogic perception's grasp of the real.

As I have noted throughout, Buddhists in Dignāga's lineage understand the object of inferences to be conceptual universals, which create the appearance of spatiotemporally extended objects and repeatable properties, while the object of perception is particulars—discrete atoms with no spatiotemporal extension. Furthermore, only particulars are real and, because they are not universals (and universals are the referents of words), they are ineffable. Nevertheless, Tsongkhapa, like Chapa, argues that yogic perception's representational capacity is warranted through its initiating concept's correspondence with reality. But to prove that this concept corresponds with reality, Tsongkhapa will have an uphill battle. How can we prove that the referents of our concepts are real if reality—that is, particulars—is beyond conceptual-linguistic thought?

Tsongkhapa could just deny that particulars are beyond thought. He could argue concepts correspond with real particulars because the properties captured by concepts *really* inhere in particulars. But this would undermine the entire Buddhist soteriological project, which problematizes conceptual thinking as distortive, as productive of suffering, and as that which must be subverted in meditative insight. Tsonkhapa thus must hedge. He claims that conceptual distortion does not undermine conceptual correspondence. This is again indicative of quasirepresentationalist realism, since, according to Tsongkhapa, (normal, nonyogic) appearances also both represent and distort reality.[12] This view is recurrent in Tsongkhapa's various analyses of yogic perception.

Falling Hairs

CANDRAKĪRTI

Tsongkhapa's *Clarifying the Intent* (*Dgongs pa rab gsal*), his famed commentary on Candrakīrti's *Introduction to the Middle Way*, gives a detailed account of the meditation on bones that I first explored in chapter 2. Tsongkhapa's analysis in this text is admittedly beyond the scope of Dignāga's and Dharmakīrti's frameworks. Nevertheless, it reflects his theory of yogic perception elsewhere, particularly on the point of why meditation on bones is *not* yogic perception. Thus, this digression is useful for understanding his views on yogic perception.

First, a quick recap. Dharmakīrti cited mediation on bones as analogous to the clear appearances in yogic perception. But he claims that they are dissimilar from yogic perception in that the bones are unreal, while the object of yogic perception is real.

Candrakīrti, on the other hand, discussed yogic meditation of bones to deny their intersubjective appearance. He offered this as a counterexample to Yogācāra's rejection of external objects. He argued that there cannot be appearances that are purely mental and exist independently of an external object, since then yogically generated bones would be seen by both yogis and nonyogis. If all phenomena are mind only, Candrakīrti claims, then mental projections should be universally shared: there would be nothing to ensure their privacy. (This argument is admittedly counterintuitive; see chapter 2 for a more detailed discussion.) Candrakīrti also noted that the appearance of bones is "just like" that of falling hairs to someone with clouded vision, or that of pus to a hungry ghost. These appearances are idiosyncratic to each of their observers—they are not intersubjective. And that privacy is ensured by individual, private external objects—so he argues.

Candrakīrti seems to suggest that these three examples—the bones, the falling hairs, and the pus—are all exemplary of the same phenomenon. That is, their having private, external referents ensures their idiosyncrasy. But Tsongkhapa argues that although these are all similar in their idiosyncrasy, they hold different epistemological weight relative to their referents. In other words, some of these referents are more real than others. He thus invokes a representationalist theory to determine which of these appearances, despite their uniform lack of intersubjectivity, are truly representative and which are not.

To do this, he appeals to a framework of the twelve sense objects (*skye mched*, **āyatana*). This describes the six senses (the eye, ear, nose, tongue, body, and mind) and their respective objects (form, sound, smell, tastes, tangible objects, and thoughts). According to Tsongkhapa, a sense cognition is accurate to the degree that the appearance presented to it represents a veritable sense object. He uses this criterion to distinguish the appearances of bones, falling hairs, and pus:

> Those bones appear clearly even though there are no bones. Thus, we must accept that they have form in the manner an apparition does. Still, because the bones appear to mental consciousness only, they, also like apparitions, are not visual forms (**rupāyatana*). And since it cannot be one of the other nine sense objects either—[the five physical senses or other four objects besides form], it is nominally a form which is the sense object of the mind (**dharmāyatana*). The appearance of a falling hair to the eye consciousness, on the other hand, is like an apparition but *is* a visual form [since it appears to sense consciousness and not mental consciousness alone, like the bones]. Lastly, since the appearance of pus and blood to a hungry ghost appears to their eye consciousness, it must be posited as a visual form [but not like an apparition].[13]

Tsongkhapa taxonomizes the bones, falling hairs, and pus using two distinctions: whether it is an external sense object and whether it is like an apparition. The bones and falling hairs are both like an apparition. The falling hairs and the pus, on the other hand, are both considered visual forms. The bones are only nominally a type of form. Like an apparition, they appear to sense consciousness *like* a form might. But that appearance is not truly an external object, since (as we saw in chapter 3) it is an object of *mental* concentration. Still, because those bones *seem* visual but do not fit into one of the other nine external sense objects, they are nominally (*kun brtags*) a type of form.

The falling hairs, on the other hand, *are* an external sense object. As we know today, to see floating hairs is to see protein strands floating in the eye's vitreous humor. Thus, they are veritable forms, not just mental concoctions. Nevertheless, they do not behave in the way we would expect from their appearance. We cannot, for example, comb these seeming hairs. Thus, they are still apparitional. Only the pus is both a type of form, since it has an external referent, and *not* like an apparition, since that pus really functions like pus for hungry ghosts as dictated by their karma.[14]

Tsongkhapa appears to take liberal interpretive license here. In chapter 2, we saw Candrakīrti analogize yogic meditation on bones both to falling hairs and pus. There, he marshalled all three examples in common to demonstrate that private external objects explain distinct observations between perceivers. Tsongkhapa, however, *differentiates* each example. In sum, he claims that representing an external object (the sense object) and functioning as expected (being nonapparitional) are individually necessary and collectively sufficient for an appearance to be truly *of* a form. Each example succeeds and/or fails on each criterion for different reasons.

Still, Candrakīrti's argument does not preclude Tsongkhapa's reading. It is possible to give these appearances differing epistemological weight without denying Candrakīrti's axiom that all appearances have external objects, which was his reason for citing each example in the first place. Tsongkhapa's key intervention, then, is his argument that *just because all appearances are of some external object does not necessitate that all appearances are authentic representations*. This again is indicative of a quasirepresentationalist view. Although all appearances refer to some object, as stipulated by Candrakīrti, Tsongkhapa contends that some representations do a better job than others. The appearance of bones refers to some liminal form, but poorly; that of fallings hairs, better, but is still distortive; while only the appearance of pus accurately captures how that pus behaves for the ghost.

Nevertheless, Tsongkhapa does seem to make an exegetical leap in arguing that the bones, hairs, and pus are epistemically distinct from each other. This is not clearly expressed by Candrakīrti. It also may be philosophically dubious. If we take it as an axiom that all appearances have referent external objects, then in what cogent sense can an appearance deviate from its object and become a poor representation? As soon as Tsongkhapa introduces the possibility of a mismatch between appearances and their objects, he undercuts the thrust of Candrakīrti's nondualist argument about the relationship between mind and world, since this mismatch depends on some aspect of the appearance *not* having an external counterpart. It is thus unsurprising that this position was extensively criticized by other Tibetan thinkers, notably Taktsang Lotsāwa (Stag tshang lo tsā ba, 1405–1477).[15]

There are larger issues at stake here than ghoulish musings on ghosts, bones, and pus. Both Candrakīrti and Tsongkhapa are trying to clear two different but interrelated epistemological hurdles. As we saw in chapter 2, Candrakīrti argues that all appearances have referent objects to stave off idealism. If we suspect *some* appearances (like that of bones) have no referent objects, and we only ever have access to appearances, then how can we confidently deny that *all* appearances are referentless? Candrakīrti thus categorically states that all appearances have referents, even private ones. But the possibility of private objects immediately brings up the possibility of relativism, a world in which there is no surefire way to differentiate personal hallucination from the veritable perception of existing objects.

Indeed, Taktsang Lotsāwa argues that Candrakīrti's analysis vitiates any robust, epistemological differentiation of this type.[16] Tsongkhapa recoils at this suggestion, since it undermines epistemic warrant and devolves into all out relativism. He thus nuances Candrakīrti's maxim and argues that having a referent object is not sufficient for being an authentic representation. Thereby, he can make distinctions between illusions and veritable cognitions. Tsongkhapa is thus trying to preserve Candrakīrti's rejection of idealism without teetering over into relativism.

The discussion thus far only tangentially concerns yogic perception: Candrakīrti's example of yogic meditation on bones. And this is not the same as yogic perception proper. Nevertheless, the differentiation that Tsongkhapa sets up here between these three examples becomes pertinent in his more explicit discussion of yogic perception. We saw that in the Buddhist *locus classicus* for yogic perception, Dharmakīrti's *Commentary*, that meditation on bones was the primary point of comparison to yogic perception—while both share the same perceptual clarity, they differ in their epistemological authenticity. Interestingly, we will see that in his own analysis, Tsongkhapa also attempts to establish yogic perception's authenticity via comparison. But in his case, he differentiates yogic perception from that of falling hairs. This choice substitution, I argue, reveals his representationalist thinking.

DHARMAKĪRTI

The source for Tsongkhapa's view on yogic perception is his *Notes on the Perception Chapter* (*Mngon sum le'u'i brjed byang*), a commentary on that chapter of Dharmakīrti's *Commentary*. Tsongkhapa picks up on the issue of falling hairs in the context of his discussion of yogic perception. An interlocutor argues that the object of yogic perception cannot be epistemically warranted because it is neither a particular nor a universal. Yogic perception cannot perceive a universal, since, according to Dharmakīrti, only conceptual thinking apprehends universals, while perception grasps particulars. Nor can it perceive a particular, since its meditative object is contrived by inference, which is conceptual. Thus, because yogic perception cognizes neither, the opponent contends, yogic perception cannot be epistemically warranted, since there is no third epistemically warranted object. The interlocutor thus likens the object of yogic perception to falling hairs. "[Objection:] When a falling hair appears clearly, it is not a particular, since it has no causal efficacy. Nor is it a universal, since it appears clearly, and clear appearances do not come after [some previous cognition]. Nevertheless, that falling hair is an object (*yul*), because it appears clearly. Therefore, it is a comprehended object that is a third option besides a particular or a universal."[17]

The opponent argues that the clear appearances in yogic perception are like the clear appearance of falling hairs. Falling hairs cannot affect anything—they do not behave like hairs—so they cannot be particulars. But because they appear clearly, they cannot be purely conceptual objects either, since only nonconceptual cognitions are clear. Appearances in yogic perception have these same qualities. The appearance of impermanence qua property is not the appearance of a functional, impermanent thing—actual particulars. But this appearance is clear, so it cannot be conceptual. Yogic perception's object is thus neither a particular nor a universal, and thus it is unwarranted, so says the interlocutor.

Tsongkhapa predictably responds with an appeal to representationalism. The appearance of falling hairs have no referent object. Therefore, it is not problematic that falling hairs are neither a universal nor a particular, since only cognitions of particulars and universals are warranted. Thus, although both yogic appearances and the appearance of falling hairs are alike in their being clear, they are distinct on the question of representation. The ability to represent and not clarity simpliciter warrants yogic perception.

> Therefore, the falling hair is not an object. If it were, then we would have to assert that an object exists however it appears (*snang*) according to its linguistic sign ["falling hairs"]. But it does not exist in the manner that it is necessarily conceived (*zhen*). On this view, while we deny that the falling hairs appearing to a sense consciousness, within which trickling falling hairs appear, are an object, what about the consciousness of the appearance of falling hairs? We do not deny that the mental image of the appearance of falling hairs is an object.[18]

Tsongkhapa uses the novel Tibetan distinction between appearing object (*snang yul*) and conceived object (*zhen yul*) to substantiate why falling hairs are illusory and unreal.[19] Namely, while their appearance qua appearance exists, their appearance qua referent, the conceived object—that is, *actual* falling hairs—does not.[20] In other words, the appearance of falling hairs exists, but that appearance fails as a representation. It is this failure that explains this appearance's epistemic inauthenticity.

There is also a subtle allusion to yogic perception. Tsongkhapa notes that the appearance of falling hairs fails to be authentic due to an incongruity between how it appears and what is suggested by its designation (*brda la byang*). They *look* like hairs but do not behave as we would expect of "hairs." But the object of yogic perception, "impermanence," does not have this incongruity. As we saw Jñānaśrīmitra argue in chapter 3, "impermanence" is unique in its capacity to correspond, since only it captures the nature of phenomena. Thus, Tsongkhapa posits criteria concerning two objects that both render the appearance of falling hairs inauthentic and those within yogic perception authentic: the ontological referent object as conceived and the corresponding conceptual-linguistic object as designated. As Dharmakīrti mentions in the *Commentary*, it is meditative fixation on *warranted* concepts that constitute yogic perception once they become clear.

Tsongkhapa's criteria also provide an epistemological account of the counter examples to yogic perception that Dharmakīrti identifies in verses 3.281–82, such as hallucinations provoked by intense emotion toward someone and the earth *kasiṇa*, (see chapter 3). These are also examples of conceptual objects that become clear with meditative practice. However, while these appearances exist *as* appearances, they fail to exist as conceived, that is, as actual people or actual earth. Those appearances thus fail as representations, unlike yogic perception, whose object exists as conceived. This is roughly the same strategy that Tsongkhapa used to differentiate the falling hairs from the pus in his *Intent*. In both texts, the inaccuracy of the appearance of hairs occurs as a failure of representation, whereas the accuracy of the appearance of pus or those in yogic perception derive from their successful representation.

So, at this point Tsongkhapa has made clear that yogic perception's object is *not* like falling hairs. While both appearances may be clear, they differ in their representational capacity. But this leaves a fundamental question unanswered: If appearances in yogic perception do have a referent object, then what is *that* object? Is *it* a universal or a particular? Tsongkhapa tackles the answers in the next section.

Sutrist Versus Mind Only

The distinction between appearing objects and conceived objects gives Tsongkhapa a criterion for defining accurate representations and thus differentiating false appearances from veridical ones. But this strategy now creates a new issue for Tsongkhapa. The object of yogic perception does seem suspiciously like the falling hair. Like the falling hair, this object cannot be a causally effective particular, since it is a negative property—impermanence, selflessness, emptiness. Nor, however, can it be a universal. It appears clearly in yogic perception, and universals, as conceptual objects, do not appear clearly. Unlike the falling hair, however, appearances in yogic perception must refer, since otherwise this would undermine its status as an epistemic warrant. Yogic perception's object therefore must be either a particular or universal, although it seems to be neither.

Dharmakīrti bites the bullet on this. He eschews representationalism for pragmatism. On his view, the appearance of selflessness need not represent some real selflessness in the world. Rather, its cognition only needs to serve pragmatic ends, namely, liberation. Tsongkhapa's representationalist framework precludes this strategy: yogic perception must represent some real object. So, is *this* object a universal or a particular?

Tsongkhapa gives two solutions, one from the perspective of the Yogācāra school and another from the realist Sutrist perspective. As we saw in chapter 4, the latter is a representationalist, external realist view. Tsongkhapa understands the former to be idealist—"Mind Only" (*cittamātra*)—much like Candrakīrti, who argues that Yogācārins deny the existence of external objects (see chapter 2).[21] Continuing in his *Notes on the Perception Chapter*, he first sets up the problem yogic perception poses for both Sutrist and Mind Only in the voice of an interlocutor.

> [Objection:] *The system of enumerating two epistemic instruments—perception and inference—is either from the perspective of the Sutrists only, or from a perspective shared with the Mind-Only school. It cannot be the first, [for four reasons]: First, from the lower [school, the Sutrist, on up], that reality is empty of the two types of persons*[22] *is thoroughly established. Thus, second, they both must explain how the enumeration of the two epistemic instruments are subsumed by the type of yogic perception that perceptually realizes those two emptinesses. Thirdly and furthermore, this is explained repeatedly [in the* Commentary*], not just in the perception chapter. Finally, these last three*

> *characteristics sufficiently determine the Unchanging Absolute* (*parinișpanna) *[as defined in Mind Only] as well. But even if the two epistemic instruments are enumerated from the perspective of both the Sutrists and Mind Only in common, [the problem persists], since although the Unchanging Absolute must be a nonfunctional entity, Mind Only does not accept it as a universal, and this makes no sense.*[23]

The Mind Only and Sutrist schools share a similar hurdle. Both assent to two types of emptinesses, the emptiness of the coarse person and that of the subtle person.[24] They also agree that these can be known both inferentially and directly in yogic perception. Lastly, both schools agree that yogic perception begins with an inference of a universal and culminates in a direct perception of a particular. Therefore, both schools must also explain how yogic perception subsumes (*ya gyal du bsdus pa*) this inferential understanding perceptually.[25] This is no small task, since perception is restricted to particulars and inference is restricted to universals. And yet, yogic perception must somehow bridge the divide, providing a continuity between conceptual inferential understanding and direct perceptual insight.[26]

Tsongkhapa further mentions that the requirements of yogic perception in the Sutrist school apply mutatis mutandis to the "Unchanging Absolute" (*'gyur med yongs grub*). This is a reference to the third of the so-called three natures (*trisvabhāva, mtshan nyid gsum*), specifically, the Absolute (*parinișpanna, yongs grub*), or emptiness as understood in Mind Only. The absolute nature is revealed once reality appears how it actually exists, that is, as *empty* of conceptual overlay, including subject-object dichotomies.[27] As the ultimate truth in this school, it must be perceived in yogic perception. But, as the interlocutor notes, it is unclear how it could be a perceptual object, since it is unchanging (*'gyur med*), which should render it a universal, a fact that the Mind Only school strangely denies.

Tsongkhapa thus clarifies: "The Mind Onlyist[28] does not agree that if something is unable to perform a function that it is necessarily a universal, nor that if it is a particular it necessarily performs a function."[29] In other words, the Mind Onlyist accepts an unchanging, nonfunctional emptiness as a particular. Thus, they argue it can be a proper object of perception. Despite being unchanging, the Absolute can thus still be an appropriate object of yogic perception.[30] Essentially, this allows Tsongkhapa to have his cake and eat it too. The conceptual universal of the Unchanging Absolute and the Unchanging Absolute itself are both permanent entities. And so, there is no perceptual hump between its initial inference and its yogic perception.

Tsongkhapa's representationalism necessities his account of the Absolute qua particular. To establish that yogic perception correctly represents reality, he must give an ontological account of ultimate reality that makes it available to perceptual instruments. Otherwise, yogic perception would mispresent how the Absolute exists. This strategy is also reflected in his construal of the Sutrist view of yogic perception. But here, the difficulty is more egregious: there is no possibility in this school for negative entities like impermanence, selflessness, or emptiness to be a particular. Only positive entities are particulars. How can impermanence, selflessness, or emptiness be an object of yogic perception, if yogic perception only grasps positive particulars? Tsongkhapa explains: "From that Sutrist perspective, yogic perception engages the selflessness of persons (*gang zag gi bdag med*) implicitly and explicitly apprehends the causally effective particular. Therefore, it says in Dignāga's *Compendium*[31] that 'yogis see just the object, independently from the guru's instructions.'"[32]

How does yogic perception realize negative entities? Tsongkhapa answers "implicitly" (*shugs rtogs*). This describes a cognition's ability to realize something about an object that does not directly appear to it. According to Gelugpas, the perception of my desk includes the implicit perception of an absence of an elephant thereupon. Similarly, apprehending selfless particulars, free of reification, is sufficient for an implicit perception of their selflessness. Furthermore, this implicit perception is not inferential—it is part of perception.[33]

This introduction of implicit cognition into Dharmakīrti's system is likely a Tibetan invention[34] and was also likely first championed by Chapa.[35] Within the context of Dharmakīrti's pragmatism, there is simply no need for such a notion. In that system, warrant is a function of pragmatic ends, not how cognitions succeed or fail to represent real objects. Likewise, how negative concepts map onto positive particulars (implicitly or otherwise) is not a problem for pragmatism. In the context of Tsongkhapa's thought, however, implicit cognition allows him to explain how the perceptual appearance of selfless particulars can represent their selflessness without selflessness directly appearing.[36]

In the next section, however, Tsongkhapa seems to pivot sharply. He compares this Sutrist theory of implicit cognition with the Middle Way philosophy championed by Candrakīrti. In Gelug doxography, Middle Way supersedes both Sutrist and Yogācāra / Mind Only views. While Sutrists are external realists, and Mind Onlyists are idealists, Middle Way posits the interdependence of mind and world. Tsongkhapa's hermeneutic shift toward Middle Way is marked by his reference to a work by Nāgārjuna (ca. 150–250 CE), thought to be the founding figure of Middle Way thought. "However, this Sutrist position is overturned in the commentary to Nāgārjuna's *Sixty Verses on Logic* (*Yuktiṣaṣṭīkā*), where he refutes this position while responding to an opponent. There, the Unchanging Absolute realized by yogic perception is an explicit realization and is *not* realized implicitly."[37]

According to Middle Way, yogic perception explicitly realizes the Absolute, so Tsongkhapa contends. The change of school here is odd. By and large, Tibetan works take strenuous efforts to be doxographically clean, making sure not to switch registers between philosophical viewpoints. Why this sudden change of philosophical framing?

To understand what Tsongkhapa is doing here, we must reintroduce the notion of a "sliding scale of analysis" from chapter 4. But it must be nuanced slightly. The sliding scale is not merely a hierarchy of views within which higher views supersede lower ones. More than this, each view must feed into the other, giving way to gradual philosophical advents with each subsequent step. Even though higher views invalidate certain aspects of lower views, each subsequent rung builds of off the foundation of the lower ones. There is thus a delicate balance between supersession and continuity. Tibetan doxography is therefore not merely a taxonomy, but a pedagogical tool that allows adherents to amass philosophical sophistication progressively.

With this in mind, I argue that Tsongkhapa's gesture toward Nāgārjuna suggests that his *Notes* is proleptically setting the groundwork for his eventual Middle Way view. In the Sutrist school, it is axiomatic that inference and perception take different objects. And so Tsongkhapa recruits implicit cognition to bridge the divide. In the context of Mind Only, he argues that emptiness is a particular, and so relinquishes implicit cognition. And once he arrives at Middle Way, he accepts that even universals, like emptiness, are perceptible.[38] Yogic perception simply sees directly what inferential thinking only knows conceptually.

While he argues that Middle Way interpretations supersede Sutrist and Mind Only views about the respective objects of perception and inference, Tsongkhapa remains consistent on representationalism.[39] His sliding scale is thus variable on the dimension of how epistemic instruments function but consistent on the view that these instruments' warrant derives from their correspondence with or representation of real objects. Yet this move is not without its critics.[40] In chapter 6 I explore how, in a similar effort to keep their sliding scale continuous, Sakya authors' rejection of representationalism within Middle Way influences their presentation of Sutrism.

In the Gelug view, however, the appeal to implicit cognition at lower levels preserves the representationalism that he argues remains in Middle Way, according to which yogic perception represents the Absolute directly.[41] Consistently through all three schools, the referent object of yogic perception is afforded by a metaphysics in excess of Dharmakīrti's pragmatism: yogic perception is not simply effective, but representative. Because this real object is both inferable and perceivable, yogic perception can "subsume" the realizations of both epistemic instruments.

The Creation Stage

Interestingly, however, this is not to say that Tsongkhapa relegates his discussion of yogic perception solely to the cultivation of appearances that appropriately refer, represent, or correspond. He also maintains that the vivid appearance of purely fictional entities, like that of the falling hairs or bones, can be beneficial—and even have soteriological value. This claim reinforces his distance from pragmatism: cognitions can be pragmatically effective and still fail to be epistemic. Thus, pragmatic efficacy is *not* sufficient for veritable yogic perception, since, according to Tsongkhapa, yogic perception is *both* pragmatic and accurately represents.[42]

Tsongkhapa affords these hallucinations a role in his formulation of the tantric Creation Stage (*utpattikrama, bskyed rim*). This stage of tantric practice focuses on deity yoga (*devatāyoga, lha'i rnal 'byor*). The practitioner visualizes a meditational deity—replete with their attendant entourage of celestial figures, comprising a "mandala," or circle of deities—until that mental image appears clearly. The creation stage reaches its zenith when the meditator can perfectly visualize a host of details about the deities and their environment, as if they were right in front of them. In the highest form of tantric practice, one even meditates that they themself are the deity, generating what is known as "divine pride" (*lha'i nga rgyal*). These vivid appearances are meant to disrupt our ordinary quotidian appearances (*tha mal pa'i snang ba*), which represent ourselves as suffering beings in a suffering world. It is a sort of bootstrapping method that helps the practitioner generate the necessary merit to reach enlightenment—a fake-it-until-you-make-it strategy.

The primary goal of both cultivating yogic perception and the Creation Stage is meditative clarity. This parallel is not lost on Tsongkhapa.[43] In his *Great Treatise on the Stages of Mantra* (*Sngags rim chen mo*), Tsongkhapa heavily relies on Dharmakīrti's *Commentary* and its discussion of yogic perception to explain the Creation Stage. Specifically, he cites the same verses 3.284–5 explored in chapter 3. First, he comments on verse 3.284, which compares meditation on real and unreal objects. This verse references meditation on bones. Although Tsongkhapa skirted this example in his analysis of yogic perception in *Notes on the Perception Chapter* (focusing instead on falling hairs), here he reintroduces it. Tsongkhapa writes:

> There are heretics who also refute what the buddhas say in scripture [about the power of meditation to generate clear appearances] and claim that freedom is impossible. Even they fail to deny the example[44] that serves as the basis for determining the entailment between the reason for and the veritable arising of yogic perception, [the probandum]. Nevertheless, this denial is leveled by others. And so, for the sake of other schools, there is an analysis of the fundamental premise that people like Noble Ones (**ārya*), etc., exist. Therefore, Dharmakīrti intends that that meditation on an object, whether real or not, will result in a clear appearance merely from that meditation.[45]

The "other schools" in this passage may be a reference to certain Mīmāṃsakas who reject the existence of meditative insight, liberation, and yogis (see chapter 2). As we also saw, these Mīmāṃsakas do not reject the possibility of creating clear meditative appearances, only that such appearances are epistemic (see chapter 3). In response, Tsongkhapa claims that the possibility of nonepistemic meditative appearances does not undermine the existence of epistemic ones sufficient for yogic insight.

While Tsongkhapa's proof of yogis is fascinating in its own right, what concerns us here is how Tsongkhapa understands yogic perception in the context of Creation Stage practice. As he notes, mere meditation on unreal objects can culminate in their clear appearance, but does *not* constitute yogic perception. So does Creation Stage practice culminate in veritable yogic perception, or a "mere" vivid meditative appearance? Tsongkhapa explores this question further on in the text, where he again quotes verse 3.285 of the *Commentary,* explaining that the Creation Stage meditator "visualizes each and every aspect of the deity in detail. Then, in addition to the mere manifestation of that meditation and its aspects, the meditator must cultivate a powerful mental certainty [of being that deity], since grasping both the clear mental image of that deity and the divine pride of being that deity are necessary."[46] Tsongkhapa therefore understands vivid appearance of oneself as the deity to be the culmination of the Creation Stage. This is coupled with the conviction that this is the case, which is described as "divine pride."

Although Tsongkhapa previously argued that the clear, meditative appearance of the Unchanging Absolute represented a real object—meaning that it was not *merely* a mental image—Tsongkhapa makes no such concession here. He first explains that the mental appearance of the deity in meditation is not the same as an actual sensorial one.

> When one has steady Deity Yoga through intense habituation [and there is a clear appearance of the deity], nothing appears to visual consciousness, nor to the other external sense consciousnesses. Because the mental consciousness needs to be fully engaged with its object, the power of the conditions for meditation are diminished as soon as the visual or other consciousnesses arise. Therefore, given that at that time those other senses are inoperative, appearances other [than the deity], like colors, etc., do not manifest. This does not mean, however, that the Creation Stage negates those sensory appearances.[47]

In other words, cognition of external sensory appearances hinders meditation, and so they cannot operate in tandem with meditation, within which mental consciousness alone apprehends the meditative object. This is consistent with Tsongkhapa's assessment of meditating on bones in *Clarifying the Intent*. There he argued that meditation on bones were a liminal type of form. They appear to be form but cannot be form strictly speaking since they appear directly to the mind and not the eye consciousness. Tsongkhapa thus consistently argues these mind-generated quasiforms are mutually exclusive with actual forms so seen by the eyes. Whether it be bones or the deity, meditative appearances can only be seen by the mind and not in tandem with the eyes. Tsongkhapa also makes use of Dharmakīrti in making this point, citing *Commentary* verse 2.112cd: "Attached to another object, the mind has no meditative power, because it can grasp nothing else."[48] If the mind is preoccupied with apprehending visual forms, it cannot generate meditative appearances. So meditation operates at the expense of any external visual cognition.

This is not just a minor point about the mutual exclusivity of meditative and visual "seeing." The ramifications are metaphysical. Tsongkhapa notes that the absence of sensory appearances during meditation does not mean the Creation Stage negates the sensory world itself. Rather, that world fails to appear to sense consciousness during meditation. He thus eschews any phenomenalism. By extension, any appearance that *is* merely phenomenal—in other words, that does not represent any external object—must be fallacious, even if such appearances are spiritually effective. "Therefore, when one achieves the power to stop ordinary appearances at the level of mental consciousness through the exceptional appearances of the deity, one gains what is necessary. *Although one will not have reached the deity in reality* [emphasis added], even when the uncontrived pride of the deity arises, one gains what is necessary thereby."[49] Tsongkhapa corroborates elsewhere that in the Creation Stage, "meditation on authentic objects for these clear appearances is not necessary, since meditation on any inauthentic object will result in its clear appearance," again citing *Commentary* verse 3.285.[50]

Tsongkhapa is therefore careful to distinguish the clear, meditative appearance of oneself as a deity from having "reached the deity in reality." There is a difference between faking it and actually making it—even if we fool ourselves in the faking. To reinvoke a distinction Tsongkhapa made earlier, while such divine appearances qua appearance are instrumental in cultivating the Creation Stage, they remain inaccurate qua referent, since one is not actually a deity. That one is not yet a deity is evinced by the fact the sense consciousnesses must be inoperable to create the illusion of being one.[51]

It is thus revealing that in this case, where the goal of deity yoga is to concoct a vivid appearance of an unreal object, Tsongkhapa cites the verses from the *Commentary* concerning meditative appearances of unreal objects like bones. Just as meditation on bones is meant to provoke disgust for the world, deity yoga is practiced to cultivate divine pride. There is thus a natural affinity between meditation on bones and deity yoga, both practices being effective—one toward renunciation and the other toward tantric progress—but fallacious. But when Tsongkhapa discusses yogic perception proper and its epistemic warrant, the stakes concern representation, not pragmatic efficacy. In this case, bones are a muddled counterexample, since they are effective despite failing to represent. The failing hairs simplify the comparison, since they are a straightforward example of an appearance without a referent. Thus, Tsongkhapa *likens* bones and deity yoga on the dimension of pragmatic efficacy, but he *differentiates* falling hairs from yogic perception on the dimension of representationalism. According to Tsongkhapa, this representationalist capacity is the ultimate measure of perceptual authenticity.[52]

Tsongkhapa thus betrays an epistemological preference for representationalism over pragmatism. Meditative appearances of objects like bones and deities may be soteriologically effective, but they do not qualify as yogic perception. This requires something more, that yogic perception represents a real object. Dharmakīrti's pragmatism offers a different view. On his position, appearances in yogic perception do not represent anything. Their clarity and pragmatic efficacy toward liberation is sufficient for their status as veritable perceptions. Dharmakīrti, therefore, might be suspect of Tsongkhapa's representationalist distinction between clear meditative appearances of a deity and clear appearances within yogic perception, since both are soteriologically efficacious. Nevertheless, Dharmakīrti vacillates, since he does not accommodate the clear appearance of bones as yogic perception, despite its spiritual efficacy.[53]

This disparity between Dharmakīrti and Tsongkhapa is put all the more in relief by a glaring difference between the Tibetan and Sanskrit editions of the *Commentary* concerning verse 2.112cd. Again, Tsongkhapa uses this verse to substantiate that the other senses shut down when one is immersed in meditation. Translated from the Tibetan, this verse reads, "Attached to another object, the mind has no meditative power, because it can grasp nothing else." The Sanskrit witness, however, puts this hemistich closer to: "When consciousness is defiled with attachment to another object, it is because it grasps no other object [than consciousness itself]."[54] Prajñākaragupta's commentary confirms this latter reading: "By no means is the arising of conceptual habits [to see] consciousness as separate [from the object] seen due to something else [besides consciousness], such as a subject under the sway of some object creating some interceding influence between them. And thus it is appropriately settled that consciousness alone comes from consciousness."[55]

In other words, Dharmakīrti does not mean (as Tsongkhapa takes it) that mental and sensory appearances cannot be simultaneous. Rather, it is only because we are "defiled with attachment" that we falsely believe in representationalist realism, where appearances seem to represent external objects. Dharmakīrti advocates, instead, that we bracket such metaphysical claims and discuss epistemic warrant only in terms of what appears to consciousness. As I mentioned in chapter 4, this amounts to a type of verificationism.

Tsongkhapa marshals the Tibetan deviation from the Sanskrit to bolster his representative realism. What Dharmakīrti intends as a rejection of external realism, Tsongkhapa takes as a cognitive limitation, such that we cannot meditate and be aware of the sensory world at the same time. By taking the claim cognitively rather than metaphysically, Tsongkhapa argues that the reality of the sensory world persists independent of what appears to consciousness. Sensory appearances are thus epistemically warranted where meditative ones (in the Creation Stage) fail because the former represents reality while the latter does not. Likewise, no appearance in and of itself can warrant oneself as a deity, since the reality behind that appearance determines its warrant.

Although it may seem as if Tsongkhapa is making some interpretive leaps to shoehorn Dharmakīrti into a representationalist framework, we ought to remember that Dharmakīrti and his Indian commentators equivocate on this issue. For example, if Dharmakīrti advocates a strong pragmatism, on what basis can he claim the bone and *kasiṇa* meditations are not epistemically warranted? This meditation also achieves desired ends—namely, gaining renunciation and the ability to control the elements—and culminates in clear appearances. So why is it not a type of yogic perception? As we saw, Jñānaśrīmitra also had to invoke representationalism to make sense of the epistemic discrepancy between these meditations and yogic perception.

We must wonder, then, what Dharmakīrti would have to say about Creation Stage practice in general. If appearances do not represent, would he consider seeing oneself as a deity equivalent to *being* a deity? We have seen Jñānaśrīmitra (in his capacity as a Yogācārin) argue something equally radical: knowledge of the past and future is a function of how phenomenal content mutually coheres, not of those appearances' accurate representation of past or future objects. If phenomenal content is sufficient for temporal omniscience, then presumably it is also sufficient for being an actual buddha. One would only need to have sufficiently convincing deity yoga. Tsongkhapa, however, strongly resists this slippery slope toward solipsism. He advocates stricter criteria for buddhahood. You can have perfect deity yoga with utter conviction and still not be a buddha. Again, Tsonkhapa's argument for the insufficiency of deity yoga is indicative of his representationalism, where appearances are distinct from facts of the matter, no matter how convincing appearances may be.

Conclusion: Moore and Quasirepresentationalism

Indian Buddhist sources leave certain ambiguities in their formulation of yogic perception. There is a general equivocation between representationalist and pragmatist formulations. Tibetan exegetes want to foreclose these vacillations in a systematic fashion. Gelugpas by and large achieve this by siding with representationalism over pragmatism. Across Sutrist, Yogācāra (Mind Only), and Middle Way contexts, Tsongkhapa consistently argues that yogic perception's epistemic warrant is a function of its appearances' accurate representation of the world.

In this chapter I first explore representationalism in Chapa's theory of the role of inference in developing yogic perception. His opponent argues that although developing yogic perception initially begins with inference, the culminating realization is a negation of any referent object, even qua absence. Chapa argues this position is self-subverting. Epistemic warrant is only cogent in relation to some corresponding object. If inference and yogic perception are epistemic warrants, they must be so in relation to some object. Therefore, he argues that this inference corresponds with the same object that yogic perception represents: reality bereft of any ultimate entities.

Similarly, Tsongkhapa establishes yogic perception's epistemic warrant by differentiating it from falling hairs, appearances that do not have a referent object. He further explains that both the Mind Only and Sutrist schools understand yogic perception's epistemic warrant in terms of its referent object. In the former, yogic perception realizes the Unchanging Absolute, a perceivable particular. In the latter, yogic perception directly perceives the momentary particular and implicitly perceives its impermanence. Tsongkhapa's distance from pragmatism is also evident in a tantric context.

Although appearances of oneself as a deity in deity yoga are clear, nonconceptual, and efficacious, they fail representationalist criteria. Since one is not actually a deity, these appearances are not yogic perception.

Representationalism is thus a consistent theme of Tsongkhapa's hermeneutic across his analysis of all Buddhist schools. It is also predicated on a degree of realism. That appearances represent entails that there is some reality they depict. But I say "degree" because Tsongkhapa cannot accept a naive realism, where the world exists *exactly* as it appears. If this were the case, then there would be no need for Buddhist practice, which is meant to correct appearances. Tsongkhapa's position is thus quasirepresentationalist, since although appearances do represent reality to some degree, globally, they are erroneous. Tsongkhapa's position is thus still a breed of error-theory, but one that admits that appearances are sufficient fodder for a workable epistemology, despite their inherent epistemic shortcomings.

It is tempting to interpret Tsonghapa as trying to have his realist cake and eat his Buddhist one too. That is, he wants to maintain representational realism but also preserve the Buddhist soteriological project, which problematizes representations. We might think then that Tsongkhapa is trying to jerry-rig two incompatible views to achieve his theological aims. But on a more generous read, Tsongkhapa is dealing with a fundamentally philosophical issue, one that recognizes this incongruity as endemic to our experience.

I illustrate this with reference to G. E. Moore (1873–1958), who dealt with the same issue.[56] In contrast to the sense data theorists (like Ayer) explored in chapter 3, Moore's earliest position was that we do not see sense data but rather the surface of objects. So, when I see a penny, I see the surface of a penny, not colors and shapes that I infer to be a penny. This seems to get us out of the problem of representationalism, since we simply see objects; there is no intermediary representation between objects and our seeing of them. But Moore quickly realized that this position was untenable. The surface of a penny does not look the same from two different perspectives. Therefore, what we see cannot be identical to the surface of penny, since that surface is singular, but perspectives on it are multiple. Moore thus speculates on what the relation is between the many perspectives on an object and that object itself, a relation he dubs "R." His concluding sentences are rather unnerving. "I was, therefore, certainly mistaken in supposing that . . . the sense-datum in question is always identical with the part of the object's surface which is being seen. . . . But I still think that no philosopher, so far as I know, has explained clearly what the relation R is, where it is not identity."[57]

On the one hand, Moore concedes that we cannot accept that what we see is identical with the object—the relation R is not one of identity. Yet, on the other hand, it is difficult to make sense of seeing objects if the relation R is not one of identity. If we concede that the multiplicity of perspectives entails some degree of representationalism, then we seem forced to accept that these representations both succeed and fail at capturing the world.

We can thus read both Moore and Tsongkhapa as quasirepresentationalists. Both are trying to explain how representations depict the world while recognizing that representations contain some type of distortion.[58] But how can we ever know which part is the distortion and which part is real if all we ever have access to is representations? We might think yogic perception gets us out of this bind, since it sees reality as it is without distortion. But recall that according to Tsongkhapa and his predecessors, yogic perception's epistemic warrant derives from a correct inference, whose warrant in turn derives from representations. Thus, we are back to the same problem.

Nevertheless, there may be a coherentist solution to the problem. Representations allow us to infer how reality exists and this inference is confirmed by yogic perception. And how do we know that yogic perception accurately shows us the world? Well, because it is substantiated by sound inference. While Moore would not accept mystical insight as such a warrant, we could adapt this solution to his conundrum. How do I know that my perspective is *of* a penny? Well, because I can also infer it is a penny, with the help of the report of other perspectives. And how do I know that I have correctly inferred that those other perspectives are of a penny? Well, because I can confirm that inference from my singular perspective by looking and seeing a penny. Thus, the relation R is not strict identity, but circular reinforcement: perception x is warranted by inference y and inference y is warranted by perception x. I know that I am perceiving a penny based on what I can infer from other perspectives, and I can confirm that inference based on a perception from any one perspective. Yogic perception's warrant functions in the same manner, where inference warrants the meditative object, and the culminating yogic perception confirms the original inference.

But here again there is a potential weakness apart from the obvious circularity. It is only by metaphysical fiat that what can be cogently inferred from perception, and what can be perceived based on inference, is necessarily real. Just because the inference of a real penny effectively explains a multitude of perspectives does not demand that this the penny is itself real. This is the entire point of Dharmakīrti's antimetaphysical pragmatism. The notion that appearances must refer to real pennies in order for those appearances to cohere merely question begs realism.

It is thus difficult to demonstrate the necessity of realism for epistemic warrant without an appeal to fiat. We might make a transcendental argument in response, arguing that *insofar* as there is such thing as knowledge, it must be *of* something real. Authors in this chapter by and large work with this assumption, such as Chapa, who argued that *insofar* as yogic perception provides knowledge of the real, its instigating concept must as well. But not all Tibetan schools understand yogic perception in this fashion. Instead, they question if yogic perception can be considered epistemic at all, and thus also bring the very possibility of epistemology into question. In place of a realism, then, these other schools favor a more thoroughgoing antirealism, one that undermines representationalism. It is to these positions that I now turn.

SIX

Sakya Antirepresentationalism

Introduction: Wittgenstein and the Limits of Language

We saw in the last chapter how Gelug thinkers appeal to representationalism to wrest yogic perception away from epistemic obscurity. Because appearances represent the world in part, albeit with distortion, they are sufficient to build sound inferences. These in turn become the starting point for cultivating yogic perception. This move, however, is in tension with another intellectual current running through yogic perception's interpretive history. We saw in chapter 3 how Asaṅga understands yogic perception as transcendent, perceiving a reality completely beyond appearances. If that reality has no continuity with appearances, then Tsongkhapa's quasirepresentationalism cannot explain how to reach this deeper insight from the starting point of our quotidian world. According to Asaṅga, therefore, yogic perception marks a complete departure with how we know the world now. Asaṅga rejects that yogic perception is simply a more direct way of understanding what we can know inferentially, a position held by Tsongkhapa.

On the flip side, however, Asaṅga's position frees up our everyday, nonyogic epistemology. Tsongkhapa had to go to great lengths to explain how appearances both represent and distort. If appearances do not represent anything at all—since reality is beyond them entirely—then reality no longer plays the role of an epistemic constraint. Because what we nonyogis call "knowledge" does not concern the real, we can define knowledge in terms of how the world appears and how we talk in common about it, however removed from "reality" those might be.

Candrakīrti, for example, gives such an epistemological account, criticizing Dignāga's theory of perception. Dignāga's theory of sense perception is causal, arguing that perception is epistemically warranted because it is caused by real, albeit ineffable, particulars. Candrakīrti rejects this theory on the grounds that it is too far afield from what we mean by perception in an everyday context. When we (nonyogis) perceive things, we *see* medium-sized dry goods, not ineffable particulars.[1] In other words, I perceive tables and chairs, not the particulars that make them up. Candrakīrti thus defines "perception" relative to our common-sense usage, not relative to its relationship to "real" particulars. In a famous line, he argues that his conventional epistemology is based upon "what is known to cowherds and women."[2] Despite the reproachable classism and sexism, Candrakīrti's point is clear: our everyday epistemology must be grounded in quotidian common sense.

Candrakīrti's appeal to common sense is strikingly similar to that of Ludwig Wittgenstein and his linguistic turn. Especially in his later period, Wittgenstein argued that it was through ordinary language usage that philosophical problems were best addressed. Thus, often what appears to be an insoluble philosophical problem is just a product of using language in nonstandard ways. For example, he argues that the long-historied metaphysical investigation on the nature of time is predicated on nonstandard and therefore nonsensical usages of the word "time." When we say "now," or "six o'clock," or "today" in our everyday usage, we are not positing metaphysically real entities like an instance, a point in time, or a date, respectively. Any cowherd, as Candrakīrti would say, can use these temporal phrases in common-sense ways in "the stream of life" to indicate when one wants to meet, when dusk will come, or when they expect to arrive home. The suspicion that there is more to time than this is just an unfortunate quirk of our language, with which we can form nonsensical questions like "What is time?"[3] Wittgenstein, by contrast, seeks "to bring words back from their metaphysical to their everyday use."[4] This is highly reminiscent of Candrakīrti's critique of Dignāga's position about perception. Candrakīrti argues that the word "perception" does not denote a direct cognition of the metaphysically real, some ineffable particular. Rather, "perception" simply means the ability to see common-sense objects.[5]

Candrakīrti and Wittgenstein thus both invoke ordinary language toward a rejection of the need for metaphysical grounding in some deeper, extralinguistic reality—be it the ineffable particular or the nature of time. But even though Candrakīrti agrees ordinary language and common sense are sufficient for our *conventional* knowledge, he also shares Asaṅga's affinity for the transcendent: something beyond the conventional world, an *ultimate* reality, that yogis realize. In other words, common sense cannot tell us everything, only what we need to know to function day to day. If we want to be liberated, however, we need yogic knowledge, a realization beyond the confines of language.

Does Wittgenstein also accept some type of extralinguistic reality of this sort? His *Tractatus* demonstrates some delicious tensions on this theme. At certain points, he hints toward an ineffable real: "There is indeed the inexpressible. This *shows* itself; it is the mystical."[6] But immediately before this passage, he suggests there is no real beyond what can be said. Once one realizes metaphysical statements are nonsensical, "there is then no question left, and just this is the answer. The solution of the problem of life is seen in the vanishing of the problem."[7] In other words, all questions about what exists outside of language are "answered" by demonstrating their meaninglessness. These are precursors to what is perhaps the most oft-quoted section of the *Tractatus* and its concluding remark: "My propositions are elucidatory in this way: he who understands me finally recognizes them as senseless, when he has climbed out through them, on them, over them. (He must so to speak throw away the ladder, after he has climbed up on it.) He must surmount these propositions; then he sees the world rightly."[8]

Wittgenstein's vacillation leading up to this passage leaves the reader with an enticing ambiguity. Once we have used language to realize its limits, do we arrive somewhere beyond it? Do we throw away the ladder (as described in a famed Buddhist parable) like a boat that we have used to cross to the other side of a river?[9] Or is Wittgenstein's arrival at the limits of language meant to demonstrate there is nowhere beyond language to go? Do we throw away the ladder after climbing back down it, realizing that it leads nowhere?

The Tibetan thinkers I explore in this chapter affirm both sides of the disjunction. They hail mainly from the Sakya (Sa skya) tradition, so-named for the eponymous monastery in Shigatse (Gzhis ka rtse) where it originated. They accept an ultimate reality beyond ordinary language and the world of appearances, one that yogis realize. Nevertheless, for us normal folk, this world of appearances is all that is available and constitutes our everyday epistemology. Sakyapas thus argue a clean split between appearances and reality, one below the ladder and the other above it, as it were. This position is in stark contrast to the Gelug position in chapter 5, which theorized yogic perception via an (imperfect) fit between appearances and reality in the form of representationalism. Just as Gelug representationalism entails realism, the division advocated by Sakyapas entails both fictionalism and antirealism. That is, appearances are fictions that allow for a shared world and its attendant epistemology, as if we were all part of a collective dream. Nevertheless, these appearances give us no information about what reality is actually like, which is only within the purview of awakened yogis.

Sönam Tsemo on Yogic Perception

In chapter 5 we saw Chapa argue a form of representationalism to rebuke an interlocutor who argued that yogic perception is objectless. According to the interlocutor, that yogis perceive the world "free from elaborations" means they see no objects at all. Chapa argued that his interlocutor's position was self-defeating. Without an inferential object, there is no way to substantiate that yogic perception is epistemically warranted, nor nothing to meditate upon, without which yogic perception could not be cultivated. Chapa's interlocutor may ventriloquize Sönam Tsemo (Bsod nams Rtse mo, 1142–1182), a founding figure of the Sakya tradition, as well as Chapa's student at Sangpu Monastery.[10] Even though they are cut from the same cloth, Chapa appears to rebut his own student, given how closely Chapa's interlocutor mirrors Sönam Tsemo's forthcoming arguments.

The section explored below hails from Sönam Tsemo's commentary on Śāntideva's (685–763) *Introduction to the Way of the Bodhisattva* (*Bodhisattvacaryāvatāra*). Where Chapa was adamant that freedom from elaborations did not vitiate epistemic objects, here we see the opposite view: once mental elaborations are eliminated, no knowable object remains.

> Though the erring mind has an intentional object, when its extremes are eliminated, one is free from elaborations. Deceptive reality is the intentional object of an erring mind, since anything that appears to such an awareness is unreal. The inferential sign (*mtshan ma*) that determines the characteristics (*mtshan*

> *nyid*) [of reality] is ultimate reality free of elaborations. It is known by yogic perception through a type of vision that only sees that there is nothing at all to see. And it is determined by an inference that negates elaborations through the negation of a negatum.[11]

Sönam Tsemo's analysis of freedom from elaborations closely parallels Chapa's interlocutor. Because the probandum is beyond elaboration—the "extremes" of either existing or nonexisting—it can only be determined through negative Modus Tollens. This negation, however, is not predictable, since to realize it in yogic perception is to "see that there is nothing at all to see." Thus, this determination leads to yogic perception of a nonepistemic object. This reflects a reproach of the representationalism championed by both Chapa and Tsongkhapa. Because appearances have no referents, then, according to Sönam Tsemo, establishing warrant relative to them is meaningless. Yogic perception thus grasps the absence of referents, not some reality behind appearances that those appearances partially represent.

Just as Chapa's representationalism informs his understanding of inference, so too does Sönam Tsemo's rejection of representationalism inform his own theory of inference. "That deceptive reality is like an illusion determined through conventional epistemic means just as it appears. That it is real is negated by the inference that negates elaborations. This determines that appearances are unreal."[12]

Sönam Tsemo argues that conventional epistemic warrants based on appearances can only, at best, reveal appearances to be illusory. Only the complete inferential denial of elaborations, synonymous with intentional objects themselves, sufficiently reject appearances. Inferential certainty is thus, according Sönam Tsemo, a necessary precursor to yogic cultivation, such that by reaching certainty that appearances are erroneous through and through, one can gradually attenuate them in meditation. Chapa, on the other hand, argued that affording this liminal role to inference, as instrumental but referentially inert, results in absurdities. On his position, inference either warrants or fails to warrant the object yogic perception perceives directly.

But Sönam Tsemo insists he can avoid this absurdity. He continues on to explain the complicated relationship between inference and direct realization. First, he gives a supersessional framework that explains a stepwise series of realizations that eventuate the Buddhist soteriological goal.

> Ultimate reality, whose characteristics are explained in scripture, is a property of the mind, which is an epistemic warrant determining the basis of those characteristics (*mtshan gzhi*). . . . This includes a supersessional progression of realizations. . . . Worldly people, who perceive the self, etc., supersede [that wrong view] through the knowledge that the self is unreal, having seen it as no self directly. Thus, the yogi who still grasps things in the world trumps the common worldly view. The wisdom of the yogi who sees nonduality, in turn, trumps that yogi, who, only aspiring to be an arhat, still sees *phenomena* as endowed with a self. [They come to see the world as mind only]. But appearanceless wisdom trumps seeing the world as mind only. Thus, through this special yogic mind, these views are superseded one after the other.[13]

Here, Sönam Tsemo explicitly employs Asaṅga's three-tiered model (see chapter 3). In tier 1 the yogi analyses objects and realizes that they do not exist as they appear. While those yogis aspiring to be arhats only realize the selflessness *of persons*, those aspiring to be buddhas realize that even the self's constituent *phenomena* are also selfless—that is, empty. But although they have deconstructed external phenomena, the yogi may still grasp to the mind as existing. This is indicative of tier 2, where the yogi understands everything as mind only. This view is superseded by tier 3, where even the mind is vitiated, and nothing appears at all. Thus, Sönam Tsemo's view that the ultimate realization is "appearanceless wisdom" echoes Asaṅga's assessment that "in nonconceptual wisdom, none of those objects appears at all."[14]

Sönam Tsemo, however, amends this framework slightly: "But, given that normal people do not see reality, how can these states of mind trump one another? This is determined through inference."[15] Thus, inferential thinking is necessary at each step to proceed to the subsequent level of direct realization. But he is clear that these inferences are only provisional heuristics.

> To say that the yogi sees the truth while the normal person does not is a lower, worldly manner of speaking, which posits some essential difference between existence and non-existence and is attached to [the distinction] between yogis and worldly folk. But it is not like this, since to say so is, from that lower perspective, to make yogis and worldly folk disputants. But, in fact, they are antithetical. And to be antithetical contradicts their being in dispute. Therefore, even

> supersession is not perceptual but understood through inference. And thus, furthermore, this model that accepts both [the worldly and yogic perspective] does not supersede the original inference, since, as has been stated, via that supersessional inference, the yogic mind supersedes the worldly one and the special yogic mind supersedes that.[16]

Not only the inferences that represent the next realization, but even the entire inferential framework of yogic progression is only a provisional framework! The very distinction between yogis and normal people is eventually elided in full-blown yogic perception. Nevertheless, such distinctions still abide at the level of inference. It would be a category mistake to reify this ultimate ecumenism between yogic and worldly perspectives as the highest rung on the superesessional ladder. Unlike Chapa, then, Sönam Tsemo argues a sharp divide between perception and inference, one where inference functions progressively to eventually perceive that there is no progression at all.

Of course, Sönam Tsemo's argument here is steeped in double talk. Is it possible to realize that there is nothing to realize? Sönam Tsemo and Chapa thus seem to be talking past each other about the content of realization. Chapa argues that it is impossible to have an objectless realization, and so that object must be warranted by epistemic instruments. Sönam Tsemo, on the other hand, argues that the appearance of any object, the presence of something *to be* realized, indicates error; if within yogic perception there were some distinction warranting its superiority, it would also be mired in ignorance. But both Sönam Tsemo and Chapa make their respective claims via fiat. They are not so much arguing with each other as working from different presuppositions about the fundamental error that yogic perception corrects.

Although Sönam Tsemo limits the warrant of inferential thinking, he does not undermine it entirely, claiming both its quotidian and spiritual instrumentality. On this point he appears a kindred spirit with Wittgenstein. On the quotidian aide, both claim that language and inference cannot approach metaphysical truth. But both also agree that these provide instrumental rungs up a progressive ladder, even if, eventually, that ladder is discarded. In Wittgenstein, it is ambiguous what lies beyond this ladder. But according to Sönam Tsemo, a new world is unveiled through the gradual deconstruction of our epistemic strictures. Chapa, by contrast, argues that this destruction of our epistemic framework makes it impossible to even begin the meditative project. And thus, he argues that whatever is realized in meditation must be expressible in language, even if only through a glass darkly.

Sakya Paṇḍita on Yogic Perception

The Treasury of Reasoning and Epistemology

During Sönam Tsemo's floruit, Sangpu was the Tibetan center for the study of logic and epistemology, but the importance of Sakya Monastery grew over time. This change was precipitated in large part by the rising notoriety of a later Sakya figure, Sakya Paṇḍita (Sa skya Paṇ ḍi ta, 1182–1251, henceforth Sapen). Sapen took issue with how traditional epistemological texts had been read by the Sangpu tradition, arguing that their interpretation had been sullied by exogenic Tibetan accretions not endemic to the Indian originals. One of few Tibetan scholars skilled in Sanskrit, Sapen thus sought to reform epistemology in Tibet by correctly reinterpreting Dharmakīrti's *Commentary.*

Like Sönam Tsemo, Sapen also describes yogic perception of ultimate truth as devoid of appearances. I argue that this position finds its Indian genesis in the works of Asaṅga, since it is not found explicitly in Dharmakīrti's work. Nevertheless, Sapen advocates appearanceless yogic perception in the context of the *Commentary.* He also recognizes two different types of yogic perception, a distinction not recognized in Gelug literature.[17] The first type is indicative of spiritual realization—namely, selflessness or emptiness. This yogic perception is devoid of appearances. The second type is akin to the yogic perception explored in chapter 1—the ability to see distant objects. In particular, he argues that yogis are able to see an increasing number of distant worlds as they spiritually progress. This type of yogic perception does have appearances.[18] Sapen's articulation of these two types are found in his *Treasury of Reasoning and Epistemology* (*Tshad ma rigs gter*):

> Because yogic perception is free of subject-object duality, it is unmistaken. When subject and object are abandoned through meditation, there is an absence of error. If there is no error, this entails that there is no conceptualization.

> Therefore, because yogic perception with and without appearances see respectively how things are deceptively and how they are ultimately, both are free of conceptualization and error.[19]

Using a Madhyamaka hermeneutic invoking the two truths (see chapter 2), Sapen offers separate epistemological criteria for two different types of yogic perception granting enumerative and spiritual knowledge respectively. This makes sense, since each type has different content. Better said, the latter *lacks* content, or any appearances. Indeed, this erasure is the precursor of its grasping the ultimate truth. But reality is so far removed from appearances, that even their lack cannot be predicated of it. Citing Dharmakīrti's remark in the *Proof of Other Minds* that final yogic wisdom is inconceivable,[20] Sapen claims that "even the assertion made by some Mādhyamikas that the continuum of appearances terminates [in Buddhahood] is at ends with this inconceivable wisdom, and so this is not Dharmakīrti's intention."[21]

Sapen thus makes a major departure from Dharmakīrti, who insisted that yogic perception, even of the highest spiritual truths, comprises clear appearances.[22] His interpretation is also at odds with that of Gelugpas. Tsongkhapa argues that yogic perception realizes selflessness "implicitly" (*shugs rtogs*) via the appearance of the selfless particular (see chapter 5). In this way, Tsongkhapa makes cogent how the appearance of an object accords with the realization of its selflessness.[23] As another example, Gyaltsab Darma Rinchen (Rgyal tshab Dar ma Rin chen, 1364–1432), one of Tsongkhapa's primary students, contends that appearances in yogic perception are responsible for one's gaining conceptual *certainty* about impermanence after that meditative realization. This certainty is also known as an "ascertainment" (*nges pa*) of impermanence. He argues that "yogic perception has a clear appearance as its object" and that this clear appearance gives rise to an "ascertainment of those appearances as momentary, etc."[24]

Again, indicative of Sapen's distancing between our everyday experience and yogic perception of reality, he rebukes the notion that yogic perception's instrumentality is derivative of its ability to generate mundane certainty of some concept. Because selflessness qua abstract property is only conceptually superimposed onto selfless particulars post facto, yogic perception, being a perception, has no innate power to induce ascertainment about appearances' being selfless or impermanent.

> First, all yogic perception must be an authentic epistemic instrument.
>
> *Because subsequent cognition* (bcad shes) *and ascertainment are both conceptual, they are not perception.*
>
> *Therefore, all yogic perception is an authentic epistemic warrant because it is perception.*
>
> Subsequent cognition and ascertainment are both conceptual, and thus not concordant with perception. This is conclusive. Therefore, whether direct perception is an epistemic instrument in terms of whether it has the capacity to induce ascertainment need not be examined.[25]

Sapen's reasoning is straightforward. Yogic perception is perceptual. Ascertainment occurs post facto to perception—that is, conceptually. (I address his reference to "subsequent cognition"—which is also conceptual—shortly.) Therefore, ascertainment must obtain at the level of conception, not perception. If certain perceptions had some innate power to induce specific forms of ascertainment, then such perceptions would have to have some conceptual content. But this would vitiate their being perceptual. Thus, perception can have no implicit power to produce some ascertainments over others.[26]

Here again we see the tension between Gelug representationalism and the general Sakya antirealist rejection of representation. According to Gelugpas, appearances in yogic perception have an implicit relationship with the conceptualization of ultimate objects such as impermanence and selflessness. On their view, yogic appearances uniquely represent these qualities in real particulars, and so, yogic perception has a unique capacity to produce conceptual certitude about such objects, since those concepts also accurately correspond with those same qualities. Sapen severs the connection between yogic perception and conceptualization. He denies that yogic perception represents the real via an appearance. And thus, furthermore, yogic perception's warrant is not a function of its inherent capacity to produce conceptual certainty about reality, since any such certainty fails to so correspond by virtue of its being conceptual—a mere overlay.

If yogic perception does not represent selflessness, then what does it mean, according to Sapen, for it to "perceive selflessness?" Sapen likely means something similar to Sönam Tsemo. Yogic perception "perceives" the vitiation of objects. In the absence of false apparitions of a self or permanence, no objects appear at all. Yogic perception thus does not represent a negative object, but removes objects entirely. By eliminating appearances, one eliminates the fodder for conceptual superimposition. Where the Gelugpa warrants yogic perception via its ability to *produce* ascertainment, Sapen warrants it via its ability to *vitiate* appearances and any subsequent conceptual designations downstream.

Sapen also makes a passing reference to "subsequent cognition." This cognition occurs when one cognizes something that has already been cognized prior. We saw in chapter 3 how Sucaritamiśra argued that yogic perception could not be an epistemic instrument because it perceived something already cognized via inference: impermanence and selflessness. Sucaritamiśra argued that yogic perception is not epistemically warranted because it is not "fresh"—it gives no new information to help achieve desired ends. Thus Sapen, like Jñānaśrīmitra, must distance yogic perception from subsequent cognitions. Sapen argues that yogic perception is mutually exclusive with any repeated cognitions because it never cognizes the same entity twice. Because perceptual particulars are in constant flux, their perception must be as well. By the contrapositive, any cognition that recognizes "the same" object entertains a reified abstraction: an enduring object. According to Sapen, then, subsequent cognitions must be conceptual, since they superimpose a sameness across otherwise discrete moments. But this also entails that yogic perception, as an authentic perception, has no capacity to recognize enduring objects. This creates a point of contention explored in the next section.

Gorampa and Sapen on Omniscience

Gorampa Sonam Senge's (Go rams pa Bsod nams Seng ge, 1429–1489) commentary on the *Treasury* expands on Sapen's discussion of subsequent cognition. Gorampa was another seminal figure in the Sakya tradition and an ardent critic of Tsongkhapa's philosophy.[27] He first raises an objection about subsequent cognition in the context of omniscience.

> There is an objection about how omniscient yogic perception is an epistemic warrant for an object in the second moment. [Objection:] *Omniscience is an*

> *authentic cognition in the first moment. In the second moment, it cannot rightly be asserted as a subsequent cognition. This is because [omniscience is perceptual and] all perception is nonconceptual and unmistaken. And thus, in the same manner that epistemic instruments are substantiated, yogic perception should be epistemically warranted.*[28]

Gorampa argues that buddhas see objects freshly in every moment. They do not have conceptual cognitions that construe an amalgam of moments into an enduring object, which is a precursor for recognition of the "same" object via a subsequent cognition. But this creates a problem. How can a Buddha be omniscient without subsequent cognition? For normal people, the world appears populated with objects that persist through time. If this appearance is vitiated for buddhas, then their knowledge is limited, since they do not know how the world appears for us. We saw a similar debate in chapter 4: How can a buddha's yogic perception know conventional objects if those objects, so conceptually constructed, are fictions?

The objection continues: "*But if direct perception does not ascertain its own object, then yogic perception could not reveal what objects are to be acquired or avoided*[29] *based on the presence or absence of certain characteristics. Therefore, it must be conceptual.*"[30] Gorampa replies that this is not a problem.

> Your qualm here poses no problem for our position. It is only *normal* epistemic instruments that . . . through ascertainment reveals what objects are to be acquired or avoided. When those Noble Ones, who are not yet free of the propensity to conceptualize, are in their normal state, they ascertain these like normal people. When they are in meditative concentration, however . . . they can acquire and avoid objects through the power of concentration, [without the need of conceptual ascertainment]. But those [buddhas] who are free of the propensity to conceptualize do this exclusively though meditative concentration.[31]

Gorampa's strategy is to differentiate ascertainment from the ability to acquire and avoid (*'jug ldog byed pa*) per one's intentions. Although normal people must conceptually ascertain an object's characteristics to obtain this knowledge, omniscience and high meditative states possess the latter without need of the former. This explanation is a fair reading of Dharmakīrti's pragmatism. The function of ascertainment is to get us what we want and keep us away from what we do not. Gorampa argues that meditation can accomplish this directly without the need of ascertainment and its associated conceptual error.

Gorampa thus appeals to Dharmakīrti's pragmatism to circumvent any need for a representationalist framework. Omniscient perception accomplishes the same aims as ascertainment without constructing conceptual objects that (falsely) represent enduring entities. It would be as if we could find a causal flux of particulars able to dose a fire without ever having the thought "water." It would be impossible to describe such an experience, since any linguistic description of it would be predicated on the very reifications of which such an experience is supposedly devoid.

Such an experience of the world is thus inherently mysterious. It is thus unsurprising that Sapen and Gorampa—like the Indian Buddhist authors cited in chapter 4—concede these meditative states are simply inconceivable (**acintya, bsam gyis mi khyab*).[32] For example, we saw Ratnakīrti appeal to inconceivability to explain how omniscience can be aware of past and future objects even though appearances only occur in the present. On that position, omniscient appearances are inconceivable because buddhas can be aware of conceptual objects through perception. Sapen's appeal to inconceivability, however, is even more radical, since he argues that buddhas are omniscient *without appearances at all*! Sapen first raises the difficultly of this position in the voice of an interlocutor. "[Objection:] *If a buddha does not know the past and the future, they cannot be said to be omniscient. But if they do know it, and they know it through appearances, the three times would only be established after the fact [conceptually and thus not through perception]. But if nothing appears, then it cannot be said that omniscient yogis have a perceptual buddha eye.*"[33]

The interlocutor's doubt is understandable. To be omniscient is to know the past, present, and future. But the interlocutor argues that if a buddha sees appearances, then temporal distinctions are only made after the fact, since appearances do not represent temporal objects. Interestingly, this is exactly the argument Ratnakīrti assents to. He argued that, indeed, because appearances have no temporal content, we can only ever verify temporal omniscience via other conceptual distinctions post facto.[34] But the interlocutor takes this position as an absurdity, since a buddha must have *perceptual* knowledge of the three times. This perceptual knowledge cannot come through appearances. But if nothing appears to a buddha at all, then how can they be said to have a perception of objects in the three times? Sapen's only recourse is to appeal to inconceivability.

> This wisdom is inconceivable and how it knows the three times is not estimable. If the mind of someone who is awake is not estimable by one impaired by sleep, surely, then, ordinary beings—whose vision on this side of samsara is impaired by subject-object duality—have no ability to speculate about wisdom when the basis is transformed (**āsraya-parivṛtti*). Therefore, because it has been transformed, awareness of the three times and that mind which is beyond are inconceivable.[35]

Unlike Ratnakīrti, who understands yogic *appearances* to be inconceivable, Sapen argues that yogic *appearanceless wisdom* is inconceivable. Sapen's rejection of appearances is thus likely inflected by Asaṅga's False Aspectarian position that ultimate realization is free of appearances (see chapter 3). A fortiori, Sapen's position would reject Tsongkhapa's, which not only accepts appearances, but is predicated on those appearances' being representations. Sapen's position thus marks the complete antithesis of Tsongkhapa's.

Sapen therefore agrees with Sönam Tsemo that ultimate reality and its yogic perception completely transcends how the world appears to us now. Sapen's insistence that it is utterly impossible for us normal folk to encounter ultimate reality, I argue, also shares sympathies with Wittgenstein's rejection of metaphysical speculation as nonsense. Sapen and Wittgenstein agree that whatever appears to us is always already entangled in concepts and language. Thus, appearances cannot signify any extralinguistic reality. And therefore, if such a reality were knowable, it could not be said to "appear." Sapen's soteriological project, however, necessitates that reality's knowability. If yogic perception is to achieve this, it thus must do so without appearances and their linguistic-conceptual trappings. Sapen would thus likely *disagree* with Wittgenstein that the real ever "shows itself" of its own accord. Its encounter is hard-won through the cultivation of yogic perception.

Gorampa Versus Kedrub

To reiterate, the consistent contrast between Chapa and camp, on the one hand, and Sönam Tsemo and his, on the other, concerns whether yogic perception has a referent object. The former advocate a type of representationalism. Yogic perception directly perceives the same referent that is garnered by sound inference. This is what it means for yogic perception to be an epistemic instrument. That warrant is derived from the authenticity of its referent object, as confirmed by inference. The latter argue that yogic perception is epistemically unique in that it transcends all referent objects. All other epistemic instruments, in being so confined to such objects, can only tell us about deceptive appearances. Yogic perception is thus uniquely an epistemic warrant for ultimate reality exactly because it is objectless.

The Sakya position on this front has two corollary points: (1) Epistemic instruments *beside* yogic perception are confined to conventional reality and its deceptive appearances. This is the Wittgensteinian point, since Sakyapas and Wittgenstein in common reject the cogency of metaphysical speculation. Sakyapas concede, however, that inferences about ultimate reality may be instrumental in cultivating yogic perception. But those inferences per se do not yield any knowledge about ultimate reality. (2) Because yogic perception is objectless, it is not warranted by its representation of an *object*. It is therefore warranted with respect to the type of "inconceivable" *mind* it generates. (3) This last point is an entailment of the first. Yogic perception is not like other types of perception, such as sensory perception, which still engage with appearances. This recapitulates the fact that yogic perception is an objectless epistemic warrant.

The Gelugpas disagree on all three points. (1) They concede that inferences about ultimate reality do not have the same soteriological power as its perception. Conceptual thinking is opaque where perception is transparent. Indeed, this is why yogic perception is necessary. But this does not negate the accuracy of inferential conclusions about ultimate reality. Reality *is* selfless and impermanent. Those attributions are not falsified by yogic perception but confirmed therein. (2) Likewise, yogic perception has an object—selflessness and impermanence. It is not objectless. Indeed, it is warranted by its object. (3) Yogic perception is the same as the other epistemic instruments in this regard. It is not categorically different from sensory perception. It merely has an epistemic capacity to capture objects that sensory perception cannot—namely, ultimate truths.

We can demonstrate the differences in interpretation between these schools through a close read of their respective commentaries on the same text, Dharmakīrti's *Commentary,* with special attention to verses 3.284–86 on yogic perception. I compare passages from Gorampa's commentary with another from one of Tsongkhapa's primary students, Kedrub Gelek Pelzang (Mkhas grub Dge legs Dpal bzang, 1385–1438). Both commentaries intersperse Dharmakīrti's root verses with their own prose, incorporating Dharmakīrti's phrases verbatim without explicitly demarcating which phrases are from the root text and which are their own commentarial additions. Much of their wording is thus the same. But the devil is in the details, and small discrepancies in their commentarial choices reveal more global disagreements. Differences salient for the discussion I mark in **bold**. These will form anchor points for comparison between the two works and are meant for the reader's reference. So, for example, when the translation of Gorampa's work reads, "**This is an epistemic warrant**," this phrase is meant to be compared with Kedrub's phrase marked by "**This is not an epistemic warrant**." I proceed in three subsections, each corresponding to the three points of comparison mentioned above.

The Limits of Epistemic Warrants

In this first section, Gorampa and Kedrub tackle the issue of clear appearances that arise in meditation. As noted, Dharmakīrti recognizes that a cognition's clarity is not sufficient for its epistemic warrant. One can meditatively fixate on anything and eventually see that object clearly in meditation—even unwarranted, unreal objects. This explains grief hallucinations, the apparitions of one's lover when one is lovesick, the appearance of bones, the earth and water *kasiṇas,* and so on (see chapter 3). Someone might then object that there is no epistemic resource to differentiate warranted yogic perception from any meditatively induced hallucination, since they are phenomenally identical. Kedrub and Gormapa both tackle this question. We start first with Gorampa's work:

> [Objection:] *If you assert that in any meditation there can arise a clear appearance, then that contradicts your assertion that yogic perception has the clear appearance of a real object* (don)*.* [Reply:] Even when you meditate on an unreal object it will appear clearly. A meditator manifests the appearance of unreal objects, such as bones and the like, repulsiveness, and the earth and water *kasiṇas* by meditating on them repeatedly. The resultant cognition is nonconceptual. They

> are seen as having a clear appearance **by an authentic epistemic instrument (*tshad ma*)**.[36]

Compare this to Kedrub's commentary:

> [Objection:] *But, if through the power of meditation, an object* (yul) *appears clearly (and that is necessarily nonconceptual), is it the case that every instance of yogic cognition—in which there is a clear appearance of an object through the power of meditation—also constitutes yogic perception?* [Reply:] When one manifests and produces an appearance of unreal objects, such as bare bones and the like, repulsiveness, and the earth and water *kasiṇas*, by meditating on them repeatedly, those objects upon which one meditates are **seen** nonconceptually and as having a clear appearance.[37]

In both sections, the topic of debate is the clear appearance of those things that are unreal—bones, the earth and water *kasiṇas*, and so on. Gorampa interestingly claims that these are seen "by an authentic epistemic instrument" (*tshad mas mthong ba*).[38] Kedrub, by contrast, just says they are "seen," not admitting them any epistemic authenticity. Gorampa's claim does seem odd, given that he admits, on the one hand, that those objects are unreal, but, on the other, also says their appearance is epistemically warranted, since they are apprehended with an authentic epistemic instrument. What, then, does he mean?[39]

There is another clue elsewhere in Gorampa's same commentary about how he understands "seeing with an epistemic instrument" (*tshad mas mthong ba*). The following comes from the beginning of his commentary on the perception chapter of Dharmakīrti's *Commentary*. In this this section, he is arguing from the point of view of the realist Sutrist against an Anti-Essentialist (*ngo bo nyid med par smra ba*), an epithet for Middle Way (see chapter 5). Like Wittgenstein, the Anti-Essentialist argues that we cannot make any metaphysical claims about ultimate (metaphysical) reality, since we never have any direct experience of it. While Gorampa's response refutes the Anti-Essentialist, he seems to give them partial concession, revealing an affinity for their position.

> The Anti-Essentialist argues that being ultimately functional cannot be the definitional basis of being a particular, since no instance of cognition is aware of

> an ultimately functional entity. But their reason is false, since we see how seeds and fire have the power to produce sprouts and smoke. They may retort that we can only accept that these observations arise *conventionally*, but not ultimately, and so if one were to define the ultimate in terms of [a conventional understanding of how things function], this would be an overreach (*khyab ches*). Thus, it is not possible to define production ultimately. But whether it is conventional or ultimate, we define the particular via its functionality as seen by an authentic epistemic instrument (*tshad mas mthong*). If they call this "conventional," then this is just quibbling about names, simply because we call a functional entity "ultimate."[40]

The Anti-Essentialist argues that we can never escape the confines of our everyday conventions. Thus, even if we say, "things must *really* abide by cause and effect, since we see things cause each other, just like how a seed causes a sprout," the Anti-Essentialist responds that even that experience is circumscribed in our conceptual framework and so cannot amount to a metaphysical truth. Again, this is the Wittgensteinian point. Gorampa "responds" by saying that this is just quibbling about names. If something functions, it is epistemically warranted. Who cares if it is warranted *ultimately* or not?

This response is sufficient for everyday pragmatic concerns. "Ultimate" just means things that function and that thus can achieve desired ends. Whether those things "really" exist as functioning things is irrelevant. Or, to invoke Wittgenstein, such a question amounts to metaphysical nonsense. Yogic perception, however, *does* purportedly reach beyond our everyday pragmatic worldview. Gorampa thus does not deny that there is an ultimate truth beyond the conventional, only that our normal epistemic warrants about functioning things have no business assessing it. Effectively, Gorampa relegates epistemic warrant to the conventional. It is only from the standpoint of how reality appears now that "real" things are defined as what "is seen by an authentic epistemic instrument." From the side of *ultimate* reality, however, such assessments fall short. Our current experience of causality does not lend some indication about how things actually exist, nor can it serve for a warrant of how they ultimately exist.

In sum, when Gorampa argues an object is "seen by an authentic epistemic instrument" (*tshad mas mthong*), he concedes that this seeing is confined to conventional appearances. And because conventional appearances are not ultimately real, they are illusory. This may explain why Gorampa, unlike

Kedrub, claims that even *unreal* objects like the bones and *kasiṇa* are "seen by an authentic epistemic instrument." Epistemic instruments *only* capture illusions like bones and *kasiṇas,* since whatever appears conventionally is illusory and vitiated ultimately. Likewise, those apparitions are pragmatically advantageous; they have soteriological *functions*, even if they are unreal. Yogic perception, however, *does* reach the real. Thus, Gorampa needs to contrast yogic perception, which transcends illusion, with (normal) epistemic instruments, which *only* grasp illusions. He does so, like Sapen, by defining yogic perception as necessarily bereft of appearances, which grants it a transcendent window into the ultimate.

This is not Kedrub's view of Sutrist philosophy. Against Gorampa, he would argue that ultimate reality is not defined by conventional fiat—it is not something we just *say*. Rather, the ability to perform a function is (in this Sutrist context) a property that real things have. And any epistemically warranted knowledge about that reality hinges on its capacity to represent that property, either directly (as in perception) or indirectly (as through inference). Yogic perception is only a special case of epistemic warrant, since it represents *how* things exist—as impermanent and selfless—rather than *what* things are. Likewise, Kedrub would thus reject Gorampa's view that we are categorically entrenched in illusion, since nonyogic epistemic instruments succeed at representing the "what" of objects. So, contra Gorampa, Kedrub contends skeletal apparitions are nothing like the appearance of real objects. Thus, to put it succinctly, where Gorampa *differentiates* yogic perception from other epistemic instruments, Kedrub *likens* them. This explains why they differ on the proximity of yogic perception to conventional appearances.

Gorampa's half-hearted rebuke of the Anti-Essentialist interlocutor likely proleptically anticipates Gorampa's final Middle Way view. Ultimately, Gorampa, like his Anti-Essentialist interlocutor, accepts that epistemic instruments cannot substantiate anything about ultimate reality. On this view, anything we can *say* about ultimate reality is still within the realm of conventions. By the contrapositive, the direct realization of ultimate reality undermines anything we can say conventionally—including our previous descriptions of it. Kedrub's presentation also bespeaks his own final, Middle Way analysis. Like Tsongkhapa, he argues inference can warrant truths about ultimate reality even if yogic perception is required to realize those truths directly. Both authors therefore subscribe to different tracks of sliding scales of analysis (see chapter 5). In each case, the progressive steps build on each other toward different ends. While Gorampa sets up his analysis at the level of the Sutrist to ultimately vitiate epistemic instruments, Kedrub presents the Sutrist in a manner that preserves the utility of epistemic instruments throughout.

Mind Versus Object as the Criterion of Authentic Perception

Another point of comparison between these two texts reveals further discrepancies between Sakya and Gelug epistemology and its implications for Middle Way philosophy. In Gorampa's Middle Way theory, ultimate and conventional truth are not two facets of the same reality, but two different dispositions. They are thus a division of the mind, not of real objects. This position is consistent with Gorampa's ontology. Because conventional objects do not exist at all, it would be nonsense to claim that our conventional talk concerns objects. Conventional "truth," according to Gorampa, is thus merely a faulty disposition, one that is not just deceived, but downright delusional.[41] The perspective from ultimate truth, however, apprehends reality.

According to Tsongkhapa and his fellow Gelugpas, on the other hand, conventional and ultimate truth describe different facets of reality. As I mentioned, they argue that conventional truth concerns *what* things are. Seeing a chair as a chair, for example, does not misrepresent reality per se. This misrepresentation involves another cognitive error entirely, our failure to perceive the chair's ultimate truth: *how* it exists. Namely, it does not exist independently of our conceptual designation that it is a chair, even though it seems that way. This truth can be perceived by yogic perception and inferred. But neither of these realizations vitiate that a chair is a chair. Thus, according to Gelugpas, the distinction between conventional and ultimate concerns different aspects of objects, not our disposition.[42]

Although this describes Gorampa's and Kedrub's contrasting views on Middle Way, it still filters down to each one's analysis in the context of Dharmakīrti's Sutrist framework. The next sections that we will compare comment on verse 3.286abc, "Among those, an informative perception arising from meditation, such as [the perception of] an object previously determined, is an epistemic warrant/instrument."[43] There is a certain ambiguity here. What about this meditative perception makes it informative? Is it informative because it gives information about *something* that is real—because it warrants something? Or is it informative because the cognitive apparatus doing the informing is accurate—because that cognition is a reliable instrument? This ambiguity is exacerbated by the fact that "*pramāṇa*" or "*tshad ma*" can have either meaning. We see Gorampa and Kedrub split on this exact polysemy. Reading *pramāṇa* as a cognitive instrument, Gorampa defines yogic perception in terms of the mind.

> Between meditation on authentic and inauthentic objects, which both produce a **nonconceptual clear appearance**, consider **any mind** that arises as a clear appearance from meditation on how real entities exist per the Four Noble Truths, which are explained previously in the second chapter of Dharmakīrti's *Commentary*. **That mind** is asserted to be an authentic perceptual epistemic instrument, since it is an awareness of an authentic object, free from conceptualizations, and informative (**avisaṃvāda, bslu med pa*).[44]

Compare this to Kedrup's commentary on the same section. Kedrub argues that yogic perception is a *pramāṇa* by virtue of the object it warrants.

> Similarly, there are two types of nonconceptual awarenesses with clear appearances that arise through the power of meditation: one with an authentic object and another with an inauthentic one. Concerning those, meditative cultivation which is a nonconceptual awareness that is informative (**avisaṃvāda, slu ba med pa*) **relative to its own epistemic object,** is asserted to be an authentic perceptual epistemic warrant. [Specifically], that awareness arises from a meditation that realizes an authentic object, such as the sixteen aspects of the Four Noble Truths,[45] beginning with real things' being impermanent, which is established previously **by an authentic epistemic instrument.**[46]

Gormapa suggests *the mind* is the locus of perceptual authenticity, citing its qualities as the determinant of its warrant: "an awareness (*shes pa*) of an actual object, free from conceptualizations, and informative." Gorampa does not deny that the presence of an "authentic object" (*yang dag pa'i don*) is necessary. But his emphasis is on the mind, which he takes as the logical subject (*chos can*) of his argument. It is yogic perception qua *awareness* of an actual object and its nonconceptuality that guarantees its authenticity. The actuality of the object is thus derivative of the authenticity of the mind.[47]

Nor does Kedrub deny that it is mind which ultimately bears (or fails to bear) the quality of being an epistemic instrument. But Kedrub, by contrast, emphasizes its warranted object as the determinant of its authenticity. He makes clear that informativity is only a quality of awareness "relative to its own epistemic object (*zhal bya*)." Furthermore, he goes into more detail about the specifics of this object, the Four Noble Truths, which serve as the guarantor of that authenticity.

Finally, each author's gloss of the Four Noble Truths coincides with their respective emphases. Gorampa argues that the Four Noble Truths are instrumental as a meditational object insofar that they produce "*a clear appearance* . . . of how real entities exist." Here, again, he emphasizes a quality of cognition. But Kedrub, on the other hand, emphasizes the authenticity of the object, as warranted by the reasoning undergirding the Four Noble Truths. Thus, those Truths are instrumental insofar that they render actual features of real things, namely their "being impermanent." Where Kedrub emphasizes the authenticity of the object as the warrant for yogic perception, Gorampa emphasizes a certain quality of mind.

This subtle distinction also traces Chapa and Sönam Tsemo's divergence on representationalism. Chapa argued that the epistemic warrant of yogic perception is corroborated by a correct inference that corresponds with the ultimate. Again, it is through this inferential object's connection with ultimate truth qua object that yogic perception's clear appearance is epistemically trustworthy. Sönam Tsemo, by contrast, argued that true yogic perception is objectless: "Awareness of innate awareness (*shes pa'i rig*) is the object of practice and since that is informative, it is ultimate. Freedom from elaborations is the truth concerning the nature of awareness, and so it is the ultimate truth."[48] On this view, the mind is the only basis for authenticity insofar that it has the capacity to rid itself of objects. In construing the epistemic warrant of yogic perception in relation to the mind, Gorampa is likely following in the tradition of Sönam Tsemo, setting the groundwork for a type of objectless yogic perception. Kedrub, by contrast, in emphasizing the authenticity of the object as the determinant of yogic perception's epistemic warrant, insists, like Chapa, that yogic perception is never objectless, since its referent is responsible for its authenticity.

Yogic Perception as Like or Unlike Other Epistemic Instruments

Gorampa's and Kedrub's contrasting views on authentic perception—whether it is substantiated by the mind or the object—are indicative of their contrasting views on the limits of epistemic instruments. According to Gorampa, yogic perception is unique in that it transcends appearances, unlike other epistemic instruments, which remain fettered to them. Kedrub, on the other hand, sees no need to distance yogic perception from the other epistemic instruments. Yogic perception may capture a special dimension of epistemically warranted objects, their ultimate nature. But otherwise, yogic perception is like the other epistemic instruments in their ability to represent existing things. All epistemic instruments, he argues, rely on appearances.

This difference between Gorampa's and Kedrub's commentaries is revealed in their analysis of illusory meditative appearances. As we noted, Gorampa does not seem to strongly differentiate illusions—like bones and the *kasiṇas*—from conventional epistemic warrants. According to him, all conventional objects are equally illusory—an illusion that yogic perception transcends. Kedrub has stronger conviction in epistemic instruments. Thus, according to him, false meditative appearances are distinct from warranted conventional appearances. This maintains yogic perception's connection to other epistemic instruments. Where Gorampa differentiates yogic perception from the other epistemic instruments, which are all based on illusory appearances, Kedrub likens yogic perception to the other epistemic instruments, which collectively obviate illusions. First, Gorampa's commentary: "Consider the rest of those meditative appearances, such as meditative concentration on the earth *kasina*, and so on. Despite being free of conceptualization, they are not **yogic perception**, since they are perceptual distortions (**upaplava, nye bar bslad pa*) and mistaken (**bhrānta, 'khrul pa*)."[49]

And now, Kedrub's: "The rest of those meditative appearances, such as the appearance of the earth *kasina*, and so on, may appear clearly and be nonconceptual, but they are not **authentic perceptual warrants**, since they are perceptual distortions (**upaplava, nye bar bslad pa*) and mistaken (*bhrānta, 'khrul pa*)."[50]

While Gorampa considers meditation on unreal objects to be inaccurate because they are "not yogic perception," Kedrub argues that these same appearances "are not authentic perceptual warrants." By distancing these illusions from yogic perception, but not epistemic instruments in general, Gorampa implicitly reconfirms the illusory nature of those instruments. This is consistent with his claim that the appearance of bones and the *kasiṇa* are "seen by an authentic epistemic instrument." Kedrub, by contrast, has no problem with conventional perception and yogic perception warranting facts about the same appearing object. Thus, Kedrub distances these illusions from authentic perception and the other epistemic instruments generally, implicitly reconfirming that yogic perception is included among them. This is consistent with his claim that those illusions are only "seen," but not by an authentic instrument.

We can illustrate these differences between Gorampa and Kedrub in the diagram below (figure 6.1):

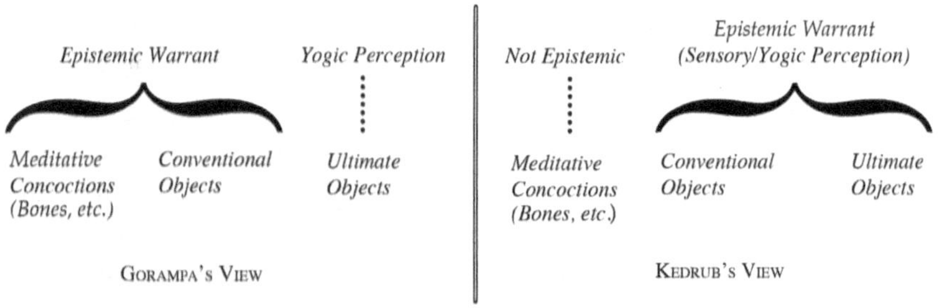

FIGURE 6.1 Gorampa Versus Kedrub

In Gorampa's view, the meditative concoction of bones is not vastly epistemically different from normal apprehension of conventional objects; both involve illusions. Yogic perception, by contrast, is beyond the epistemic instruments, and so grasps ultimate reality. In Kedrub's view, both conventional and ultimate objects are within the ken of epistemic warrant. While yogic perception gleans the ultimate truth of those objects, the other epistemic warrants, like sensory perception, are instrumental for gleaning their conventional truth. Meditative concoctions are outside the scope of epistemic warrant, simply because those objects do not exist.[51]

Within the sphere of Dharmakīrtian exegesis, these distinctions between Gorampa and Kedurb may only be inchoate—they are only gestural, not necessarily philosophically incongruent. But to be sure, once Gorampa and Kedrub get to the level of Middle Way, these differences become much more pronounced.[52] My more circumspect argument, then, is that each author makes subtle differences in commentarial choice that proleptically anticipate more pronounced differences at the level of Middle Way, even though they are constrained to a Sutrist framework within their respective texts. Indeed, Gorampa seems to vacillate to some degree about how he understands epistemic authenticity, appearing sympathetic to his Anti-Essentialist opponent's argument about the limits of linguistic correspondence. This vacillation is understandable within the context of how he eventually develops his sliding scale, the zenith of which reveals (like his own interlocutor) that epistemic instruments cannot warrant ultimate truth. Kedrub, on the other hand, betrays no such vacillation, since the reliability of epistemic instruments remain consistent at each level of analysis.

Each author's analysis of epistemic instruments has further consequences for their final theory of appearances. On Gorampa's construal of Middle Way, appearances are completely vitiated within the direct experience of ultimate reality.[53] According to Tsongkhapa's view, on the other hand, yogic perception does not transcend appearances. While it is true that nonbuddhas cannot see appearances and ultimate reality at the same time, they eventually occur together once one has reached full enlightenment.[54] While Gorampa's view problematizes quotidian appearances as something to be eliminated, Kedrub's retains them as something to be refined and nuanced through yogic insight.

Gorampa's Sakya view on appearances has certain affinities with Wittgenstein. Sakyapas argue that appearances and epistemic instruments are irreconcilably entangled, barring their access to deeper metaphysical truths. This is similar to Wittgenstein's appeal to ordinary language and his rejection of metaphysical statements. But Wittgenstein argues that the ineffable still "shows" itself. Gorampa and his fellow Sakyapas seem to reject even this showing. The ultimate truth realized in yogic perception does not appear at all, not even to yogic perception, which grasps it (somehow) without appearances—not even qua the absence of appearances.

Gelugpas agree that reality does indeed show itself, albeit through a glass darkly. Although appearances misrepresent how things exist, they still carry sufficient information for an inference of their correct mode of existence. This conceptual understanding in turn suffices for a meditative procedure through which we can come to see the world as it is, vouchsafing certainty. At no point are appearances elided and, indeed, developing yogic perception is a process of refining those appearances' representative capacity. Gelugpas would thus reject Wittgenstein's position that metaphysical realism is nonsense, siding with Russell's realism and the representative capacity of perception—at least, perception sufficiently refined.

Śākya Chokden Versus Tsongkhapa

The previous section analyzed these issues within a Sutrist framework with implications for Middle Way. But these Sakya-Gelug distinctions also percolate within each school's analysis of Yogācāra. In chapter 5, I covered Tsongkhapa's analysis of yogic perception within the Yogācāra school, where he made extensive efforts to illustrate that yogic perception represents an epistemically warranted object. He argued that within this school, yogic perception has a particular as its object, the Unchanging Absolute (*'gyur med yongs grub*). Tsongkhapa insisted that that this object was ontologically robust. Although from the point of view of the Sutrist it was problematic to claim that a particular could be unchanging, this is accepted within Yogācāra, so he argued. Thus, Tsongkhapa preserves the representational capacity of yogic perception relative to an epistemically warranted particular.

It is unsurprising that this position is at odds with that of another famed Sakyapa, Śākya Chokden (Shākya Mchog ldan, 1428–1507). Śākya Chokden was undeniably an independent thinker, one who broke with the Sakya party line on many occasions. But his analysis of yogic perception of the Unchanging Absolute seems simpatico with that of Sapen and Gorampa, and thus, his position is also antithetical to Tsongkhapa's representationalist theory of yogic perception. In the following section, Śākya Chokden, like Tsongkhapa, refers to the Yogācāra school as "Mind Only."

> As Dignāga says in the *Compendium*, "Yogis see just the object, independently from the guru's instructions."[55] Later commentators explained this as a nonimplicative negation (*med dgag*). But this cannot be known, since a nonimplicative negation must either be a universal [in which case it would not be perceptual] or an independent object [in which case it could not be a nonimplicative negation, which is conceptual]. Therefore, according to the Sutrists, yogic perception

> with and without appearances are both acceptable. Both necessarily take the particular as their object, since ultimate truth is necessarily constituted by particulars [and yogic perception must see the ultimate truth]. According to the tenets of Mind Only,[56] perception with appearances is necessarily constituted by particulars, while vision within yogic perception without appearances is defined as seeing just one specific particular, since it only sees the unmistaken Absolute. This Unchanging Absolute (*'gyur med yongs grub)* is a nonimplicative negation. But since to see the Absolute is really to see nothing, it is only nominally called seeing. Thus, it is difficult to posit exactly what ultimate truth is, since it is not truly established.[57]

First, we see that Śākya Chokden's view of negations strongly contrasts that of Chapa. Chapa, argues that negations are always true *of* some knowable object (see chapter 5), that the property "absent of a self," for example, is only predictable of some positive entity, and positive entities are accessible by epistemic instruments. He rejects a view of authentic negations that establish nothing at all, since pure nothingness per se is not predictable. Negations therefore imply epistemic objects. Śākya Chokden, on the other hand, like Sönam Tsemo before him, argues that these negations vitiate knowability—they implicate nothing.[58] Śākya Chokden is thus in a line of Sakya thinkers that understand yogic perception as objectless.

This is again reflected in his appeal to the distinction between yogic perception with and without appearances, a distinction not accepted by Tsongkhapa. While Śākya Chokden and Tsongkhapa agree that in both Sutrist and Mind Only thinking, yogic perception takes a particular as its object, they strongly disagree about what this means. Tsongkhapa takes this particular as yogic perception's referent object. In the Sutrist context, its appearance leads to an implicit cognition that allows one to ascertain impermanence. In a Mind Only context, yogic perception perceives the Unchanging Absolute *qua* particular directly.

Śākya Chokden, on the other hand, argues the opposite conclusions from the same premise. First, he describes the Sutrist system. Because the particular is ineffable, it cannot properly be considered an "object" of yogic perception. The particular is *not* a knowable object at all, since all knowledge is conceptual. Thus, it can only be realized without appearances. At the next level, that of Mind Only, yogic perception not only lacks an object, but it is not even a type of seeing. Because the Unchanging Absolute is a total negation, to "see it" is "really to see nothing." Thus, while Tsongkhapa attempts to keep representationalism consistent between Sutrist and Mind Only levels, Śākya Chokden describes its gradual erosion: concerning the first, he denies that yogic perception grasps some knowable object, and on the second, he denies that yogic perception grasps anything at all. Again, this is reminiscent of Asaṅga's tripartite procedure, which understands yogic insight as the gradual erosion of appearances. In Śākya Chokden's text, this progression is reflected first in the Sutrist rejection of a particular cum object and then of yogic perception cum seeing.

In sum, Śākya Chokden problematizes appearances as something that must be transcended to afford insight, while for Tsongkhapa, the challenge is to show how appearances accord with yogic perception's insight. This difference is consistent across both thinker's interpretations of Sutrism and Mind Only. While Śākya Chokden attempts to exacerbate the gulf between appearances and ultimately real particulars, Tsongkhapa consistently maintains a bridge between them. These tendencies magnify across each thinker's progressive interpretations of Buddhist doxography.

Conclusion: Laruelle and the Limits of Representation

The authors considered in this chapter have strikingly different understandings of yogic perception from those of the previous chapter. In the previous chapter, Gelugpas argued that yogic perception's warrant derives from its representation of an epistemically warranted object. Yogic realization may be qualitatively different from a premeditative inference of the same object. Nevertheless, sound inference and yogic perception do not apprehend different objects. They simply realize the same object differently. The Tibetan exegetes in this chapter, however, all argue that yogic perception is defined by its *discontinuity* with those objects realized by other epistemic instruments. It is thus objectless. I identified these different understandings of yogic perception as paralleling Dharmakīrti's and Asaṅga's contrasting theories of meditative insight. Dharmakīrti's representationalist presentation (in contrast to his pragmatist one) is preserved in the Gelug interpretation. The object is first inferred and then realized directly. Asaṅga's interpretation is preserved in the Sakya contingent. Meditation involves a whittling away of objects until they disappear entirely.

Sönam Tsemo described this progression explicitly. In contrast to Chapa, he argued the starting point of yogic perception is an inference denying objects. The meditator then focuses on the mind as the basis of their contemplation. This leads to a realization of nonduality and a final elimination of all appearances. Sapen echoes yogic perception's realization as appearanceless. Although he admits appearances in the context of remote seeing, yogic perception about reality is categorically bereft of appearances. Unlike the Gelugpa, then, he does not understand yogic perception as having some innate power to produce ascertainment of some object. That is not its goal. Like Sönam Tsemo, Sapen understands yogic perception as a method to escape (conventional) epistemically warranted objects entirely. If the purpose of yogic perception were to produce conceptual determinations, then, according to Sapen, it would be counterproductive, only further ensnaring the yogi in conceptions.

Sapen's theory of appearanceless yogic perception at the Sutrist level likely anticipates his final Middle Way view. This continuity is especially salient in Gorampa's commentarial analysis of yogic perception. There, he suggests that illusions (like the earth *kasiṇa* and bones seen in meditation) are seen by an epistemic instrument. This seems to anticipate his final Middle Way position that conventional objects are simply illusions. Although we might have conventional epistemic procedures to "know" such objects, they are patently unreal.

This view is in sharp contrast to the Gelug view, which argues that, although conventional objects have an illusory aspect—they appear to be permanent, endowed with a self, and independent—their appearance is not illusory simpliciter. Tsongkhapa thus argues that conventional epistemic instruments can warrant these nonillusory aspects: what those objects are. Gorampa, on the other hand, insists that these epistemic instruments *only* grasp at illusions. The apparitions of the *kasiṇa* or meditative bones are ultimately no more accurate than the appearance of conventional objects we interact with every day.

Gorampa thus also argues that yogic perception's authenticity is based on the mind. This anticipates his Middle Way view that the two truths are dispositional. Gorampa contends that because ultimate reality only manifests in the absence of appearances and because appearances are purely a mental phantasm, we can only describe yogic perception as a type of perspectival shift—one that, like turning our head in another direction, reveals a completely different world. Kedrub, by contrast, argues that yogic perception is warranted by its object. This is consistent with the Gelug view that the two truths are aspects of every existing object, not a change in perspective that would vitiate those objects.

This difference also determines each author's understanding of the relationship between yogic perception to the other epistemic instruments. Because Gorampa argues that yogic perception does not have an object, he distances it from epistemic instruments, whose function is to warrant objects. According to Kedrub, yogic perception does have an object. Thus, it is not dissimilar from other epistemic instruments.

Finally, Śākya Chokden has a completely different theory of particulars from Tsongkhapa. Because yogic perception apprehends particulars, it does not entertain appearances and "really sees nothing." Tsongkhapa, on the other hand, argued that particulars appear in yogic perception. Thus, he must explain how this appearance implicitly leads to the realization of an absence—impermanence and selflessness. For Śākya Chokden, there is no such problem, since he does not need to bridge any such gap; appearances eventually disappear entirely.

In sum, the Sakya thinkers in this chapter deny that our normal epistemic instruments have any capacity to represent ultimate reality. This is why yogic perception must, according to those thinkers, be understood in a nonrepresentationalist, antirealist framework. I suggest that this rejection is indicative of a certain Wittgensteinian rejection of metaphysics. Just as Wittgenstein argues that our language cannot render metaphysical truths, Sakyapas argue that ultimate reality is out of bounds of what can be known to us now. Still, Sakyapas insist that, consistent with the general Buddhist promise of liberation, an encounter with a nonlinguistic reality is possible. This is the role of yogic perception. Wittgenstein may admit such a possibility as well when he notes the ineffable can "show" itself.

Both Wittgenstein and the Sakya position, however, betray a certain tension. They agree that conceptual-linguistic thinking cannot bootstrap beyond itself. We cannot think our way to mystic revelation. According to Sakyapas, whatever yogic perception realizes, it cannot be inferred. Likewise, Wittgenstein reminds us, "Whereof one cannot speak, thereof one must be silent."[59] But silence does not necessitate that there is nothing to be done. Indeed, according to the Sakyapa, silence is the starting point for meditative practice.

But what epistemological possibility do Sakyapas leave for such practice? If not only how we think, but also how the world appears to us, are erroneous through and through, where do we begin? The Gelugpas offer a starting point, suggesting we can build off sound inference. Sakyapas also seem to concede some role for conceptual thinking. But it is vague. How can inference be a starting point for practice if it fails to represent even a modicum of reality? Likewise, if, according to Wittgenstein, our world is one of "facts, not of things,"[60] where within such a world could the mystical "show" itself, since the factual world is always at the behest of language?

Perhaps this is just the nature of mystical experience. If we could give a cogent account about the transition from conceptual understanding to direct insight, that experience would not be particularly mystical. But there are other ways we might mine the Sakya, antirepresentationalist schema to give an expressible answer to this question. On this point, I borrow from the nonphilosophy of François Laruelle (1937–) to make an enticing parallel. Like the Sakyapas contra Gelugpas, Laruelle argues that philosophy fails to recognize its own representational limit. Philosophy is a *product* of the Real and therefore is only part of it—it cannot represent the whole of which it is only a part.[61]

As an analogy, we might say that no knot in a string could be pulled so tight as to become an unknotted piece of string. The knot is a made of the string. But it cannot fold itself into the straight piece of string from which it is formed. Of course, we can untie the knot. But then then there is just the piece of string. There is no longer a knot. The knot is like our philosophical representations of the world and the string itself the Real. The string can accommodate many different knots. But each knot is only ever part of the whole. Just so, Laruelle argues that "the Real excludes that it can be given as a thing in a mirror, that it can be alienated into an image that would be its representation."[62]

To what would be the chagrin of the Gelugpas, Laruelle argues that we can never hope to represent reality. Representations themselves are real, but they cannot serve as a stand-in for the Real. But this does not mean, however, that the Real is therefore something that lies beyond thought and appearances, "as it is in Wittgenstein."[63] Rather, it is radically immanent. "The mystical is not in front of us, far from us, or close behind, virtual or potential. . . . It is in us or rather it is us who are actually in it. . . . Moreover immanence (to) itself, not being a property or a relation, is the Real itself insofar as it is absolutely distinct from and even indifferent to empirico-ideal reality, which is to say to what we call effectivity."[64]

Laruelle argues that the mystical is our most intimate encounter with the world, before it is synthesized via relations to other constructs and thus loses its immanence. In many ways, his description appears close to the True Aspectarian Yogācāra view of appearances. Appearances are immediate, and it is only after the fact that they are construed as representative or phenomenal (Laruelle's "empirico-ideal reality"), or as pragmatically effective (*arthakriyā*) relative to certain conceptualized desires (Laruelle's "effectivity"). The Yogācārin theory of appearances echoes Laruelle's account of representations.

Like Sapen, however, Laruelle argues that even to construe the Real as a type of appearance places it too far downstream. "Vision-in-One" of the Real is "the Given-before-all-givenness, the Manifested-before-all-manifestation."[65] In other words, even to say the Real "appears" suggests some separation between phenomena and noumena, mind and world—a representational vestige. This is irresistibly close to Sapen's understanding of yogic perception as appearanceless, within which the Real is manifested without any manifestation. Both Sapen and Laruelle thus agree that the direct encounter with the Real cannot be represented *even as a referentless appearance*, since any representation "forecloses"[66] the Real in piecemeal terms that can never encompass its entirety. Thus, even appearance talk is too distant from the immanently Real.

I offer this parallel between Laruelle and Sapen not merely to demonstrate similarities, but to offer a rational reconstruction of how we might confront Sapen's bootstrapping problem, without just dismissing his position as mystical obscurantism. In contrast to the representationalism inherent in philosophy, Laruelle describes his nonphilosophy as a *practice*. One element of this practice accords with Sapen's understanding of conventional truth. In "reflection according to the real," one realizes that all philosophy is "autopositional." That is, it takes some position as axiomatically true, from which it derives its entire system, foreclosing the Real. Nonphilosophy, however, resists this "philosophical Decision." That is, it never takes any position, even its own, as autopositional. Any position is just one part of the whole. In other words, Laruelle does not say "nonphilosophy is 'antispeculative'—it is never the negation or reversal of philosophy—but that it is nonspeculative."[67] Likewise, Sapen's theory of conventional truth accommodates epistemic warrant relative to a given position or set of conventions. Like Laruelle, he merely faults any conventional positionality that claims to represent the Real. Sapen is not opposed to conventional truth, merely insistent that the Real is nonconventional.

What of ultimate truth? Here, Laruelle's theory of practice strongly accords with Sapen's. Laruelle distinguishes "the action of the intellectuals"[68] from the "practice" of non-philosophy: "Finally, action reproduces images or doubles of itself, it produces representation, while practice destroys representations."[69] In other words, the purpose of nonphilosophy is to eradicate the conceit of thinking that it represents the Real. Likewise, Sapen understands yogic perception as a method to see the world without appearances, that is (perhaps) to experience the world without experiencing it *as* appearance. Through the practice of "destroying representations," we atrophy the impulse to take our inevitable foreclosures of the Real as an appearance representing it.

To be sure, there is not a perfect fit between Sapen and Laruelle here. By and large, the Tibetan Buddhist milieu within which Sapen was writing does not understand enlightenment as a realization of radical immanentism. There is also, admittedly still the problem posed by Chapa. How can one seek to "destroy representations" without *representing* the Real as inherently non-auto-positional? In response, Laruelle claims that non-philosophy is "performative" rather than representational, with its own "self-destruction" built in.[70] Conceivably, as a performative practice, nonphilosophy destroys both philosophical representations and nonphilosophical representations of those representations' destruction. But how exactly this occurs seems just as mysterious as the transition from conceptual understanding to yogic perception. Indeed, they are part of the same axiological hurdle: how do we move toward nonrepresentational thinking, or even practice, without representing it?

Sorting these philosophical questions would require a book in itself. But, at this juncture, I merely wish to illustrate that these Sakya thinkers are dealing with difficult questions about the limits of thought, anticipating many of the conclusions of their Western counterparts. A close analysis and comparison to Laruelle illustrates that they are engaged in a profound critique of representationalism. And their project is not just negative. Like Laruelle, they are invested in developing a practice to overcome our tendency to think in a representationalist manner.

This practice has real-world consequences. According to Laruelle, the destruction of representation undoes philosophy's authoritarian character, since, in claiming to represent the Real, philosophy can easily become weaponized through the conceit that it describes the natural order.[71] Similarly, in a Buddhist context, the eradication of representations culminates in a buddha's compassion. Although hailing from the Gelug tradition, this is beautifully rendered in a prayer traditionally offered to Tsongkhapa, the Migtsema Mantra (*Dmigs brtse ma*). It begins, "O Bodhisattva of Compassion, who looks upon us with a treasure trove of love that sees no one at all."[72] Just as removing representations from philosophy nullifies authoritarianism, yogic perception's eradication of representation leads to universal love.[73]

Conclusion

Delimitations and Future Directions

BY NOW, I hope to have presented a clear picture of yogic perception's intellectual development over the *longue durée*. The discussions in this book have taken us from the *Bṛhadāraṇyaka Upaniṣad*, well before the common era, to Śākya Chokden in the sixteenth century, from Buddhaghoṣa in Sri Lanka to Tsongkhapa born in present-day northeast China. Despite this vast spatial and temporal swathe, there appear to be several consistent themes that run across yogic perception's intellectual history. The intellectual evolution of yogic perception proves to be layered, like accruing strata of geological sediment, with old facets of yogic perception persisting alongside new interpretations, rather than serial, where later theories would supersede older ones.

The earliest conceptions of yogic perception as a type of remote seeing—especially evinced by sustained references to *Yogasūtra* 3.25—appears preserved at every stage, sometimes more prominent, other times more vestigial, but always there. Verse 3.25 itself adopts even older conceptions of yogic perception as projective or extramissive. Although Buddhist deny extramissive theories of vision outright, they retain some of these notions implicitly when describing yogic perception as a type of projective, mental, luminous entity. Most of the traditions explored in these pages also formed a united front against the Mīmāṃsā rejection of yogic remote seeing, which was predicated on the fear that it would render Vedic authority superfluous. These debates began just after Patañjali with Śabara's critique and persisted in

India up until at least the turn of the millennium in the form of Vācaspatimiśra and Jñānaśrīmitra's exchange.

But it appears to be around the sixth century CE, in works such as those by Praśastapāda and Dignāga, that yogic perception receives its earliest epistemological exegesis. This analysis only deepened with time, culminating in long, multipartnered exchanges by the end of the first millennium. In this later period, we saw debates between Buddhists and Naiyāyikas, Naiyāyikas and Mīmāṃsakas, and Mīmāṃsakas and Buddhists, with additional input from Jain, Śaiva, and Vedāntan schools. Because yogic perception evolved to become an agreed-upon epistemic instrument of spiritual insight, it makes sense that it would become a flashpoint for debate, as each school had vastly different conceptions of what spiritual insight entails and how it is achieved. By the time of Śāntarakṣita in the eighth century, yogic perception became not just a source of insight, but the means by which a buddha knows everything. This inventive interpretation did not, however, arise ex nihilo. We considered how it was an extension of yogic perception's capacity for remote seeing. Omniscience is simply the capacity for remote seeing taken to its logical extreme.

Tibetan exegetes were charged with synthesizing these disparate understandings of yogic perception into a cohesive framework. In addition to yogic perception as remote seeing, they had to negotiate three theories: (1) Asaṅga's theory of yogic meditation as transcending worldly objects entirely, so that they do not appear at all; (2) Dharmakīrti's theory of yogic perception as spiritual insight into the Four Noble Truths, which concerns the flux of appearances; and (3) Kamalaśīla's theory of yogic perception as a type of omniscience. The Gelug school emphasizes Dharmakīrti's (2) over Asaṅga's (1). Yogic perception may transcend normal ways of seeing, but it still sees directly what can be substantiated by sound inference. The Sakya school, we saw, emphasized Asaṅga's (1) over Dharmakīrti's (2). Yogic perception grasps something completely ineffable that cannot be corroborated by other epistemic instruments like inference—it is beyond appearances. These different hermeneutic strategies informed how each school understands Kamalaśīla's (3). Because Sakyapas argue that appearances and yogic insight are antithetical, they are forced to conclude that omniscience is "inconceivable"—it paradoxically includes knowledge about mundane objects without those objects' appearing. For Gelugpas, there is no such hurdle, since yogic insight is not incompatible with appearances.

Throughout these debates, I highlighted their philosophical dimensions. The historical persistence of yogic perception as projective demonstrates the power of intuitions. I argued that these intuitions can override the philosophical desire for logical consistency, and that even the most rational minds may have a high tolerance for incongruity and cognitive dissonance. I argued that this provides an important lesson for philosophical analysis: we should be wary of the extent to which we can invoke a systematic analysis of a philosopher to interpret their thinking in every instance.

Indian debates on yogic perception and scriptural authority are directly relevant to contemporary epistemological debates on testimony. Most Indian traditions rejected the Mīmāṃsā position that there can exist authentic testimony in the absence of a direct experience that serves as its ultimate foundation, a position similar to that of Robert Audi. Also, like Audi, these traditions differentiate criteria for justified belief in testimony from when it transmits knowledge, though avant la lettre. Debates about these criteria raise interesting questions about which types of experiences count as testimonial foundations. If determining these criteria requires an inference, then these experiences cannot constitute unilateral foundations. Coherentism seems unavoidable to make sense of how and which experiences warrant different instances of testimony.

The question of coherentism is also prevalent in Buddhist theories of yogic perception. I identified that thinkers like Dharmakīrti are often described as foundationalist in secondary scholarship. However, his view on yogic perception complicates this picture. On the one hand, he argues that perception is epistemically warranted by virtue of its nonconceptual clarity, a seemingly foundationalist view. But in the context of yogic perception, he argues that this clarity is insufficient. Yogic perception gains its warrant from being guided by an accurate inference, a coherentist move where perception and inference must mutually cohere. We saw subsequent Buddhist struggle with this vacillation. Jñānaśrīmitra thus equivocates between pragmatism and correspondence theories, while Gelugpas appear to opt squarely for the latter. These debates reveal general difficulties in determining the relationship between mind and world.

One possible solution to this problem is an appeal to the mystical and the ineffable. We saw resonances of this strategy in Dharmakīrti as well in works where he was not bound by a representationalist, Sutrist framework. Because anything we can say about thinking already presupposes it, we can never get behind thinking enough to articulate its relationship to the world. But this itself raises two possible responses. Either, therefore, there is *nothing* beyond thinking, or there is *something* that cannot be thought. Jñānaśrīmitra again appears to equivocate between these two possibilities, while Sakyapas appear to lean toward the latter, tending toward global antirealism. Although our epistemic instruments may be pragmatically useful in the context of mutual consensus about how the world appears, they are erroneous through and through relative to a reality that can only be perceived at their expense. Yogic perception describes this transcendent state and, as such, cannot be evaluated by any other epistemic instruments.

Placing these debates on yogic perception in the context of contemporary Euro-American philosophy thus generated some novel insights. The first concerned philosophical hermeneutics. Acknowledging the power of intuitions, we need clearer delineations between philosophical exegesis and rational reconstruction, since local arguments often conflict with a thinker's global framework. In chapter 2 I demonstrated that debates on yogic perception have ramifications for how we understand experts. Hume's reductionism is too strict, and so we need more capacious trust of experts. This is especially pertinent in the age of "fake news" polemics, but it may also open up a wider range of attestable phenomena. In chapter 3 I demonstrated how yogic perception in the "reverse direction" forces us to rethink conceptual thinking: that it is not just *responsive* to perceptual input, but *generative* of it.

These concerns gave way to a discussion of phenomenology in chapter 4. I argued that in contrast to the first-person-centric views of traditional Euro-American phenomenology, Buddhist discussions of omniscient yogic perception suggest an omniphenomenology with this structure elided. Tibetan thinkers, however, seemed compelled to reengage with the metaphysical speculations that omniphenomenology is meant to skirt. Philosophers in chapter 5 thus offered an important nuance to representational realism, quasi-representational realism, which can better account for representational distortion. Thinkers in chapter 6, on the other hand, opted for a limits-of-language argument. But unlike the linguistic turn in the Euro-American context, these thinkers also attempted to theorize the mystical and transcendent in ways that test the cogency of linguistic-turn arguments. Through a rational reconstruction, I argued that their analysis may, in fact, suggest a radical immanentism.

As a final concluding exercise, I want to borrow from a framework used in scientific writing—the custom of ending with delimitations and directions for further study. I appreciate this convention, since it preserves epistemic humility, reminding us that no study is ever conclusive and always has possibilities for expansion. Concerning the first, the present study—in culling from a broad range of sources over long stretches of time—is undeniably patchwork. This has the advantage of being expansive in scope, offering a textual analysis over the *longue durée*. It also risks, however, the possibility of insufficient contextualization. In the juxtaposition of several textual selections against each other, the meaning of each text within this gestalt may deviate from that of original authorial intention. One solution to this problem is to double down on a hermeneutics championed by Hans-Georg Gadamer (1900–2002). On this approach, there is no text in and of itself with an inherent meaning independent of its readership and their exegetical aims. All hermeneutics involves a "fusion of horizons" between that of the text and the interpreter.[1] Thus, my comparative interpretation of these texts is just one among many valid readings, each relative to the perspective and agenda of their readers.

I appreciate this approach insofar as it reminds us that interpretation is always a dialogue with a text, not the study of some object seen transparently and objectively. Nevertheless, I fear its creep toward relativism.[2] The conflation of interpretation with dialogue can easily metastasize into monologuing. Although the interpreter's voice is inextricable, there is still a cogent sense in which these texts are speaking *to* us more so than *with* us. I am thus not interested in eliding authorial intention. This means that it is still important to "get it right" when presenting Indian and Tibetan materials. There is a "there" there that I want to communicate. And so, I have done my best to make sure that I am translating with the larger historical and philosophical context of these works in mind. Still, the more disparate data points one works with, the higher the risk that comparative interpretation can become cobbled more so than felicitous. I leave it to other scholars to evaluate where I have succeeded and where I have failed.

Nevertheless, I maintain that this comparison is a fruitful enterprise. For example, the continuity of *Yogasūtra* 3.25 through a broad range of texts would have been impossible to see without this wide and disparate sampling.[3] I therefore envision more scholarship of this kind, which embraces thematic analyses across a broad range of texts.[4] I argue this intertextual approach is a particularly powerful way to understand what is implicit in these authors' thinking, especially those presuppositions that they do not feel necessary to articulate. While such presuppositions may be counterintuitive to a modern audience, they were likely so obvious to these authors to not be worthy of mention. They thus can only be revealed through triangulated intertextual reading.

For example, our broad analysis of Buddhist theories of yogic perception revealed a picture of consciousness that is not nonspatial but spatially unbounded, expansive, able to move about in ways that physical objects cannot. This is a presupposition that persists to this day. Recently, I was having a conversation with a friend who is a Tibetan Buddhist monk in the Kagyü (*Bka' rgyud*) tradition. He argued that the mind is different than matter. For example, when I think about the food in my fridge, my mind is unimpeded by the wall separating my living room from the kitchen, or by the refrigerator door hiding the food, while physical objects are so impeded. Implicitly, he suggested that when we think about objects, there is some sense in which the mind actually *goes* to those objects. This is vastly different from a Cartesian model, which informs the way many English speakers think about the mind. In that model, only physical objects are res extensa—having physical extension in space—while the mind is a res cogitans without extension. Buddhist informed intuitions, by contrast, do not differentiate mind and matter by virtue of extension—mind in fact has an even *greater* extensive capacity, able to take up large amounts of space uninhibited. Thus, mind is differentiated from matter, not on the axis of extension, but on the axis of physical obstruction.

This vignette evinces the fruits of the comparative project. We not only gain an insight into the fundamental philosophical assumptions of other traditions, but we become aware of the fundamental presuppositions in our own thinking. That the mind is nonextended is just as axiomatic as the assumption that it is spatially boundless. The former is closest to us (English speakers) but remains most hidden and might have failed to show itself without this point of contrast. In the language of Heidegger, the comparative enterprise "breaks" equipment in our intellectual toolkit, disclosing it to us for the first time, "announcing itself afresh."[5] Armed with this new understanding, we can engage in better philosophical interpretation overall, better able to recognize (what Laruelle called) the "autopositional" premises that inform a given system of thought. Such premises, though foundational to philosophy, are often the hardest to unearth. Indeed, as Novalis (1772–1801) said, one of the most important functions of education is to render the familiar strange as much as the strange familiar.[6]

As I also argued in chapter 1, however, there are many intuitions we can identify that span cultures and epochs. Technically, of course, from the point of view evolutionary psychology, intuitions are *only* those ways of thinking that are pan-human, since they are the result of our shared evolutionary pedigree. But culturally contingent ways of thinking can become as deeply ingrained as intuitions, even if they are not the product of hard-wired cognitive processes.[7] This is why cognitive science is all the more vital in large comparative projects such as these. We need sophisticated tools to decipher what philosophical presuppositions are ubiquitous and which are learned. This is rarely prima facie obvious. But I propose that making these differentiations are a crucial element of good philosophical interpretation. And again, it is only through comparative philosophy, both cross-cultural and over the *longue durée,* that such differentiations can be made.

I expect more comparative scholarship of this sort will continue to confirm its philosophical value. As I argued in this book, this is especially (and counterintuitively) the case for comparative material that is not stereotypically philosophical in nature. Of course, there is undeniable benefit in continuing to explore tried and true philosophical themes in Indian and Tibetan works, such as Buddhist *Higher Knowledge* (*Abhidharma*) concerning philosophy of mind, metaphysics, and ontology, or Tibetan *Mind Training* (*Blo sbyong*) texts that teach applied ethics, or the *Commentary on Politics* (*Nītiśāstra*) that focuses on political philosophy.

But what about sexual fluids consumed in Tantric rituals? Could this offer a philosophy of materiality? What about the Tibetan notion of Mind Treasures (*dgongs gter*), texts that are deposited in the minds of practitioners from previous lives? Might this offer a philosophy of textuality? And consider the pantheon of fierce female deities in both Buddhist and Hindu traditions, often considered preeminent and the most propitiated divinities. Could this lend itself to its own feminism? These explorations will require both reading through and behind texts, both with a deep respect for their intended meaning and a willingness (with the requisite sophistication) to explore their unintended entailments. To draw on a distinction championed by Wayne Proudfoot (1939–), what is required is both deep description and rich explanation, an effort to "get it right" but also demonstrate consequences beyond the text.[8] I believe these efforts will be expansive for philosophy writ large, demonstrating not just the philosophical sophistication of Indian and Tibetan traditions, but even redefining what we think of as philosophical and how we go about looking for it, analyzing it, and developing it.[9]

Notes

Introduction

1. J. W. de Jong, "Book Review: Outline of Indian Philosophy," *Indo-Iranian Journal* 16, no. 2 (1974): 147–49; Paul Williams, *Yogācāra, The Epistemological Tradition and Tathāgatagarbha*, vol. 5. Buddhism: Critical Concepts in Religious Studies (London: Routledge, 2005), 262.
2. I use the term "Indo-Tibetan" like "Euro-American" in a broad sense, meaning traditions from *either* India or Tibet or from *both*. This is different from other works which use the term exclusively to mean traditions that came from India and survive in Tibet, namely, Buddhism simpliciter.
3. Evan Thompson, *Why I Am Not a Buddhist* (New Haven, CT: Yale University Press, 2020), https://doi.org/10.2307/j.ctvt1sgfz.
4. Charles Taylor, *Sources of the Self: The Making of the Modern Identity* (Cambridge, MA: Harvard University Press, 1989), chap. 20; Robert N. Bellah, "Rousseau on Society and the Individual," in *The Social Contract: And, The First and Second Discourses*, ed. Susan Dunn and Gita May. Rethinking the Western Tradition (New Haven, CT: Yale University Press, 2002), 266–87.
5. Mary Wollstonecraft and Janet Todd, *A Vindication of the Rights of Men A Vindication of the Rights of Woman Historical and Moral View of the French Revolution*. Oxford World's Classics (Oxford: Oxford University Press, 1999), 7.
6. Jay Garfield gives an illuminating retrospective on this disparity. Jay L. Garfield, "Practicing Without a License and Making Trouble Along the Way: My Life in Buddhist Studies" (2018), https://jaygarfield.files.wordpress.com/2018/10/practicing-without-a-license.pdf.
7. Here, I draw on Wayne Proudfoot's distinction between description and explanation. Wayne Proudfoot, *Religious Experience* (Berkeley: University of California Press, 1985), 196–99.

8. It should be noted that (perhaps) unlike other epistemological traditions, Indo-Tibetan epistemology theorizes epistemic warrant (*pramāṇa*) as contingent and relative to a given epistemic object (*prameya*). Thus, *what* yogic perception perceives has direct consequences for an account of how it yields knowledge, and so is highly contested among these traditions.
9. The distinction between Buddhism and Hinduism in India is somewhat artificial, especially during the first millennium CE. David N. Lorenzen, "Who Invented Hinduism?," *Comparative Studies in Society and History* 41, no. 4 (1999): 630–59. Nevertheless, the distinction has some cogency, since Buddhists distinguished themselves from other Indian traditions in their rejection of Vedic authority, the Vedas being the earliest extant Sanskrit corpus of hymns to have flourished in India. Those traditions that accept Vedic authority I group under "Hinduism." And although they have some shared philosophical traits, these Veda-sympathetic lineages should not en masse be understood to constitute a self-conscious philosophical school of some sort.
10. Robert E. Buswell, ed., *Encyclopedia of Buddhism*, vol. 1 (New York: Macmillan Library Reference, 2003), 856.

1. Extramission, Remote Seeing, and Intuitions

1. Bertram R. Forer, "The Fallacy of Personal Validation: A Classroom Demonstration of Gullibility," *The Journal of Abnormal and Social Psychology* 44, no. 1 (1949): 118–23, https://doi.org/10.1037/h0059240.
2. For an overview, see Joshua Cuevas, "Is Learning Styles-Based Instruction Effective? A Comprehensive Analysis of Recent Research on Learning Styles," *Theory and Research in Education* 13, no. 3 (November 1, 2015): 308–33, https://doi.org/10.1177/1477878515606621.
3. The American Philosophical Association, for example, defines philosophy as "a reasoned pursuit of fundamental truths." Robert Audi, "Philosophy: A Brief Guide for Undergraduates," The American Philosophical Association, 2017, https://www.apaonline.org/page/undergraduates.
4. My thanks to Harunaga Isaacson for his suggestions on how to best translate *prāpyakārin* (personal communication, January 2, 2022).
5. Richard King, *Indian Philosophy: An Introduction to Hindu and Buddhist Thought* (Washington, DC: Georgetown University Press, 1999), 147–48.
6. Śaṅkara, *The Bṛhadāraṇyaka Upaniṣad: With the Commentary of Śaṅkarācārya*, trans. Madhavananda Swami, 3rd ed. (Mayavati, Almora: Advaita Ashrama, 1950), 599 v. 4.3.3.
7. Arion Rosu, *Les conceptions psychologuqes dans les texts médicaux indiens* (Paris: De Boccard, 1978), 201; Jan Gonda, *Eye and Gaze in the Veda* (Amsterdam: North Holland Publishing Company, 1969), 19–20.
8. Jwala Prasad Mishra, ed., *Śiva Māhapurāṇa*, vol. 1 (Mumbai: Sri Venkateswar Steam Press, 1920), v. 17.1.100.

9. Lawrence A. Babb, "Glancing: Visual Interaction in Hinduism," *Journal of Anthropological Research* 37 (1981): 396–99.
10. Oliver Hellwig, ed., *Matsyapurāṇa, 1-176* (Göttingen: Göttingen Register of Electronic Texts in Indian Languages (GRETIL), 2020), vv. 154.248–49, http://gretil.sub.uni-goettingen.de/gretil/corpustei/transformations/html/sa_matsyapurANa1-176.htm.
11. Diana L. Eck, *Darśan: Seeing the Divine Image in India*, 3rd ed. (New York: Columbia University Press, 1998), 7.
12. Saṃyutta Nikāya SN 12.64, *Atthirāgasuttaṃ*, 103.13–104.4. Note that all citations of the Pāli Canon, including commentaries and Buddhaghoṣa's *Visuddhimagga*, use the Pali Text Society pagination. Léon Feer and Caroline A. F. Rhys Davids, eds. *Saṃyutta-nikāya* (London: Pali Text Society, 1960), vol. 2.
13. Alex Watson, "Light as an Analogy for Cognition in Buddhist Idealism (Vijñānavāda)," *Journal of Indian Philosophy* 42, no. 2–3 (2014): 406.
14. Akṣapāda Gautama and Vātsyāyana, *Savātsyāyanabhāṣyaṃ Gautamīyaṃ Nyāyadarśanam with Bhāṣya of Vātsyāyana*, ed. Anantalāla Ṭhakkura (New Delhi: Bhāratīyadārśanikānusandhānapariṣatprakāśitam, 1997), 154 v. 3.1.34.
15. Technically, *yojana*, unit of distance about 12–15 km.
16. Vālmīki, *Rāmāyaṇa*, ed. Muneo Tokunaga (Göttingen: Göttingen Register of Electronic Texts in Indian Languages, 2020), vv. 4.57.22–23 and 28cd–29. http://gretil.sub.uni-goettingen.de/gretil/corpustei/transformations/html/sa_rAmAyaNa.htm.
17. Siddheswar Jena, ed., *[Śrīnarasiṃhapurāṇam] = The Narasiṃha Purāṇam: Text with English Translation and Notes* (Delhi: Nag Publishers, 1987), 213 v. 50.147.
18. Narayana Godabole Balakrishna and Kāśīnātha Pāṇḍuraṅga Paraba, eds., *Hitopadeśa*, 5th rev. ed. (Bombay: Tukârâm Jâvajî, 1904), 96.8.
19. David White remarks that secondary scholarship in general has failed to acknowledge the role of the *Yogasūtras*' third chapter in forming notions of yogic perception. David Gordon White, "How Big Can Yogis Get? How Much Can Yogis See?," in *Yoga Powers: Extraordinary Capacities Attained Through Meditation and Concentration*, ed. Knut A. Jacobsen (Leiden: Brill, 2012), 61.
20. Pantañjali, *Pantañjali's Yoga-Sūtras with the Yoga-Bhāṣya Attributed to Veda-Vyāsa and the Explanation Entitled Tattva-Vāiçāradī of Vacaspati-Miçra and the Brief Explanation of Bālarāma*, ed. Svāmi Bālarāma of Saṁvat (Varanasi: Svāmi Bālarāma of Saṁvat, 1908), 235.6–9.
21. Mark Singleton and James Mallinson, *Roots of Yoga*, Penguin Classics (London: Penguin, 2017); Pradeep P. Gokhale, *The Yogasutra of Patañjali: A New Introduction to the Buddhist Roots of the Yoga System* (London: Routledge, 2020).
22. Also see Jed Forman, "Subtle, Hidden, and Far-Off: The Intertextuality of the Yogasūtras," *The Journal of Hindu Studies*, April 10, 2023, 1–24, https://doi.org/10.1093/jhs/hiad013.
23. Rāma Prasāda takes this as a clear instance of projective light, arguing the yogi sees those objects "by directing the light of higher sense-activity towards them." Pantañjali, *Pātañjali's Yoga Sūtras: With the Commentary of Vyāsa and the Gloss of Vāchaspati Miśra*, trans. Rāma Prasāda (New Delhi: Munshiram Manoharlal, 1998),

224. Trevor Leggett takes a similar reading, arguing that the yogi does so "by projecting the light of supernormal radiant perception." Pantañjali, *The Complete Commentary by Śaṅkara on the Yoga Sūtras: A Full Translation of the Newly Discovered Text*, trans. Trevor Leggett (London: Kegan Paul International, 1990), v. 3.25. Shyam Ranganathan, on the other hand, does not take the *āloka* as literal light, describing it as a type of "illumination" of those objects, such that yogis see them "by directing effort towards illumination." Pantañjali, *Patañjali's Yoga Sūtra*, trans. Shyam Ranganathan (London: Penguin, 2009), v. 3.25.

24. There are other instances in the text where there is no doubt that Pantañjali advocates *prāpyakārin*, such as in *Yogasūtra* 3.21, where he says yogis can become invisible by obstructing the eye-light (*cakṣuḥ-prakāśa*) of potential onlookers. Pantañjali, *Pantañjali's Yoga-Sūtras with the Yoga-Bhāṣya Attributed to Veda-Vyāsa*, 232.

25. Pantañjali, *Pantañjali's Yoga-Sūtras with the Yoga-Bhāṣya Attributed to Veda-Vyāsa* 218 v. 3. 16cd.

26. Patañjali describes these three in *Yogasūtra* 3.13. Pantañjali, *Pantañjali's Yoga-Sūtras with the Yoga-Bhāṣya Attributed to Veda-Vyāsa*, 201. These are transformation of the substrate of an object (*dharma*), the transformation of its characteristics (*lakṣaṇa*), and the transformation of its state (*avasthā*).

27. Praśastapāda and Śrīdhara, *The Praśastapāda Bhāshya, With the Commentary Nyāyakandali of Sridhara*, ed. Vindhyeśvarīprasāda Dvivedī, 2nd ed. (Delhi: Sri Satguru Publications, 1984), 187.7–13; Praśastapāda and Śrīdhara, *Nyāyakandalī: Being a Commentary on Prasastapadabhasya with Three Sub-Commentaries*, ed. J. S. Jetly and Vasant G. Parikh (Vadodara: Oriental Institute, 1991), 455.1–4.

28. Fourfold contact as a condition of external sense cognition is also first articulated by Praśastapāda: "Without the connection between the *ātman* and the mind, the mind and the senses, and the senses and the object, there is no perception. Thus, this fourfold contact is the cause [of perception]." See a discussion and citation of the pertinent root verses from the *Nyāyakandalī* in Satkari Mookerjee, *The Buddhist Philosophy of Universal Flux. An Exposition of the Philosophy of Critical Realism as Expounded by the School of Dignāga* (Calcutta: University of Calcutta, 1935), 152n1.

29. Praśastapāda and Śrīdhara, *The Praśastapāda Bhāshya, With the Commentary Nyāyakandali of Sridhara*, 187.7–11; Praśastapāda and Śrīdhara, *Nyāyakandalī: Being a Commentary on Prasastapadabhasya with Three Sub-Commentaries*, 455.1–3; also see Anna-Pya Sjödin, "The Girl Who Knew Her Brother Would Be Coming Home: Ārṣajñāna in Praśastapādabhāṣya, Nyāyakandalī and Vyomavatī," *Journal of Indian Philosophy* 40, no. 4 (2012): 473–74.

30. Praśastapāda and Śrīdhara, *Nyāyakandalī: Being a Commentary on Prasastapadabhasya with Three Sub-Commentaries*, 455.12.

31. Praśastapāda and Śrīdhara, *Nyāyakandalī: Being a Commentary*, 72.10–13.

32. Praśastapāda and Śrīdhara, *Nyāyakandalī: Being a Commentary*, 456.7–10.

33. Praśastapāda and Śrīdhara, *Nyāyakandalī: Being a Commentary*, 457.3–4.

34. Praśastapāda and Śrīdhara, *Nyāyakandalī: Being a Commentary*, 457.5–8.

35. David White makes this connection explicit: "Yogi perception arises when one's own self [i.e., soul] or mind is yoked, via a ray of perception, to another being's

self inside that other being's body." David Gordon White, *Sinister Yogis* (Chicago: University of Chicago Press, 2009), 160.

36. Also see White, "How Big Can Yogis Get? How Much Can Yogis See?," 70–73; White, *Sinister Yogis*, 159–61.

37. Jadunath Sinha, *Indian Psychology: Perception* (London: Kegan Paul, Trench, Trubner and Co., 1934), 16–25; K. N. Hota, "Is Sense-Organ Prāpyakārin in Perception?," *Bulletin of the Deccan College Research Institute* 75 (2015): 255–62.

38. Kundakunda, Amṛtacandra, and Jayasena, *Srī Kundakundācārya's Pravacanasāra (Pavayaṇasāra): A Pro-canonical Text of the Jainas*, ed. and trans. A. N. Upādhye (Agas: Srimad Rajachandra Ashrama, 1964), 35.7–10.

39. Akṣapāda Gautama and Vātsyāyana, *Savātsyāyanabhāṣyaṃ Gautamīyaṃ Nyāyadarśanam with Bhāṣya of Vātsyāyana*, 9.5–9.

40. Later Buddhists, however, came to reject this position. Dignāga's position, as we will see, argues that each epistemic instrument has its own, unique object. Thus, inferred fire is not the same object as directly perceived fire. Lawrence McCrea and Parimal Patil describe this difference between Nyāya and Buddhist views as "convergence of the sources of knowledge" (*pramāna-samplava*) versus "differential application of the sources of knowledge (*pramāna-vyavasthā*)." Lawrence J. McCrea and Parimal G. Patil, *Buddhist Philosophy of Language in India: Jñānaśrīmitra on Exclusion* (New York: Columbia University Press, 2010), 10. As I discuss in chapter 3, this creates a unique problem for Buddhist in Dignāga's lineage to explain the relationship between inference and yogic perception. But is also interesting to note that both Vātsyāyana and Dignāga describe yogic perception (*pratyakṣam yoga-samādhijam* and *yogīnām pratyakṣam*) as the direct perception of inferential teachings (*upadeśa* and *nirdeśa*). Akṣapāda Gautama and Vātsyāyana, *Savātsyāyanabhāṣyaṃ Gautamīyaṃ Nyāyadarśanam with Bhāṣya of Vātsyāyana*, 9.8 and 9.11; Dignāga, *Dignāga's Pramāṇasamuccaya, Chapter 1: A Hypothetical Reconstruction of the Sanskrit Text with the Help of the Two Tibetan Translations on the Basis of the Hitherto Known Sanskrit Fragments and the Linguistic Materials Gained from Jinendrabuddhi's Ṭīkā*, ed. Ernst Steinkellner (Vienna: Österreichische Akademie der Wissenschaften, 2005), 3.11. This may reflect a shared desire to substantiate yogic perception as the direct realization of scriptural truth against Mīmāṃsā, as we will see in the next chapter.

41. Jayanta Bhaṭṭa, *Nyāyamañjarī of Jayanta Bhaṭṭa with the Commentary of Granthibhaṅga by Cakradhara*, ed. Gaurinath Sastri (Varanasi: Sampurnanand Sanskrit Vishvavidyalaya, 1982), 1:157.1–7.

42. Jayanta Bhaṭṭa, *Nyāyamañjarī of Jayanta Bhaṭṭa*, 1:162.2–3.

43. Sjödin, "The Girl Who Knew Her Brother Would Be Coming Home: Ārṣajñāna in Praśastapādabhāṣya, Nyāyakandalī and Vyomavatī," 469–88.

44. Nāgas are mythical, serpent-like creatures that live in subterranean realms.

45. Bhāsarvajña, *Nyāyabhūṣaṇam*, ed. Śvāmī Yogīndrānanda (Varanasi: Ṣaḍdarśana Prakāśana Pratiṣṭhānam, 1968), 170.19–24.

46. Patañjali also discusses omniscient yogis in *Yogasūtra* 3.33. But this is described as a type of intuition (*prātibha*) rather than a perception (*pratyakṣa*). Pantañjali, *Pantañjali's Yoga-Sūtras with the Yoga-Bhāṣya Attributed to Veda-Vyāsa*, 243. The point

of this chapter is to analyze when abilities such as omniscience were first attributed to yogic perception, not the first advent of these abilities, which clearly precede theories of yogic perception.

47. Bhāsarvajña, *Nyāyabhūṣaṇam*, 170.27–71.4.
48. The divine eye is by no means unique to Buddhist texts, and later it becomes effectively synonymous with yogic perception in the larger Indian milieu. One example is the *Compendium of Caraka* (*Carakasaṃhitā*) (ca. 100 BCE–100 CE), the seminal text on Āyurveda, where it is said that transmigrating souls are seen with the divine eye. Agniveśa and Cakrapāṇidatta, *The Charakasaṃhitā by Agniveśa, Revised by Charaka and Dṛidhabala, with the Āyurveda-Dīpikā Commentary of Chakrapāṇidatta, Ed. Vaidya Jādavaji Trikamji Āchārya*, ed. Jādavaji Trikamji (Bombay: Satyabhāmābāi Pāndurang, 1941), 305 v. 2.31. Buddhist sources, we will see, say the same. Cakrapāṇidatta's eleventh-century commentary on this text, *The Light on Āyurveda* (*Āyurvedadīpikā*), makes explicit that "divine sight is the yogic eye." Agniveśa and Cakrapāṇidatta, 305.29–31 col. b. David White also confirms these passages specifically concern yogic perception. White, *Sinister Yogis*, 161.
49. Bradley S. Clough, "The Cultivation of Yogic Powers in the Pāli Path Manuals of Theravāda Buddhism," in *Yoga Powers: Extraordinary Capacities Attained Through Meditation and Concentration*, ed. Knut A. Jacobsen (Leiden: Brill, 2012), 91.
50. Buddhaghoṣa, *Visuddhimagga* 2.12, "Iddhividhaniddeso," 404.15–17. Buddhaghoṣa, *The Visuddhi-magga of Buddhaghosa*, ed. Caroline A. F. Rhys Davids (London: Pali Text Society, 1920), vol. 2.
51. Buddhaghoṣa, *Visuddhimagga* 2.13, "Abhiññāniddeso," 423.23–24.
52. Buddhaghoṣa, *Visuddhimagga* 2.13, "Abhiññāniddeso," 409.13–18.
53. David White also notes similarities between the divine eye and yogic perception. White, *Sinister Yogis*, 131. He especially notes these similarities in Buddhism. White, 157. I will argue in chapter 3, however, that Buddhist descriptions of yogic perception are more commonly informed by the *dharma* eye (*dhamma-cakkhu*). The distinction between the divine and dharma eye here may be similar to the distinction between unabsorbed and absorbed yogic perception in other traditions. David White explains such differentiations as a type of soteriologization strategy, in which traditions distinguish the mere clairvoyant version of yogic perception from its role in spiritual insight. White, *Sinister Yogis*, 41. The clairvoyant type of yogic perception likely predates the sanitized, spiritual type that was appropriated by religious institutions as a type of soteriological device. Early Buddhists may have made a similar distinction between the divine and dharma eye: the ability to read minds and see remote objects versus insight into reality. We will see Dharmakīrti (b. 660 CE) adopt a similar strategy.
54. Joseph Walser argues, however, that *anātman* is not a universal Buddhist doctrine, at least in its form as a rejection of the soul's existence. Joseph Walser, "Buddhism without Buddhists? Academia & Learning to See Buddhism Like a State," *Pacific World*, 4, no. 3 (2022): 103–70.

55. We see both readings in secondary literature. Thus, Bradley Clough translates this phrase as "it greatly illuminates with discerning light." Clough, "The Cultivation of Yogic Powers in the Pāli Path Manuals of Theravāda Buddhism," 91. This is a *prāpyakārin*-suggestive reading ("with" suggests an instrument, a light which discerns). But Ñāṇamoli Bhikkhu opts for "it greatly illuminates by discerning light," as in by taking in light, it illuminates objects. Buddhaghoṣa, *The Path of Purification*, trans. Ñāṇamoli Thera, 4th ed. (Kandy, Sri Lanka: Buddhist Publication Society, 2010), 416.
56. Clough, "The Cultivation of Yogic Powers in the Pāli Path Manuals of Theravāda Buddhism," 92.
57. It is interesting to note that even modern-day Hindi speakers colloquially say, "Give me the light of your eyes" (*āṃkhoṃ ke rośnī mujhe de dījiye*) to ask for someone's help if they are visually impaired. This may be vestigial of an old *prāpyakārin* cultural intuition that understands the eyes as containing projective light.
58. Going forward, I will stay concise and say that Buddhists simply reject *prāpyakārin*, meaning they reject it as an account of *visual* sensation. But this is not necessarily the case for other senses, like taste and touch, which, Buddhists agree, *do* reach out and touch their sense objects.
59. Buddhaghoṣa, *Visuddhimagga* 2.14, "Khandhaniddeso," 445.19–20; also see Chandaratana Pilasse, "Divergent Doctrinal Interpretations on the Nature of Mind and Matter in Theravāda Abhidhamma: A Study Mainly Based on the Pāli and Siṃhala Buddhist Exegetical Literature" (Diss., University of Hong Kong, 2011), 310.
60. Vasubandhu, *Abhidharmakośabhāṣyam*, ed. Prahlad Pradhan (Patna: K. P. Jayaswal Research Institute, 1975), 32 v. 1.43c and ll. 7–8.
61. Udayana wrote a long polemic against the Buddhist rejection of visual *prāpyakārin*. Kaṇāda, Praśastapāda, and Udayana, *The Aphorisms of the Vaiśeshika Philosophy by Kaṇâda, with the Commentary of Praśastapâda, and the Gloss of Udayanâchârya*, ed. Vindhyeśvarīprasāda Dvivedī (Varanasi: Braj Bhushan Das, 1919), 74.3–76.6; also see Forman, "Subtle, Hidden, and Far-Off," sec. 2.
62. Chandaratana Pilasse discusses a Buddhist *prāpyakārin* position found in the *Siṅhala Commentary* (*Sīhaḷāṭṭhakathā*), a text which in the Theravāda tradition is believed to have originated in the third century BCE. Pilasse, "Divergent Doctrinal Interpretations on the Nature of Mind and Matter in Theravāda Abhidhamma, 40–42. The text seems to suggest that the eye sees its object by reaching out to make physical contact with it (311).
63. Dharmakīrti, *Pramāṇavarttika-kārikā: (Sanskrit and Tibetan)*, ed. Yūshō Miyasaka, vol. 2, Acta Indologica (Narita: Naritasan Shinshōji, 1972), v. 2.33; Dharmakīrti, "*Pramāṇavārttikakārikā, Tshad ma rnam 'grel gyi tshig le'ur byas pa," in *Sde dge bstan 'gyur*, ed. Tshul khrims rin chen, Toh. no. 4210, vol. Tshad ma, ce (Delhi: Delhi Karmapae Choedhey, Gyalwae Sungrab Partun Khang, 1744), fol. 108b6–7.
64. Shinya Moriyama, "Pramāṇapariśuddhasakalatattvajña, Sarvajña and Sarvasarvajña," in *Religion and Logic in Buddhist Philosophical Analysis Proceedings of the Fourth International Dharmakīrti Conference Vienna, August 23-27, 2005*, ed. Helmut

Krasser et al. (Vienna: Verlag der Österreichischen Akadmie der Wissenschaften, 2011), 329–39; also see Raffaele Torella, "Observations on Yogipratyakṣa," in *Saṁskṛta-Sādhutā: Goodness of Sanskrit. Studies in Honour of Professor Ashok N. Aklujkar*, ed. Chikafumi Watanabe, Michele Desmarais, and Yoshichika Honda, (Delhi: D.K. Printworld, 2012), 475.

65. Prajñākaragupta, *Pramāṇavārtikabhāshyam or Vārtikālaṅkaraḥ of Prajñākaragupta (Being a Commentary on Dharmakīrti's Pramāṇavārtikam)*, ed. Rāhula Sāṅkṛtyāyana (Patna, India: Kashi Prasad Jayaswal Research Institute, 1943), 53.4–5; Prajñākaragupta, "*Pramāṇavārttikālaṅkāra, Tshad ma rnam 'grel gyi rgyan," in *Sde dge bstan 'gyur*, ed. 'Phags pa shes rab, trans. Paṇḍita skal ldan rgyal po, Blo ldan shes rab, and Paṇḍita Kumāraśrī, Toh. no. 4221, vol. Tshad ma, te (Delhi: Delhi Karmapae Choedhey, Gyalwae Sungrab Partun Khang, 1744), fol. 46a5–6.

66. Prajñākaragupta, *Pramāṇavārtikabhāshyam or Vārtikālaṅkaraḥ of Prajñākaragupta (Being a Commentary on Dharmakīrti's Pramāṇavārtikam)*, 460.17; Prajñākaragupta, "*Pramāṇavārttikālaṅkāra, Tshad ma rnam 'grel gyi rgyan," in *Sde dge bstan 'gyur*, ed. 'Phags pa shes rab, trans. Paṇḍita skal ldan rgyal po, Blo ldan shes rab, and Paṇḍita Kumāraśrī, Toh. no. 4221, vol. Tshad ma, the (Delhi: Delhi Karmapae Choedhey, Gyalwae Sungrab Partun Khang, 1744), fol. 120a4.

67. Prajñākaragupta, *Pramāṇavārtikabhāshyam or Vārtikālaṅkaraḥ of Prajñākaragupta (Being a Commentary on Dharmakīrti's Pramāṇavārtikam)*, 440.5–6; Prajñākaragupta, "*Pramāṇavārttikālaṅkāra, Tshad ma rnam 'grel gyi rgyan," vol. Tshad ma, the, 1744, fol. 103a7.

68. Though tangential to my discussion, there are clear parallels here with Laura Mulvey's theorization of the male gaze as phallocentric and penetrative, especially given the patriarchal milieu of these texts. Laura Mulvey, "Visual Pleasure and Narrative Cinema," *Screen* 16, no. 3 (September 1, 1975): 6–18, https://doi.org/10.1093/screen/16.3.6.

69. Biology teachers commonly deny seeds are alive. April N. Wynn et al., "Student Misconceptions about Plants—A First Step in Building a Teaching Resource," *Journal of Microbiology & Biology Education*, April 2017, https://doi.org/10.1128/jmbe.v18i1.1253. Even professional biologists respond more slowly when tasked to identify whether plants are alive as compared to animals, suggesting a tension between intuitions and reflective knowledge. Robert F. Goldberg and Sharon L. Thompson-Schill, "Developmental 'Roots' in Mature Biological Knowledge," *Psychological Science* 20, no. 4 (April 1, 2009): 480–87, https://doi.org/10.1111/j.1467-9280.2009.02320.x.

70. Dan Sperber, *Explaining Culture: A Naturalistic Approach* (Malden, MA: Blackwell, 1996), 98–118.

71. Jean Piaget, *The Child's Conception of the World*, trans. Joan Tomlinson and Andrew Tomlinson (London: Routledge & Kegan Paul Ltd., 1971), 48.

72. Jane E. Cottrell and Gerald A. Winer, "Development in the Understanding of Perception: The Decline of Extramission Perception Beliefs," *Developmental Psychology* 30, no. 2 (1994): 218–28.

73. Gerald A. Winer et al., "Fundamentally Misunderstanding Visual Perception," *American Psychologist* 57, no. 6/7 (2002): 423.

74. Arvid Guterstam et al., "Implicit Model of Other People's Visual Attention as an Invisible, Force-Carrying Beam Projecting From the Eyes," *Proceedings of the National Academy of Sciences—PNAS* 116, no. 1 (2019): 328–33, https://doi.org/10.1073/pnas.1816581115.
75. Reginald B. Adams et al., "Effects of Gaze on Amygdala Sensitivity to Anger and Fear Faces," *Science* 300, no. 5625 (2003): 1536; Nouchine Hadjikhani et al., "Pointing with the Eyes: The Role of Gaze in Communicating Danger," *Brain and Cognition* 68, no. 1 (2008): 1–8, https://doi.org/10.1016/j.bandc.2008.01.008; Yi-Chia Chen and Su-Ling Yeh, "Look into My Eyes and I Will Wee You: Unconscious Processing of Human Gaze," *Consciousness and Cognition* 21, no. 4 (2012): 1703–10, https://doi.org/10.1016/j.concog.2012.10.001.
76. George Lakoff and Mark Johnson, *Metaphors We Live By* (Chicago: University of Chicago Press, 2003); George Lakoff, *Women, Fire, and Dangerous Things: What Categories Reveal About the Mind* (Chicago: University of Chicago Press, 1990).
77. Gerald A. Winer, Aaron W. Rader, and Jane E. Cottrell, "Testing Different Interpretations for the Mistaken Belief That Rays Exit the Eyes During Vision," *The Journal of Psychology* 137, no. 3 (2003): 243–61, https://doi.org/10.1080/00223980309600612.
78. Leonard Talmy, "Fictive Motion in Language and 'Ception," in *Speech, Language, and Communication*, ed. Joanne L. Miller and Peter D. Eimas (San Diego, CA: Academic Press, 1995), 224–26.
79. Watson, "Light as an Analogy for Cognition in Buddhist Idealism (Vijñānavāda)," 408–10; Dan Lusthaus, "A Pre-Dharmakīrti Indian Discussion of Dignāga Preserved in Chinese Translation: The Buddhabhūmy-Upadeśa," *Journal of Buddhist Studies* 6 (2009): 28. There is some further nuance between these terms that need not concern us here.
80. Dharmakīrti, "*Saṃtānāntarasiddhi, Rgyud gzhan grub pa zhes bya ba'i rab tu byed pa," in *Sde dge bstan 'gyur*, ed. Tshul khrims rin chen, Toh. no. 4219, vol. Tshad ma, ce (Delhi: Delhi Karmapae Choedhey, Gyalwae Sungrab Partun Khang, 1744), fol. 359a5, http://gretil.sub.uni-goettingen.de/gretil/1_sanskr/6_sastra/3_phil/buddh/bsa059_u.htm; Dharmakīrti and Vinītadeva, *Santānāntarasiddhiḥ of Ācārya Dharmakīrti and Santānāntarasiddhiḥ Ṭīkā of Ācārya Vinītadeva: Restored and Ed. J. S. Negi*, ed. J. S. Negi, Bibliotheca Indo Tibetica Series 37 (Varanasi: Central Institute of Higher Tibetan Studies, 1997), l. 92.
81. Śāntarakṣita and Kamalaśīla, *Tattvasaṅgraha of Ācārya Śāntarakṣita with the "Pañjika" Commentary of Ācārya Śrī Kamalaśīla*, ed. Dvārikādāsa Śāstrī, vol. 2 (Varanasi: Bauddha, 1981), 719 v. 3268 and ll. 13–4.
82. Paul A Klaczynski and Kristen L Lavallee, "Domain-Specific Identity, Epistemic Regulation, and Intellectual Ability as Predictors of Belief-Biased Reasoning: A Dual-Process Perspective," *Journal of Experimental Child Psychology* 92, no. 1 (2005): 1–24, https://doi.org/10.1016/j.jecp.2005.05.001; Martin Kerwer and Tom Rosman, "Epistemic Change and Diverging Information: How Do Prior Epistemic Beliefs Affect the Efficacy of Short-Term Interventions?," *Learning and Individual Differences* 80 (2020), https://doi.org/10.1016/j.lindif.2020.101886; Krista R. Muis, Lisa D. Bendixen, and Florian C. Haerle, "Domain-Generality and Domain-Specificity in

Personal Epistemology Research: Philosophical and Empirical Reflections in the Development of a Theoretical Framework," *Educational Psychology Review* 18, no. 1 (2006): 3–54; Ivar Bråten, Helge I. Strømsø, and Marit S. Samuelstuen, "Are Sophisticated Students Always Better? The Role of Topic-Specific Personal Epistemology in the Understanding of Multiple Expository Texts," *Contemporary Educational Psychology* 33, no. 4 (2008): 814–40, https://doi.org/10.1016/j.cedpsych.2008.02.001.

83. Jñānaśrīmitra, "Yoginirṇayaprakaraṇa," in *Jñānaśrīmitranibandhavāli: Buddhist Philosophical Works of Jñānaśrīmitra*, ed. Anantalāla Ṭhakkura, 2nd. ed. (Patna: Kashi Prasad Jayaswal Research Institute, 1987), 334.7–10.
84. Jñānaśrīmitra, "Yoginirṇayaprakaraṇa," 334.17–20.
85. Jayanta Bhaṭṭa, *Nyāyamañjarī of Jayanta Bhaṭṭa with the Commentary of Granthibhaṅga by Cakradhara*, 1:157.1–7. Arguments for extramission via an appeal to night vision are not isolated to Indian texts. The European medieval scholastic Roger Bacon (1220–1292) claimed that extramission explained feline night vision. Dominique Raynaud, "Les normes de la rationalité dans une controverse scientifique: le cas de l'optique médiévale," *L'Année sociologique* 48, no. 2 (1998): 451. This also suggests that extramission is a cross-cultural, pan-human intuition.
86. Jñānaśrīmitra, "Yoginirṇayaprakaraṇa," 329.25–26.
87. Praśastapāda and Śrīdhara, *Nyāyakandalī: Being a Commentary*, 457.4-7.
88. Jñānaśrīmitra, "Yoginirṇayaprakaraṇa," 329.12.
89. Jñānaśrīmitra, "Yoginirṇayaprakaraṇa," 333.27–334.3.
90. Robert Stern, *Hegelian Metaphysics* (New York: Oxford University Press, 2009), 45–76.
91. Robert Stern gives a convincing argument as to how these idealist and realist elements are philosophically compatible and not incongruous. Stern, *Hegelian Metaphysics*, 45–76. But we might go another route and relinquish the demand that any good interpretation of Hegel reveal consistency, allowing us to see the variety in his thinking. Indeed, Paul Livingston argues that Hegel purposely includes contradiction as part of his dialectical method. Paul M. Livingston, *The Politics of Logic: Badiou, Wittgenstein, and the Consequences of Formalism*, Routledge Studies in Contemporary Philosophy 27 (New York: Routledge, 2012), 253–54.
92. There are parallels here to Maurice Merleau-Ponty's phenomenology of perception, according to which the notion of sensation is a *post facto*, scientific superimposition on our perceptual experience of the Gestalt. Maurice Merleau-Ponty, *Phenomenology of Perception*, trans. Colin Smith, Routledge Classics (London: Routledge, 2002), chap. 1. Likewise, we might think of intromission as a scientific superimposition on our embodied experience of the extramissive gaze.

2. The Epistemology of Authority and Testimony

1. Serendipitously, during revisions to my manuscript, a congressional subcommittee heard the testimony of several intelligence officers about UFOs or UAPs, one of whom claimed to have seen evidence of extraterrestrial life. "Unidentified

Anomalous Phenomena: Implications on National Security, Public Safety, and Government Transparency" (2154 Rayburn House Office Building, Washington, DC, July 26, 2023).

2. Also see John Taber, "Yoga and Our Epistemic Predicament," in *Yogic Perception, Meditation and Altered States of Consciousness*, ed. Eli Franco and Dagmar Eigner (Vienna: Verlag der Österreichischen Akademie der Wissenschaften, 2009), 71–92. He gives a sophisticated comparison of Hume's view on testimony with Indian debates about yogic perception.
3. David Hume, *An Enquiry Concerning Human Understanding*, ed. Tom L. Beauchamp, Oxford Philosophical Texts (Oxford: Oxford University Press, 1999), 174.
4. Karen Jones, "The Politics of Credibility," in *A Mind of One's Own: Feminist Essays on Reason and Objectivity*, ed. Louise M. Antony and Charlotte Witt, 2nd ed., Feminist Theory and Politics (Boulder, CO: Westview Press, 2001), 157.
5. Hume, *An Enquiry Concerning Human Understanding*, 171.
6. Hume, *An Enquiry Concerning Human Understanding*, 170.
7. This is the majority consensus in scholarship. Frederick F. Schmitt, "Justification, Sociality, and Autonomy," *Synthese* 73, no. 1 (1987): 43–85; C. A. J. Coady, *Testimony: A Philosophical Study* (New York: Clarendon Press, 1992), 79; Mark Owen Webb, "Why I Know About as Much as You: A Reply to Hardwig," *The Journal of Philosophy* 90, no. 5 (1993): 263; Elizabeth Fricker, "Against Gullibility," in *Knowing from Words: Western and Indian Philosophical Analysis of Understanding and Testimony*, ed. Bimal Krishna Matilal and Arindam Chakrabarti (Dordrecht: Kluwer Academic, 1994), 125–61; Elizabeth Fricker, "Trusting Others in the Sciences: A Priori or Empirical Warrant," *Studies in History and Philosophy of Science* 33, no. 2 (2002): 373–83, https://doi.org/10.1016/S0039-3681(02)00006-7; Alvin I. Goldman, *Pathways to Knowledge: Private and Public* (Oxford: Oxford University Press, 2002), 173; Joseph Shieber, "Locke on Testimony: A Reexamination," *History of Philosophy Quarterly* 26, no. 1 (2009): 21–41; Jennifer Lackey, *Learning From Words: Testimony as a Source of Knowledge* (Oxford: Oxford University Press, 2008), 142; Benjamin McMyler, *Testimony, Trust, and Authority* (Oxford: Oxford University Press, 2011), 23–24; Dan O'Brien, *Hume on Testimony*, 1st ed. (New York: Routledge, 2023), sec. 2.4.
8. Fricker, "Against Gullibility;" O'Brien, *Hume on Testimony*, sec. 2.4. Hume is likely drawing from John Locke (1632–1704), who explicitly delineates these two requirements for justified belief in testimony. John Locke, *An Essay Concerning Humane Understanding, Volume 2 MDCXC, Based on the 2nd Edition, Books 3 and 4*, ed. Steve Harris and David Widger (Chapel Hill, NC: Project Gutenberg, 2004), bk. 4, chap. 16, sec. 9.
9. George Campbell, *A Dissertation on Miracles* (Edinburgh: Bell & Bradfute, 1797), sec. 6.
10. John Stuart Mill, *A System of Logic, Ratiocinative and Inductive; Being a Connected View of the Principles of Evidence, and the Methods of Scientific Investigation*, ed. J. M. Robson, vol. 1 (Toronto: University of Toronto Press, 1973), 627; Coady, *Testimony*, 178–79.
11. Campbell's criticism has been reiterated several times in modern scholarship. Coady, *Testimony*, chap. 4; Axel Gelfert, "Hume on Testimony Revisited," *History*

of Philosophy & Logical Analysis 13, no. 1 (April 5, 2010): 60–75, https://doi.org/10.30965/26664275-01301004; Alexander George, *The Everlasting Check: Hume on Miracles* (Cambridge, MA: Harvard University Press, 2016), 52; O'Brien, *Hume on Testimony*, sec. 2.4.

12. Several scholars have identified this potential problem with Humean reductionism and proposed various solutions. Alvin I. Goldman, "Experts: Which Ones Should You Trust?," *Philosophy and Phenomenological Research* 63, no. 1 (July 2001): 85–110, https://doi.org/10.1111/j.1933-1592.2001.tb00093.x; Fricker, "Trusting Others in the Sciences: A Priori or Empirical Warrant;" Kristina Rolin, "Trust in Science," in *The Routledge Handbook of Trust and Philosophy*, ed. Judith Simon. Routledge Handbooks in Philosophy (London: Routledge, 2020), sec. 27.4; Jeroen de Ridder, "How to Trust a Scientist," *Studies in History and Philosophy of Science* 93 (June 2022): 11–20, https://doi.org/10.1016/j.shpsa.2022.02.003.
13. As Jay Garfield rightly points out, however, the global requirement includes customs for its own revision. For example, once there is customary consensus about quantum phenomena, there is no reason to assume that they would remain counterintuitive to our collective understanding of the world. *The Concealed Influence of Custom: Hume's Treatise From the Inside Out* (New York: Oxford University Press, 2019), 43–46. Still, what are the customs that would permit a such a revision? Quantum phenomena and miracles are equally counterintuitive to common observation. Thus, if they are to lead to customary revision, they must at first be accepted prima facie, assuming the local requirement (trustworthiness) is fulfilled. This effectively suspends the global requirement, at least initially. And if this is the case, then there is no a priori guarantee that quantum but not miraculous testimony would lead to such revision, since, in the context of that suspension, the content of the testimony is not relevant to the local requirement. Therefore Hume must either loosen a foundationalist hold on common observation, opening up a range of testifiable phenomena, or adhere to it, severally limiting testimony's epistemic currency.
14. Jones, "The Politics of Credibility."
15. Cynthia Townley makes a similar point in the context of epistemic justice. She states that communication of veritable knowledge cannot be the sole criteria of justified trust, since the disproportionate tendency to disbelieve the testimony of marginalized groups constitutes an epistemic failing, independent of the veracity of their claims. Cynthia Townley, *A Defense of Ignorance: Its Value for Knowers and Roles in Feminist and Social Epistemologies* (Lanham, MD: Lexington Books, 2011), 46–50. For a similar debate in the Indian context, see Rosanna Picascia, "Our Epistemic Dependence on Others: Nyāya and Buddhist Accounts of Testimony as a Source of Knowledge," *Journal of Hindu Studies*, April 18, 2023, hiad003, https://doi.org/10.1093/jhs/hiad003.
16. Robert Audi, *The Place of Testimony in the Fabric of Knowledge and Justification, Rational Belief* (Oxford University Press, 2015), 224.
17. Audi, *The Place of Testimony*, 233–34.
18. Audi, *The Place of Testimony*, 227.
19. Audi, *The Place of Testimony*, 225.

20. Audi, *The Place of Testimony*, 233–35.
21. My discussion of "Mīmāṃsā" is restricted to the Pūrva Mīmāṃsā, which argues that the Vedic precepts or injunctions (*codanā*) are the path to liberation. This is in contrast to Uttara Mīmāṃsā, which argues that knowledge (*jñāna*) provides the path to liberation. C. Ram-Prasad, "Knowledge and Action I: Means to the Human End in Bhāṭṭa Mīmāṃsā and Advaita Vedānta," *Journal of Indian Philosophy* 28, no. 1 (2000): 1.
22. Dan Arnold does a superb job of illustrating the general epistemological disagreement between Mīmāṃsakas and Buddhists in this regard. He identifies the Buddhist position as foundationalist in the way I have described. That is, they argue that all instances of knowledge reduce to some perceptual warrant. Mīmāṃsakas argue that this incurs a regress problem, since as soon as we demand that some beliefs have extrinsic validation by another warrant, then we have no footing by which to suspend that requirement for the so-called warranting foundation. Thus, to the degree that we have knowledge at all, we must accept that perception and Vedic testimony are intrinsically (*svatas*) warranted, since making one the foundation for the other devolves into an infinite regress. Dan Arnold, *Buddhists, Brahmins, and Belief: Epistemology in South Asian Philosophy of Religion* (New York: Columbia University Press, 2005), 59–114. Relevant for the discussion here: Mīmāṃsakas argue that perception, yogic or otherwise, cannot warrant scriptural testimony, since both are intrinsically warranted, neither foundational to the other.
23. Jaimini and Śabarasvāmī, *The Aphorisms of the Mīmāmsa with the Commentary of Sāvarasvāmin*, ed. Maheśacandra Bhaṭṭācārya, Bibliotheca Indica 45 (Calcutta: Asiatic Society of Bengal, 1873), vv. 1.1.2–4.
24. Jaimini and Śabarasvāmī, *The Aphorisms of the Mīmāmsa*, 4.3–5 and 6.22–23.
25. Jaimini and Śabarasvāmī, *The Aphorisms of the Mīmāmsa*, 538.17.
26. Arnold, *Buddhists, Brahmins, and Belief*, 63–65; Śaśipridā Kumāra, *Categories, Creation and Cognition in Vaisesika Philosophy* (New York: Springer Berlin Heidelberg, 2018), 3–4.
27. Arnold, *Buddhists, Brahmins, and Belief*, 61–63.
28. Audi, *The Place of Testimony*, 227.
29. Again, this is endemic to the Mīmāṃsā theory of "intrinsic" (*svatas*) authenticity. Arnold, *Buddhists, Brahmins, and Belief*, 59–114.
30. Praśastapāda and Śrīdhara, *The Praśastapāda Bhāshya, With the Commentary Nyāyakandali of Sridhara*, ed. Vindhyeśvarīprasāda Dvivedī. 2nd ed. (Delhi: Sri Satguru Publications, 1984), 98.4.
31. Praśastapāda and Śrīdhara, *The Praśastapāda Bhāshya*, 258.21–29.2; Praśastapāda and Śrīdhara, *Nyāyakandalī: Being a Commentary on Prasastapadabhasya*, 602.2–5.
32. Praśastapāda's position also resembles Vātsyāyana's position (explored in chapter 1) that the soul can be both perceived in yogic perception and inferred. Praśastapāda likewise argues that dharma can be both inferred and perceived.
33. Candrakīrti, whom I explore shortly, cribs his own definition of testimony from this *Nyāyasūtra*. He writes "Testimony (*āgama*) is the speech of those people who are authoritative, having direct knowledge of things beyond the senses

(*atīndriya*)." Candrakīrti, *In Clear Words: The Prasannapadā, Chapter One 1: Introduction, Manuscript Description, Sanskrit Text*, ed. Anne MacDonald, vol. 1 (Vienna: Verlag der Österreichischen Akademie der Wissenschaften, 2015), 275, §121. It would seem that Candrakīrti agrees with Uddyotakara that sound testimony is grounded in direct perceptions of realized yogis. But also see Sonam Thakchoe, "Candrakīrti's Theory of Perception: A Case for Non-Foundationalist Epistemology in Madhyamaka," *Acta Orientalia Vilnensia* 11, no. 1 (2010): 93–98. There is debate about how much Candrakīrti aligns himself with Nyāya here. Indeed, I will argue that, on Candrakīrti's view, yogic testimony is always epistemically incomplete.

34. Akṣapāda Gautama and Vātsyāyana, *Savātsyāyanabhāṣyaṃ Gautamīyaṃ Nyāyadarśanam with Bhāṣya of Vātsyāyana*, 14.3–5.
35. It should be noted, however, that (at least concerning the Euro-American epistemological distinction between justified and true belief) "reliability" is ambiguous. It can mean both trustworthy and true. If Naiyāyikas mean the latter, then their position is close to Audi's. But if they mean the former, then they give little account of justified belief in false claims. In that case, we are back to the problem of how one could trust a testifier without already being privy to the knowledge they are testifying.
36. Akṣapāda Gautama and Uddyotakara, *Nyāyabhāṣyavārttikam of Bhāradvāja Uddyotakara*, ed. Anantalāla Ṭhakkura (New Delhi: Bhāratīyadārśanikānusandhānap ariṣatprakaśitam, 1997), 54.20–55.2, 55.3–4, and 55.5.
37. This is also confirmed by Vācaspatimiśra's (ca. 900–980) commentary. Akṣapāda Gautama and Vācaspatimiśra, *Nyāyavārttikatātparyaṭīkā*, ed. Anantalāla Ṭhakkura (New Delhi: Bhāratīyadārśnikanusandhāna Pariṣatprakāśitā, 1996), 167.21–168.6.
38. As Rosanna Picascia notes, there is no clear equivalent to the notion of justified belief in a Nyāya context (personal communication, December 11, 2023).
39. Arnold, *Buddhists, Brahmins, and Belief*, 63–65.
40. Harold G. Coward and K. Kunjunni Raja, *The Philosophy of the Grammarians* (Princeton, NJ: Princeton University Press, 1990), 27–28, https://doi.org/10.1515/9781400872701.
41. Bhartṛhari specifically mentions "seers" (*ṛṣi*). As I mentioned in chapter 1, there is considerable overlap between yogic and *ṛṣic* perception, to the point that any distinction between the two is fuzzy.
42. Bhartṛhari, *Versuch Einer Vollständigen Deutschen Erstübersetzung Nach Der Kritischen Edition Der Mūla-Kārikās*, ed. and trans. Wilhelm Rau (Mainz: Steiner, 2000), 12 v. 1.38–39; Marco Ferrante, "On Ṛṣis and Yogins: Immediate and Mediate Extraordinary Cognitions in Early Brahmanical Thought," *Proceedings of the Meeting of the Italian Association of Sanskrit Studies* 89 (2016): 51.
43. Bhartṛhari, *Versuch Einer Vollständigen Deutschen*, 12 v. 1.37c; Ferrante, "On Ṛṣis and Yogins," 51.
44. Bhartṛhari, *Versuch Einer Vollständigen Deutschen*, 13 v. 1.41ab; Ferrante, "On Ṛṣis and Yogins," 51.
45. Audi, *The Place of Testimony*, 225.
46. Bhartṛhari, *Versuch Einer Vollständigen Deutschen*, 12 v. 1.40; Ferrante, "On Ṛṣis and Yogins," 51.

47. Bhartṛhari, *Versuch Einer Vollständigen Deutschen*, 12 v. 1.41cd; Ferrante, "On Ṛṣis and Yogins," 51.
48. Audi, *The Place of Testimony*, 218–19.
49. Audi, *The Place of Testimony*, 227–30.
50. But see Paul Dundas "Haribhadra," *Brill's Encyclopedia of Jainism Online*, February 14, 2020, https://referenceworks.brillonline.com/entries/brill-s-encyclopedia-of-jainism-online/haribhadra-COM_034908. This includes a summary of what his known of him and his works.
51. Frank Van Den Bossche, "God, the Soul and the Creatrix: Haribhadra Sūri on Nyāya and Sāṃkhya," *International Journal of Jaina Studies* 6, no. 6 (2010): 1.
52. Haribhadrasūri, *The Śāstravārtāsamuccaya: With Hindi Translation, Notes and Introduction*, ed. Jitendra B. Shah, trans. Krsna Kumara Diksita. Lalbhai Dalpatbhai Series 22 (Ahmedabad: Lalbhai Dalpatbhai Bharatiya Sanskriti Vidyamandira, 1969), 171–72 vv. 538–39. The meaning is opaque from the Sanskrit alone, but Diksita's Hindi commentary is helpful. "There is no epistemic warrant for the position that the yogi sees worldly objects as distinct from each other and not as undifferentiated from each other. And as for the teachings—that is, that in the teachings of some actual yogis it is said that they see worldly objects as distinct from each other—these may be given with particular disciples who have particular aptitudes in mind" (172.6–11). See a similar verse from Haribhadra in Haribhadrasūri and Municandrasūri, *Anekāntajayapatākā by Haribhadra Sūri with his own Commentary and Municandra Sūri's Supercommentary*, ed. H. R. Kapadia, vol. I (Baroda: Oriental Institute, 1947), 118.7–8.
53. Haribhadrasūri's target here is likely the Buddhist, who argues that yogis see things as momentary and thus distinct. Again, with the help of Diksita's Hindi commentary, "Haribhadra's intention is that if yogic experience tells us that each worldly object is momentary, then every instance of spiritual recognition will be erroneous. But determining what conclusion yogic experience gives on this question is no simple matter." Haribhadrasūri, *The Śāstravārtāsamuccaya*, 170.27–171.3. Haribhadrasūri's noncommittal stance here is indicative of his larger theory of Jain "non-onesidedness" (*anekāntavāda*). On this view, contradictory predicates can be true of a single object. More generally, it accepts that all religious views are tenable within certain contexts. At the conclusion of his *Victory Banner of Non-Onesidedness (Anekāntajayapatākā),* he confesses a strikingly nondogmatic pragmatism: "Having completed this analysis, I now accept whatever is beneficial. Thereby, through uprooting dissatisfaction and suffering, may the world adhere to good qualities!" Haribhadrasūri and Municandrasūri, *Anekāntajayapatākā*, vol. II, 239 v. 6.10. I am indebted to Anil Mundra for this reference. Anil Mundra, "Engaging Religious Difference: The Case of Haribhadrasūri" (Santa Barbara: University of California, Santa Barbara, 2023).
54. Haribhadrasūri, *The Śāstravārtāsamuccaya*, 190 v. 593.
55. Haribhadrasūri, *The Śāstravārtāsamuccaya*, 191 v. 596. On these verses, also see Piotr Balcerowicz, "Extrasensory Perception (Yogi-Pratyakṣa) in Jainism, Proofs of Its Existence and Its Soteriological Implications," in *Yoga in Jainism*, ed. Christopher Key Chapple (London: Routledge, 2016), 357–58.

56. "Mīmāṃsā" here has nothing to do with the eponymous tradition. Rather, it just means "analysis" or "investigation." The title is thus "Investigation of Epistemology."
57. I am tempted here to translate this term as something like "luminous cognition," since it fits nicely with salient themes in chapter 1. Hemacandra is clearly drawing on *Yogasūtra* 3.25 here with his reference to "subtle" objects, etc., and Vyāsa's commentary on *Yogasūtra* 3.25, we will recall, glosses this "higher sense ability" (*pravṛtti*) as "luminous" (*jyotiṣmatī*). Pantañjali, *Pantañjali's Yoga-Sūtras with the Yoga-Bhāṣya Attributed to Veda-Vyāsa and the Explanation Entitled Tattva-Vāiçāradī of Vacaspati-Miçra and the Brief Explanation of Bālarāma*, ed. Svāmi Bālarāma of Saṁvat (Varanasi: Svāmi Bālarāma of Saṁvat, 1908), 235.6–8. It is unclear, however, if this is what Hemacandra means. It is more likely he means *jyotis* as "the heavens," since the verses discuss knowledge of transmigration, and the Vedic opponent argues that yogic perception cannot perceive distant objects, else one could perceive how beings are born in the heavens.
58. Hemacandra, *Pramāṇamīmāṃsā: With the Commentary Pramāṇamīmāṃsāvṛtti*, ed. Sukhlalji Saṅghavi (Ahmedabad: The Sañcālaka-Siṅghī Jaina Granthamālā, 2016), 13, §55. Akalaṅka's verse comes from Akalaṅka and Anantavīrya, *Siddhiviniścaya With the Commentaries Siddhiviniścayavṛtti, Siddhiviniścayaṭīkā*, ed. Liudmila Olalde, SARIT: Enriching Digital Text Collections in Indology (Baden-Württemberg, Germany: University of Heidelberg, 2018), 647 v. 8.2, https://sarit.indology.info/siddhiviniscayatika.
59. Hemacandra, *Pramāṇamīmāṃsā*, 14, §56.
60. Śākyabuddhi (ca. 700 CE) identifies Dharmakīrti's allusion to "one person who knows" as Jaimini, the author of the *Mīmāṃsāsūtras*, and these "others"—who are denied such authority by the interlocutor—as Buddhists. Vincent Eltschinger, *Can the Veda Speak? Dharmakīrti Against Mīmāṃsā Exegetics and Vedic Authority: An Annotated Translation of PVSV 164,24–176,16*, ed. Helmut Krasser and John Taber (Vienna: Verlag der Österreichischen Akademie der Wissenschaften, 2012), 34n11.
61. Dharmakīrti, *The Pramanavarttikam of Dharmakīrti: The First Chapter with the Autocommentary*, ed. Raniero Gnoli (Roma: Instituto italiano per il medio ed estremo oriente, 1960), 165.13–19. Śubhagupta (eighth century CE), likely inspired by Dharmakīrti, makes a similar argument. Margherita Serena Saccone, "Of Authoritativeness and Perception: The Establishment of an Omniscient Person (Against the Mīmāṃsakas)," in *Wind Horses: Tibetan, Himalayan and Mongolian Studies*, ed. Giacomella Orofino (Napoli: Università degli studi di Napoli "L'Orientale," 2019), 455–83, esp. 462.
62. Dharmakīrti, *The Pramanavarttikam of Dharmakīrti*, 165 v. 1.312.
63. Dharmakīrti, *Pramāṇavarttika-kārikā: (Sanskrit and Tibetan)*, vol. 2, v. 2.33; Dharmakīrti, "*Pramāṇavārttikakārikā, Tshad ma rnam 'grel gyi tshig le'ur byas pa," in *Sde dge bstan 'gyur*, ed. Tshul khrims rin chen, Toh. no. 4210, vol. Tshad ma, ce (Delhi: Delhi Karmapae Choedhey, Gyalwae Sungrab Partun Khang, 1744), fol. 108b6–7.
64. Śāntarakṣita and Kamalaśīla, *Tattvasaṅgraha of Ācārya Śāntarakṣita with the "Pañjika" Commentary of Ācārya Śrī Kamalaśīla*, ed. Dvārikādāsa Śāstrī, vol. 2

(Varanasi: Bauddha, 1981), 498.10–11. The quote from Śabara is found in Jaimini and Śabarasvāmī, *The Aphorisms of the Mīmāmsa*, 5.13.

65. Śāntarakṣita and Kamalaśīla, *Tattvasaṅgraha of Ācārya Śāntarakṣita*, 2:498.31.
66. Śāntarakṣita and Kamalaśīla, *Tattvasaṅgraha of Ācārya Śāntarakṣita*, 2:631 vv. 2808–9.
67. Śāntarakṣita and Kamalaśīla, *Tattvasaṅgraha of Ācārya Śāntarakṣita*, 2:631.30–31.
68. Śāntarakṣita and Kamalaśīla, *Tattvasaṅgraha of Ācārya Śāntarakṣita*, 2:692 ff. For those who are interested in the details of his arguments, see their careful analysis in Jeson Woo, "Kamalaśīla on 'Yogipratyakṣa,'" *Indo-Iranian Journal* 48, no. 1–2 (2005): 116.
69. Śāntarakṣita and Kamalaśīla, *Tattvasaṅgraha of Ācārya Śāntarakṣita*, 2:760 vv. 3451–52.
70. Jñānaśrīmitra, "Yoginirṇayaprakaraṇa," 329.22–24.
71. Though I have yet to sufficiently explore the possibility, I suspect my coherentist picture may be closer to Susan Haack's foundherentism. Haack uses the analogy of a crossword puzzle. While the clues are like experiential evidence, already-filled-in entries are like reasons. Because the clues are independent of other entries, they serve as an asymmetrical warrant. But because the entries themselves must cohere, no "knowledge" of any one entry is noninferential or foundational. Susan Haack, *Evidence and Inquiry: Towards Reconstruction in Epistemology* (Cambridge, MA: Blackwell, 1993), 81–93. In the case of yogic perception, we might think of testimony as the already filled-in entries and one's own reproduction of the experience as the clue. While that yogic experience serves as an asymmetrical warrant, it still must cohere with previous testimony.
72. Yāmuna's *Proof of God* (*Īśvarasiddhi*) also discusses the Mīmāṃsā criticism of yogic perception. Yāmunācārya and Dāmodara Prapanācārya, "Īśvarasiddhiḥ," in *Siddhitrayam: Ātma-Īśvara-Saṃvitsiddhayaḥ*, Prathama saṃskaraṇa, Caukhambā surabhāratī granthamālā 587 (Vārāṇasī: Caukhambā Surabhāratī Prakāśana, 2015), 248.9–23.
73. It is worth noting that Veṅkaṭanātha's description of yogic perception is likely indebted to Dharmakīrti: both specifically cite meditation as instrumental in its cultivation (*bhāvanā-[bala]-ja*). Dharmakīrti, *Pramāṇavarttika-kārikā: (Sanskrit and Tibetan)*, vol. 2, v. 3.286c; Veṅkaṭanātha and Nivāsa, *Nayâyaparishuddhi by Venkatnath Vedântâchârya: Nyāyapariśuddhiḥ. With a Commentary Called Nyayasar(a) by Niwâsachârya [Nivāsa Ācārya]. Edited with Notes by Vidyabhushan Laksńmanàchàrya*, ed. Vidyabhuṣana Lakṣmanācārya (Varanasi: Chowkhambâ Sanskrit Series Office, 1918), 73.1. The importance of meditation will be made clear in the next chapter and seems to be Dharmakīrti's advent.
74. Veṅkaṭanātha and Nivāsa, *Nayâyaparishuddhi by Venkatnath Vedântâchârya: Nyāyapariśuddhiḥ*, 72.6-9.
75. Veṅkaṭanātha and Nivāsa, *Nayâyaparishuddhi by Venkatnath Vedântâchârya: Nyāyapariśuddhiḥ*, 72.9–73.4.
76. In the Catholic catechisms, for example, visionary experiences of the Virgin Mary or other saints are deemed authentic to the degree they adhere with accepted doctrine. Veronika Nela Gašpar, "Le apparizioni mariane nel nostro tempo. Il significato e i criteri del discernimento nella teologia," *IKON* 6 (2013):

17–26. This is epistemically conservative, since no one can have an authentic perceptual experience that does not already agree with scripture.

77. For a thorough analysis of the shortcomings of this analogy, see Chad A. Middleton and Michael Langston, "Circular Orbits on a Warped Spandex Fabric," *American Journal of Physics* 82, no. 4 (April 2014): 287–94, https://doi.org/10.1119/1.4848635.

78. Majjhima Nikāya MN 10, *Mahāsatipaṭṭhānasuttaṃ*, 58.9–59.10. V. Trenckner, Robert Chalmers, and T. W. Rhys Davids, eds, *The Majjhima Nikaya*, vol. 1 (Oxford: Pali Text Society, 1991).

79. Vasubandhu, *Abhidharmakośabhāṣyam*, ed. Prahlad Pradhan (Patna: K. P. Jayaswal Research Institute, 1975), 337.7–338.15; Vasubandhu, "*Abhidharmakośabhāṣya, Chos mngon pa'i mdzod kyi bshad pa," in *Sde dge bstan 'gyur*, ed. Tshul khrims rin chen, Toh. no. 4090, vol. Mngon pa, khu (Delhi: Delhi Karmapae Choedhey, Gyalwae Sungrab Partun Khang, 1744), 19a2.

80. Buddhaghoṣa, *Visuddhimagga* 1.6, "Asubhakammaṭṭhānaniddeso," 178–196. Buddhaghoṣa, *The Visuddhi-magga of Buddhaghosa*, ed. Caroline A. F. Rhys Davids (London: Pali Text Society, 1920), vol. 1.

81. Dharmakīrti, *Pramāṇavarttika-kārikā: (Sanskrit and Tibetan)*, 2:v. 3.284.

82. Candrakīrti, "*Madhyamakāvatārabhāṣya, Dbu ma la 'jug pa'i bshad pa," in *Sde dge bstan 'gyur*, ed. Tshul khrims rin chen, Toh. no. 3862, vol. Dbu ma, 'a (Delhi: Delhi Karmapae Choedhey, Gyalwae Sungrab Partun Khang, 1744), fol. 271a7.

83. Candrakīrti, " 'Madhyamakāvatāra-Kārikā' Chapter 6," ed. Li Xuezhu, *Journal of Indian Philosophy* 43, no. 1 (2015): 13 vv. 6.70cd–71ab; Candrakīrti, "*Madhyamakāvatārabhāṣya, Dbu ma la 'jug pa'i bshad pa," fol. 271a6–271b2; also see Jed Forman, "What Is the World? Neckties, Ghosts, Falling Hairs, and Celestial Cities in a Coherentist Epistemology," *Philosophy East and West* 70, no. 4 (2020): 909, https://doi.org/10.1353/pew.2020.0066. Jayānanda (ca. eleventh century)—Candrakīrti's sole Indian commentator on this text—corroborates this reading. Candrakīrti and Jayānanda, "*Madhyamakāvatāraṭīkā, Dbu ma la 'jug pa'i 'grel pa," in *Sde dge bstan 'gyur*, ed. Tshul khrims rin chen, Toh. no. 3870, vol. Dbu ma, ra (Delhi: Delhi Karmapae Choedhey, Gyalwae Sungrab Partun Khang, 1744), fols. 189b4-190b4.

84. Candrakīrti, "'Madhyamakāvatāra-Kārikā' Chapter 6," v. 6.54; Candrakīrti, "*Madhyamakāvatārabhāṣya, Dbu ma la 'jug pa'i bshad pa," fol. 265b6.

85. Candrakīrti, "'Madhyamakāvatāra-Kārikā' Chapter 6," v. 6.71ab; Candrakīrti, "*Madhyamakāvatārabhāṣya, Dbu ma la 'jug pa'i bshad pa," fol. 271b1.

86. There are some obvious parallels here with the debate on qualia. Daniel C. Dennett, "Quining Qualia," in *Consciousness in Contemporary Science*, ed. A. J. Marcel and E. Bisiach (New York: Oxford University Press, 1992), 42–77, https://doi.org/10.1093/acprof:oso/9780198522379.003.0003. Candrakīrti, I argue, would agree that yogic perception involves a type of incommunicable qualia.

87. Nāgārjuna and Candrakīrti, *Madhyamakasāstra of Nāgārjuna with the Commentary: Prasannapadā by Candrakīrti*, ed. Paraśurāma Lakshmaṇa Vaidya, Buddhist Sanskrit Texts 10 (Darbhanga: Mithila Institute, 1960), 49.8–11.

88. Candrakīrti, "*Mūlamadhyamakavṛttiprasannapadā, Dbu ma rtsa ba'i 'grel pa tshig gsal ba," in *Sde dge bstan 'gyur*, ed. Kanakavarman and Pa tshab lo tsā ba nyi

ma grags, trans. Mahāsumati and Pa tshab lo tsā ba nyi ma grags, Toh. no. 3860, vol. Dbu ma, 'a (Delhi: Delhi Karmapae Choedhey, Gyalwae Sungrab Partun Khang, 1744), fol. 119b6-7. This phrase is not found in P. L. Vaidya's Sanskrit edition. Nāgārjuna and Candrakīrti, *Madhyamakasāstra of Nāgārjuna with the Commentary: Prasannapadā by Candrakīrti*, 159.4–7. Nevertheless, find the Sanskrit reconstructed in Louis de la Vallé Poussin's edition. Nāgārjuna and Candrakīrti, *Mūlamadhyamakakārikās (Mādhyamikasūtras) de Nāgārjuna Avec Le Prasannapadā Commentaire de Candrakīrti*, ed. Louis de la Valle Poussin, Bibliotheca Buddhica IV (Saint Petersburg: l'Académie Imperiale des sciences, 1903), 373n1. Also see Mattia Salvini's analysis and translation of this section. Mattia Salvini, "Etymologies of What Can(Not) Be Said: Candrakīrti on Conventions and Elaborations," *Journal of Indian Philosophy* 47, no. 4 (September 2019): 681–82, https://doi.org/10.1007/s10781-019-09402-4.

89. For a detailed analysis of this, see Salvini, "Etymologies of What Can(Not) Be Said."
90. I should offer some nuance here. My position is that Candrakīrti argues that bones, hairs, and yogic insight are all *ontologically* individual. That is, they obtain independently of conventional strictures. Nevertheless, they are not all *epistemically* individual. The metaphysical truths that yogis perceive obtain *for everyone* even if only they realize it. Bones and hairs, on the other hand, are also real, but only *for* their perceivers.
91. My view here largely accords with Anne MacDonald's analysis of Candrakīrti's view of yogic perception. Anne MacDonald, "Knowing Nothing: Candrakīrti and Yogic Perception," in *Yogic Perception, Meditation and Altered States of Consciousness*, ed. Eli Franco and Dagmar Eigner (Vienna: Verlag der Österreichischen Akademie der Wissenschaften, 2009), 133–68.
92. Abhinavagupta and Utpaladeva, *Īśvara-Pratyabhijñā-Vimarśinī of Abhinavagupta: Doctrine of Divine Recognition*, ed. K.A. Subramania Iyer, K. C. Pandey, and Rāma Candra Dvivedī, vol. 2 (Delhi: Motilal Banarsidass, 1986), 175.9–76.5. Also see Isabelle Ratié, *Le soi et l'autre: identité, différence et altérité dans la philosophie de la Pratyabhijñā*, Jerusalem studies in religion and culture, vol. 13 (Leiden: Brill, 2011), 416n117.
93. For a discussion, see James B. Hartle, *Gravity: An Introduction to Einstein's General Relativity*, 1st ed. (Harlow, UK: Pearson, 2014), chap. 6.
94. Abhinavagupta and Utpaladeva, *Īśvara-Pratyabhijñā-Vimarśinī of Abhinavagupta*, 2:177.1–4.
95. Audi, *The Place of Testimony*, 227.

3. Pragmatism and Coherentism

1. I should make clear, however, that Candrakīrti's account of perception differs from Dignāga's and Dharmakīrti's in one key respect. All agree that special perceptual feats, like those of yogis, transcend what can be conceptualized. But while Dignāga and Dharmakīrti say this is true of *all* perception, Candrakīrti

argues that normal, sensory perception is conceptual through and through. I will discuss this more in chapter 6, but see Sonam Thakchoe, "Candrakīrti's Theory of Perception: A Case for Non-Foundationalist Epistemology in Madhyamaka," *Acta Orientalia Vilnensia* 11, no. 1 (2010): 107.

2. There are compelling arguments, however, as to why they may be unbridgeable. Ethan Mills, "On the Coherence of Dignāga's Epistemology: Evaluating the Critiques of Candrakīrti and Jayarāśi," *Asian Philosophy* 25, no. 4 (October 2, 2015): 339–57, https://doi.org/10.1080/09552367.2015.1102694.
3. For example, there is growing evidence that the brain uses predictive coding to fill in the perceptual gestalt from minimal information. Kevin S. Walsh et al., "Evaluating the Neurophysiological Evidence for Predictive Processing as a Model of Perception," *Annals of the New York Academy of Sciences* 1464, no. 1 (March 2020): 242–68, https://doi.org/10.1111/nyas.14321; Amirali Shirazibeheshti et al., "Placing Meta-Stable States of Consciousness within the Predictive Coding Hierarchy: The Deceleration of the Accelerated Prediction Error," *Consciousness and Cognition* 63 (2018): 123–42, https://doi.org/10.1016/j.concog.2018.06.010; Ryota Kanai et al., "Cerebral Hierarchies: Predictive Processing, Precision and the Pulvinar," *Philosophical Transactions of the Royal Society B: Biological Sciences* 370, no. 1668 (May 19, 2015): 20140169, https://doi.org/10.1098/rstb.2014.0169. Also see Jed Forman, "Believing Is Seeing: A Buddhist Theory of Creditions," *Frontiers in Psychology* 13 (August 3, 2022): 938731, https://doi.org/10.3389/fpsyg.2022.938731.
4. For a summary, see Lawrence J. McCrea and Parimal G. Patil, *Buddhist Philosophy of Language in India: Jñānaśrīmitra on Exclusion* (New York: Columbia University Press, 2010), 144n77.
5. Bertrand Russell, *The Problems of Philosophy* (London: Oxford University Press, 2001), 75.
6. Bertrand Russell, *Human Knowledge: Its Scope and Limits* (Routledge, 2009), 140, https://doi.org/10.4324/9780203875353.
7. A. J. Ayer, "Has Austin Refuted the Sense-Datum Theory?," *Synthese* 17, no. 2 (1967): 129.
8. Charles Sanders Peirce, *Philosophical Writings of Peirce*, ed. Justus Buchler (New York: Dover Publications, 1955), 304.
9. Peirce, *Philosophical Writings of Peirce*, 302.
10. For a discussion of this debate in Buddhist sources, see Robert H. Sharf, "Knowing Blue: Early Buddhist Accounts of Non-Conceptual Sense," *Philosophy East & West* 68, no. 3 (2018): 826–70, https://doi.org/10.1353/pew.2018.0075.
11. Dan Arnold, "The Philosophical Works and Influence of Dignāga and Dharmakīrti," *Oxford Research Encyclopedia of Religion*, July 27, 2017, para. 24, https://doi.org/10.1093/acrefore/9780199340378.013.198; also see Dan Arnold, "Givenness as a Corollary to Non-Conceptual Awareness: Thinking About Thought in Buddhist Philosophy," in *Wilfrid Sellars and Buddhist Philosophy: Freedom from Foundations*, Google Play Edition (New York: Routledge, 2019), 227–28.
12. Dignāga, *Dignaga: On Perception, Being the Pratyakṣapariccheda of Dignaga's Pramāṇasamuccaya from the Sanskrit Fragments and the Tibetan Versions*, ed. and trans. Masaaki Hattori. Harvard Oriental Series 47 (Cambridge, MA: Harvard University Press, 1968) 24 and 81n1.19.

13. Peirce, *Philosophical Writings of Peirce*, 304.
14. Dignāga, *Dignaga: On Perception*, 82–83n1.25.
15. Chien-Hsing Ho, "Saying the Unsayable," *Philosophy East and West* 56, no. 3 (2006): 410.
16. Dharmakīrti, *The Pramanavarttikam of Dharmakīrti: The First Chapter with the Autocommentary*, ed. Raniero Gnoli. Roma: Instituto Italiano per il Medio ed Estremo Oriente, 1960), 42.13–14.
17. Dharmakīrti, *Pramāṇavarttika-kārikā: (Sanskrit and Tibetan)*, ed. Yūshō Miyasaka. Acta Indologica. (Narita: Naritasan Shinshōji, 1972), vol. 2, vv. 3.54–58.
18. Dharmakīrti, *Pramāṇavarttika-kārikā*, vol. 2, v. 2.1; also see Esho Mikogami, "Some Remarks on the Concept of Arthakriyā," *Journal of Indian Philosophy* 7, no. 1 (1979): 79–94.
19. Indeed, I think that Dignāga and Dharmakīrti are more consistent than Kant on this point. In the same breath that Kant concedes that without conceptual unity there would be "no experience," he contends that that unity "subjects appearances to itself" to create that experience. Immanuel Kant, *Critique of Pure Reason*, trans. Paul Guyer and Allen W Wood (Cambridge: Cambridge University Press, 1998), A112. But if there is no experience of appearances before their being subjected to concepts, how could we ever be aware of them to deem them so subjected? Kant may have some recourse to a transcendental argument on this point, but it seems to me that his account of intuitions and appearances is too theoretically detailed for them to constitute unsayable noumena. Jed Forman, "Timeless Visions: Prajñākaragupta on Futureless Precognition and Temporal Intuitions," in *The Handbook of Intuitions*, Logic, Epistemology, and the Unity of Sciences (New York: Springer, forthcoming). Dignāga and Dharmakīrti, on the other hand, contend that because perception is a transcendental precursor, we cannot theorize its constituents, try as Kant might.
20. Those Buddhist practitioners who have achieved nirvana, or liberation from samsara, the cycle of birth and death across reincarnations.
21. See, for example, Dīgha Nikāya (DN) 12, *Lohiccasuttaṃ*, 224.24–25.3. Caroline A. F. Rhys Davids and Estlin Carpenter, eds, *The Dīgha Nikāya*, vol. 1 (London: Pali Text Society, 1890). Also see Majjhima Nikāya (MN) 27, *Cūḷahatthipadopamasuttaṃ*, 179.4–8. V. Trenckner et al., eds. *The Majjhima Nikaya*, vol. 1 (Oxford: Pali Text Society, 1991).
22. These are: (1) life is suffering, (2) it has a cause, (3) that stopping suffering is possible, and (4) there is a cause that puts an end to suffering—namely, following the Buddhist path. By actualizing each of these truths, one is liberated. SN 4, *Dha mmacakkappavattanasuttaṃ*, 420–24. Léon Feer et al., eds. *Saṃyutta-nikāya*, vol. 5 (London: Pali Text Society, 1960).
23. DN 5, *Kūṭadantasuttaṃ*, 148.13–24. Davids and Carpenter, *The Dīgha Nikāya*, vol. 1 (London: Pali Text Society, 1890).
24. See an explanation in Ñāṇamoli Thera and Bodhi Bhikkhu, eds., *The Middle Length Discourses of the Buddha: A [New] Translation of the Majjhima Nikāya*, 4th ed. (Boston: Wisdom, 2009), 91 and 1169n35.
25. See an explanation in Ñāṇamoli Thera and Bodhi Bhikkhu, *The Middle Length Discourses of the Buddha*, 485 and 1259n588.

26. See an explanation of each of these respectively in Ñāṇamoli Thera and Bodhi Bhikkhu, *The Middle Length Discourses of the Buddha*, 118–19 and 1180n89; 418 and 1245n490; 929 and 1326n1088.
27. Other Hindu traditions, as we also saw in chapter 1, adopted a similar accommodation strategy by subsuming these abilities under unabsorbed and absorbed yogic perception respectively.
28. It is unclear whether Vasubandhu's *Abhidharmakośa* or Buddhaghoṣa's (ca. fifth century CE) *Visuddhimagga* was the first to formalize the notion of paths (Skt. *mārga*, Pāli *magga*). Nevertheless, Vasubandhu's text is undoubtedly the source text for the traditions I explore. Rupert Gethin, *The Foundations of Buddhism* (Oxford: Oxford University Press, 1998), 55–56.
29. Vincent Eltschinger, "On the Career and the Cognition of Yogins," in *Yogic Perception, Meditation and Altered States of Consciousness*, ed. Eli Franco and Dagmar Eigner (Vienna: Verlag der Österreichischen Akademie der Wissenschaften, 2009), sec. 3.2.
30. This three-tiered model (with some variation) has been identified by Christian Lindtner as a general feature of Mahāyāna mediation theory. Kambala, *A Garland of Light: Kambala's Ālokamālā*, trans. Christian Lindtner (Fremont, CA: Asian Humanities Press, 2003), 115 ff. Alan Sponberg also identifies it as the "progressive model" in Yogācāra specifically. Sponberg contrasts this three-tiered model with the "pivot model," which carries the idealist features that Candrakīrti criticizes. Alan Sponberg, "The Trisvabhāva Doctrine in India & China: A Study of Three Exegetical Models," *Bulletin of Buddhist Cultural Institute, Ryukoku University* 21 (November 30, 1982): 97–119. But Joy Brennan reveals that the pivot model is actually far less prevalent among Yogācārin exegetes. Joy Cecile Brennan, "The Three Natures and the Path to Liberation in Yogācāra-Vijñānavāda Thought," *Journal of Indian Philosophy* 46, no. 4 (September 2018): 621–48, https://doi.org/10.1007/s10781-018-9356-4. Interestingly, then, Asaṅga is closer to Candrakīrti than the latter gives credit, both seeking to deconstruct any claim about ultimate reality, idealist or otherwise.
31. Oddly, however, he does not describe them in order, addressing steps (2) and (3) before returning to (1).
32. Unlike arhats, who only aspire toward nirvana, bodhisattvas practice to gain full enlightenment (*samyakṣaṃbodhi*), which includes omniscience, so that they can benefit all beings. Bodhisattvas practice the Mahāyāna path, which leads to full enlightenment.
33. Asaṅga, "*Mahāyānasaṃgraha, Theg pa chen po bsdus pa," in *Sde dge bstan 'gyur*, ed. Tshul khrims rin chen, Toh. no. 4048, vol. Sems tsam, ri (Delhi: Delhi Karmapae Choedhey, Gyalwae Sungrab Partun Khang, 1744), fol. 25a3–6. I take "*'dres pa'i chos*" as likely "**miśradharma*," and thus "various teachings." See John Powers, trans., *Wisdom of Buddha: The Saṁdhinirmocana Sūtra*. Tibetan Translation Series 16 (Berkeley: Dharma Publications, 1995), 343n17.
34. Asaṅga, "*Mahāyānasaṃgraha, Theg pa chen po bsdus pa," fol. 24b7–25a2.
35. Asaṅga, "*Mahāyānasaṃgraha, Theg pa chen po bsdus pa," fols. 15b6–16a4.
36. Yūichi Kajiyama, "Controversy between the Sākāra- and Nirākāra-Vādins of the Yogācāra School-Some Materials," *Journal of Indian and Buddhist Studies*

(Indogaku Bukkyogaku Kenkyu) 14, no. 1 (1965): 429–418, https://doi.org/10.4259/ibk.14.429.

37. There is some debate here, however. See Eli Franco, "Did Dignāga Accept Four Types of Perception?," *Journal of Indian Philosophy* 21, no. 3 (1993): 295–99.
38. Dignāga, *Dignāga's Pramāṇasamuccaya, Chapter 1: A Hypothetical Reconstruction of the Sanskrit Text with the Help of the Two Tibetan Translations on the Basis of the Hitherto Known Sanskrit Fragments and the Linguistic Materials Gained from Jinendrabuddhi's Ṭīkā*, ed. Ernst Steinkellner (Vienna: Österreichische Akademie der Wissenschaften, 2005), 3.10; Dignāga, "*Pramāṇasamuccaya, Tshad ma kun las btus pa zhes bya ba'i rab tu byed pa," in *Sde dge bstan 'gyur*, ed. Tshul khrims rin chen, Toh. no. 4203, vol. Tshad ma, ce (Delhi: Delhi Karmapae Choedhey, Gyalwae Sungrab Partun Khang, 1744), fol. 2a1.
39. Dignāga, *Dignāga's Pramāṇasamuccaya, Chapter 1*, 3.11; Dignāga, "*Pramāṇasamuccayavṛtti, Tshad ma kun las btus pa'i 'grel pa," in *Sde dge bstan 'gyur*, ed. Tshul khrims rin chen, trans. Vasudhararakṣita and Zha ma seng rgyal, Toh. no. 4204, vol. Tshad ma, ce (Delhi: Delhi Karmapae Choedhey, Gyalwae Sungrab Partun Khang, 1744), fol. 15b7.
40. Dharmakīrti, *Pramāṇavarttika-kārikā: (Sanskrit and Tibetan)*, vol. 2, vv. 3.281–82; Dharmakīrti, "*Pramāṇavārttikakārikā, Tshad ma rnam 'grel gyi tshig le'ur byas pa," fol. 129a4–5.
41. Dharmakīrti, *Pramāṇavarttika-kārikā: (Sanskrit and Tibetan)*, vol. 2, v. 3.282a; Dharmakīrti, "*Pramāṇavārttikakārikā, Tshad ma rnam 'grel gyi tshig le'ur byas pa," fol. 129a5.
42. Dharmakīrti, *Pramāṇavarttika-kārikā: (Sanskrit and Tibetan)*, vol. 2, vv. 3.284–85; Dharmakīrti, "*Pramāṇavārttikakārikā, Tshad ma rnam 'grel gyi tshig le'ur byas pa," 129a6–7. Also see these verses translated in John D. Dunne "Realizing the Unreal: Dharmakīrti's Theory of Yogic Perception," *Journal of Indian Philosophy* 34, no. 6 (2007): 516, https://doi.org/10.1007/s10781-006-9008-y.
43. Dharmakīrti, "*Pramāṇaviniścaya, Tshad ma rnam par nges pa," in *Sde dge bstan 'gyur*, ed. Tshul khrims rin chen, Toh. no. 4211, vol. Tshad ma, ce (Delhi: Delhi Karmapae Choedhey, Gyalwae Sungrab Partun Khang, 1744), fol. 161a5–161b1.
44. Dharmakīrti, *Pramāṇavarttika-kārikā: (Sanskrit and Tibetan)*, vol. 2, v. 3.286; Dharmakīrti, "*Pramāṇavārttikakārikā, Tshad ma rnam 'grel gyi tshig le'ur byas pa," fol. 129a7–129b1.
45. Namely, yogic perception is a perceptual warrant and all perceptual warrants are unmistaken. Dharmakīrti, "*Pramāṇaviniścaya, Tshad ma rnam par nges pa," fols. 161a7–161b1 and 154a7–154b1.
46. Dharmakīrti, *The Pramanavarttikam of Dharmakīrti*, 50.20.
47. Dharmakīrti, *Pramāṇavarttika-kārikā: (Sanskrit and Tibetan)*, vol. 2, v. 3.123a.
48. Dharmakīrti, vol. 2, v. 3.288cd; also see Catherine Prueitt, "Shifting Concepts: The Realignment of Dharmakīrti on Concepts and the Error of Subject/Object Duality in Pratyabhijñā Śaiva Thought," *Journal of Indian Philosophy* 45, no. 1 (2017): 31. This appears to be a departure from Dignāga, according to whom distortions are categorically conceptual. Eli Franco, "Once Again on Dharmakīrti's Deviation from Dignāga on 'Pratyakṣâbhāsa,'" *Journal of Indian Philosophy* 14, no. 1 (1986): 82–83.

49. Dharmakīrti, *Pramāṇavārttika of Acharya Dharmakirtti: With the Commentary "Vritti" of Acharya Manorathanandin*, ed. Dvārikādāsa Śāstrī, Bauddha Bharati Series 3 (Varanasi: Bauddha Bharati, 1968), 186.7–22.
50. Dharmakīrti, *Pramāṇavarttika-kārikā: (Sanskrit and Tibetan)*, vol. 2, v. 3.286.
51. See John Dunne, "Pac-Man to the Rescue? Conceptuality and Non-Conceptuality in the Dharmakīrtian Theory of Pseudo-Perception," *Philosophy East & West* 70, no. 3 (2020): 571–93, https://doi.org/10.1353/pew.2020.0045. For an excellent analysis of these issues, also see Prueitt, "Shifting Concepts," pt. I.
52. This tension is born out in the secondary sources as well, where there is debate about whether Dharmakīrti meant to construe yogic perception as epistemically warranted solely by its pragmatic efficacy, such that it still misrepresents reality, or by its accurate representation. While John Dunne argues the former, Vincent Eltschinger opts for the latter. Dunne, "Realizing the Unreal: Dharmakīrti's Theory of Yogic Perception," 515; Eltschinger, "On the Career and the Cognition of Yogins," 169n1.
53. This is correctly emended by Eli Franco, "Variant Readings from Tucci's Photographs of the Yoginirṇayaprakaraṇa Manuscript," in *Sanskrit Texts from Giuseppe Tucci's Collection* (Rome: Istituto italiano per l'Africa e l'Oriente, 2008), 332.11.
54. Jñānaśrīmitra, "Yoginirṇayaprakaraṇa," in *Jñānaśrīmitranibandhavāli: Buddhist Philosophical Works of Jñānaśrīmitra*, ed. Anantalāla Ṭhakkura, 2nd. ed. (Patna: Kashi Prasad Jayaswal Research Institute, 1987), 332.10–13.
55. Despite its title, this text is not a commentary on the Nyāya tradition.
56. Since at least Vasubandhu, Buddhists have argued that the realizations of impermanence and selflessness are included as two of four "moments" within that realization. This includes the understanding that all phenomena are in constant flux and, relatedly, because of that flux, it has no stable identity, or self. Our failure to recognize these facts and our false conviction in their opposites—that phenomena endure and have a self—are two of the primary causes of suffering. With four moments belonging to each truth, there are a total of sixteen moments. Eltschinger, "On the Career and the Cognition of Yogins," sec. 3.1 and 5.2. Asaṅga discusses these sixteen moments. Rāmaśaṅkara Tripāṭhī, ed., *Prajñāpāramitopadeśaśāstre Abhisamayālaṅkāravṛttiḥ Sphuṭārthā* (Varanasi: Central Institute of Higher Tibetan Studies, 1977), v. 4.23.
57. Maṇḍanamiśra and Vācaspatimiśra, *Vidhiviveka of Śrī Maṇḍana Miśra: With the Commentary Nyāyakaṇikā of Vāchaspati Miśra*, ed. Mahāprabhu Lāla Gosvāmī (Varanasi: Tara Publications, 1978), 105.24–28.
58. Admittedly, it is unclear why chanting "Om," an important syllable in Hindu ritual and practice, should produce a vivid cognition of fire.
59. Maṇḍanamiśra and Vācaspatimiśra, *Vidhiviveka of Śrī Maṇḍana Miśra*, 105.28–6.3.
60. Jñānaśrīmitra, "Yoginirṇayaprakaraṇa," 323.14-5.
61. Jñānaśrīmitra, "Yoginirṇayaprakaraṇa," 323.18–20.
62. Although the emphasis on pragmatics is not as explicit here, we also find it elsewhere in Jñānaśrīmitra's text. For example, he argues that cultivating the habit of seeing things as momentary is like developing a taste for neem fruit. Its pleasant taste is not a quality of the neem per se—indeed, neem juice is sour. But as one develops their taste, they begin to find it pleasant. So too is realizing

momentariness garnered by habit. And like the pleasant taste of the neem, the habit is salutary even if it is not representative strictly speaking. Jñānaśrīmitra, "Yoginirṇayaprakaraṇa," 324.25–326.20. Also see Davey Tomlinson's excellent essay on this section. His analysis also bespeaks a tension between pragmatist and representationalist accounts. Davey K. Tomlinson, "A Buddhist's Guide to Self-Destruction: Jñānaśrīmitra on the Structure of Yogic Perception," *Religious Studies* 60, no. 2 (2023): esp. 7-8. https://doi.org/10.1017/S003441252300032X. Further see my own forthcoming chapter on this. Jed Forman, "Developing Good Taste: Jñānaśrīmitra's Theory of Imagination and Aesthetic Epistemology," in *The Imagination and Imaginal Worlds in the Mirror of Buddhism*, Karin Meyers and Hugh Joswick, eds. (Berkeley: Mangalam Press, forthcoming).

63. Jñānaśrīmitra, "Yoginirṇayaprakaraṇa," 324.5-12.
64. Dharmakīrti, *Pramāṇavarttika-kārikā: (Sanskrit and Tibetan)*, vol. 2, v. 2.3.
65. Kumārila Bhaṭṭa and Sucaritamiśra, *The Mîmâmsāślokavârtika with the Commentary Kāśikā of Sucaritamiśra*, ed. K. Sambasiva Sastri, Trivandrum Sanskrit Series 99 (Trivandrum: Superintendent, Gov. Press, 1929), 217.19–28.
66. Ratnakīrti, "Sarvajñasiddhiḥ," in *Ratnakīrtinibandhavāli: Buddhist Philosophical Works of Ratnakīrti*, ed. Anantalāla Ṭhakkura, 2nd ed. (Patna: Kashi Prasad Jayaswal Research Institute, 1975), 18.18-22.
67. The reference to "exclusion" here invokes Dignāga's and Dharmakīrti's *apoha* theory. I will not burden reader with the details, but in short, *apoha* explains conceptual thinking as apprehending a double negation of the object. In this way, concepts capture the object while distorting it, since the mind in this case has the object of an exclusion rather than the positive particular from which that exclusion is constructed. John D. Dunne, "Key Features of Dharmakīrti's Apoha Theory," in *Apoha: Buddhist Nominalism and Human Cognition*, ed. Mark Siderits, Tom Tillemans, and Arindam Chakrabarti (Columbia University Press, 2011), 84–108.
68. Ratnakīrti, "Sarvajñasiddhiḥ," 18.32–19.3.
69. This is also suggested by the Sanskrit word *sparśana* used here, which can mean—in addition to "touch" or "contact"—"affecting." In the Sautrāntika framework within which Jñānaśrīmitra writes here, this contact also occurs even before sensory consciousness. Kuala Lumpur Dhammajoti, *Abhidharma Doctrines and Controversies on Perception*, 3rd ed. (Hong Kong: Centre of Buddhist Studies, University of Hong Kong, 2007), 160; Sharf, "Knowing Blue: Early Buddhist Accounts of Non-Conceptual Sense," 834. This further corroborates that Ratnakīrti does not define perception's distinct epistemic power in terms of the pragmatic knowledge it affords but through its having a special causal connection to its object, granting it superior representational capacity.
70. Wilfrid Sellars, "Empiricism and The Philosophy of Mind," in *Knowledge, Mind, and the Given: Reading Wilfrid Sellars's "Empiricism and the Philosophy of Mind," Including the Complete Text of Sellars's Essay*, ed. Willem A. DeVries and Timm Triplett (Indianapolis, IN: Hackett Pub, 2000), sec. 1.
71. Sellars, "Empiricism and The Philosophy of Mind," sec. 18.

72. Dan Arnold, "Candrakīrti on Dignāga on Svalakṣaṇas," *Journal of the International Association of Buddhist Studies* 26, no. 1 (2003): 155 and 171; Christian Coseru, "Buddhist 'Foundationalism' and the Phenomenology of Perception," *Philosophy East and West* 59, no. 4 (2009): 409–39; John D. Dunne, *Foundations of Dharmakīrti's Philosophy*, 1st ed. (Boston: Wisdom, 2004), 326–30; Āryadeva, Dharmapāla, and Candrakīrti, *Materials for the Study of Āryadeva, Dharmapāla, and Candrakīrti: The Catuḥśataka of Āryadeva, Chapters XII and XIII, With the Commentaries of Dharmapāla and Candrakīrti: Introduction, Translation, Sanskrit, Tibetan, and Chinese Texts, Notes*, trans. Tom J. F. Tillemans, Wiener Studien Zur Tibetologie Und Buddhismuskunde; Heft 24 (Wien: Arbeitskreis für Tibetische und Buddhistische Studien, Universität Wien, 1990), 41 ff.; Tom J. F. Tillemans, "Metaphysics for Madhyamikas," in *The Svātantrika-Prāsaṅgika Distinction: What Difference Does a Difference Make?*, ed. Georges B. J. Dreyfus and Sara L. McClintock, Studies in Indian and Tibetan Buddhism (Boston: Wisdom, 2002), 98.
73. Peirce, *Philosophical Writings of Peirce*, 378.
74. Dharmakīrti, *Pramāṇavarttika-kārikā: (Sanskrit and Tibetan)*, vol. 2, vv. 3.57–58; Devendrabuddhi, "*Pramāṇavārttikapañjikā, Tshad ma rnam 'grel kyi dka' 'grel," in *Sde dge bstan 'gyur*, ed. Tshul khrims rin chen, trans. Subhutiśrī and Dge ba'i blo gros, Toh. no. 4217, vol. Tshad ma, che (Delhi: Delhi Karmapae Choedhey, Gyalwae Sungrab Partun Khang, 1744), fols. 145b6–146a3.
75. Dharmakīrti, *The Pramanavarttikam of Dharmakīrti: The First Chapter with the Autocommentary*, 42.13–15.
76. Again, for a more in-depth discussion, see Forman, "Believing Is Seeing."
77. Dharmakīrti, *Pramāṇavarttika-kārikā: (Sanskrit and Tibetan)*, vol. 2, v. 3.282a; Dharmakīrti, "*Pramāṇavārttikakārikā, Tshad ma rnam 'grel gyi tshig le'ur byas pa," fol. 129a5.
78. A. Castelnovo et al., "Post-Bereavement Hallucinatory Experiences: A Critical Overview of Population and Clinical Studies," *Journal of Affective Disorders* 186 (2015): 266–74, https://doi.org/10.1016/j.jad.2015.07.032; Daniel Collerton, Elaine Perry, and Ian McKeith, "Why People See Things That Are Not There: A Novel Perception and Attention Deficit Model for Recurrent Complex Visual Hallucinations," *Behavioral and Brain Sciences* 28, no. 6 (December 2005): 737–57, https://doi.org/10.1017/S0140525X05000130.
79. Oliver W. Sacks, *Hallucinations* (New York: Vintage Books, 2013), chap. 13; A. Grimby, "Bereavement Among Elderly People: Grief Reactions, Post-Bereavement Hallucinations and Quality of Life," *Acta Psychiatrica Scandinavica* 87, no. 1 (1993): 72–80.
80. Rima Abou-Khalil and Lealani Mae Y Acosta, "A Case Report of Acquired Synesthesia and Heightened Creativity in a Musician after Traumatic Brain Injury.," *Neurocase*, 2023, 1–4, https://doi.org/10.1080/13554794.2023.2208271; Andy D Mealor, Julia Simner, and Jamie Ward, "Does Synaesthesia Protect against Age-Related Memory Loss?," *Journal of Neuropsychology* 14, no. 2 (2020): 197–212, https://doi.org/10.1111/jnp.12182; Jamie Ward, "Synaesthesia: A Distinct Entity That Is an Emergent Feature of Adaptive Neurocognitive Differences," *Philosophical Transactions of the Royal Society of London. Series B, Biological Sciences* 374, no. 1787 (2019): 20180351, https://doi.org/10.1098/rstb.2018.0351; Émilie A. Caspar and Régine

Kolinsky, "Review of an Unusual Phenomenon: Synesthesia," *L'Année psychologique* 113, no. 4 (2013): 629, https://doi.org/10.3917/anpsy.134.0629.

81. Peirce, *Philosophical Writings of Peirce*, 375–78. Peirce's more well-known pragmatist compatriot, Williams James (1842–1910), makes a similar argument. William James, "The Will to Believe," in *William James: Writings 1878–1899: Psychology: Briefer Course, The Will to Believe, Talks to Teachers and Students, and Essays* (New York: Library of America, 1992), 457–79. Interestingly, James dedicates the collection of essays of which this one is a part to none other than Charles Peirce (446).
82. Lorraine Code, *Epistemic Responsibility*, 2nd ed. (Albany: State University of New York Press, 2020), chap. 7.

4. Omniphenomenology

1. I should note that my use of "conceptual categories" differs from Kant's notion of "categories." Kant makes a clear demarcation between intuitions, as necessary for appearances, and categories as necessary for judgments. Immanuel Kant, *Critique of Pure Reason*, trans. Paul Guyer and Allen W. Wood (Cambridge: Cambridge University Press, 1998), 172–92 and 202–66. I, on the other hand, simply mean "conceptual categories" as those cognitive processes, however basic, that synthesize sense data in a manner not given empirically. This may include Kant's intuitions. Mapping Kant's framework on Dignāga's or Dharmakīrti's requires further analysis, but see Jed Forman, "Timeless Visions: Prajñākaragupta on Futureless Precognition and Temporal Intuitions," in *The Handbook of Intuitions.* Logic, Epistemology, and the Unity of Sciences (New York: Springer, forthcoming).
2. According to Heidegger, this anticipation is specifically our anticipation that eventually we will no longer have our being to be. Our anticipation of death is the wellspring of our experience of living in time. Martin Heidegger, *Being and Time*, trans. John Macquarrie and Edward Robinson (Cambridge, MA: Blackwell, 2001), 296–311. Animals, for example, may not have the same anticipation and so do not live in the same temporal world.
3. Heidegger, *Being and Time*, 456–88.
4. In many ways, my critique of these traditions parallels that of Hajime Tanabe, who argues that they are focused on "self-power" over "other-power." Hajime Tanabe, *Philosophy as Metanoetics*, trans. Takeuchi Yoshinori, Valdo Viglielmo, and James W. Heisig. Nanzan Studies in Religion and Culture (Berkeley: University of California Press, 1986), 151–92.
5. Edmund Husserl, *The Crisis of European Sciences and Transcendental Phenomenology: An Introduction to Phenomenological Philosophy*, trans. David Carr, 6th printing. Studies in Phenomenology & Existential Philosophy (Evanston, IL: Northwestern University Press, 1984), 157–58.
6. Pierre Keller, *Husserl and Heidegger on Human Experience* (Cambridge: Cambridge University Press, 1999), 111–31.

7. For example, Irene McCullin argues that Heidegger's Dasein possesses an irreducible "mineness." Irene McCullin, *Time and the Shared World: Heidegger on Social Relations*. Northwestern University Studies in Phenomenology and Existential Philosophy (Evanston, IL: Northwestern University Press, 2013), chap. 2. There is also a long history of this sort of criticism in the lineage of Emmanuel Levinas (1906–1995), dubbing Heidegger's theory of Dasein "solipsistic" and "egoist," as well as criticizing its assumption that "solitude" is ontologically prior to "sociality." François Raffoul, "The Question of Responsibility Between Levinas and Heidegger," in *Between Levinas and Heidegger*, ed. John E. Drabinski and Eric S. Nelson. SUNY Series in Contemporary Continental Philosophy (Albany: State University of New York Press, 2014), 179–80 and passim; Irina Poleshchuk, "Heidegger and Levinas: Metaphysics, Ontology and the Horizon of the Other," *Indo-Pacific Journal of Phenomenology* 10, no. 2 (October 2010): 1–10, https://doi.org/10.2989/IPJP.2010.10.2.4.1085; Tina Chanter, *Time, Death, and the Feminine: Levinas with Heidegger* (Stanford, CA: Stanford University Press, 2001), 106. There is ample resistance to these characterizations, however. See John Haugeland and Joseph Rouse, *Dasein Disclosed: John Haugeland's Heidegger* (Cambridge, MA: Harvard University Press, 2013), 121–36; Joan Stambaugh, *Thoughts on Heidegger*, Current Continental Research 217. Washington, DC: Center for Advanced Research in Phenomenology and University Press of America, 1991), chap. 2; Hiroshi Abe, "Haidegā no tasharon," *Kinsei tetsugaku kenkyū* 5 (February 10, 1999): 47–63, https://doi.org/10.14989/189800. Nevertheless, these nondual interpretations are often influenced by none other than Buddhism itself. The latter two thinkers rely heavily on Buddhism to interpret Heidegger's Dasein in this way, especially with the help of the Japanese Buddhist master Dōgen (1200–1253).
8. For a lucid analysis of the fundamentality of this structure in Heidegger, see Harrison Hall, "The Other Minds Problem in Early Heidegger," *Human Studies: A Journal for Philosophy and the Social Sciences* 3, no. 1 (1980): 247–54, https://doi.org/10.1007/BF02331812.
9. Heidegger, *Being and Time*, 294.
10. Heidegger, *Being and Time*, 296–99.
11. For a similar critique, see Alphonso Lingis, "The First Person Singular: Missteps on Heidegger's Path," *Philosophy Today* 61, no. 1 (2017): 85–97, https://doi.org/10.5840/philtoday2017320148.
12. Heidegger, *Being and Time*, 296.
13. As Levinas nicely puts it, "Everything that takes place here 'between us' concerns everyone, the face that looks at it places itself in the full light of the public order, even if I draw back from it to seek with the interlocutor the complicity of a private relation and a clandestinity." Emmanuel Levinas, *Totality and Infinity: An Essay on Exteriority*. Martinus Nijhoff Philosophy Texts, vol. 1 (The Hague: Martinus Nijhoff Publishers, 1979), 212. However, unlike Levinas, my interpretation of the texts explored does not construe this public as an Other that is irreducible in Dasein's stead. Levinas, 79–81.
14. Jean-Paul Sartre, *Being and Nothingness: A Phenomenological Essay on Ontology*, trans. Hazel E. Barnes (New York: Washington Square Press, 1978), 73–74.

15. Maurice Merleau-Ponty, *Phenomenology of Perception*, trans. Colin Smith. Routledge Classics (London: Routledge, 2002), 92.
16. Merleau-Ponty, *Phenomenology of Perception*, 94.
17. Although I will not explore it in detail here, the Buddhist Śāntideva (685–763) gives a rich critique of the notion that our experience is limited to our body. Śāntideva and Prajñākaramati, *Bodhicaryāvatāra of Śāntideva with the Commentary Pañjika of Prajñākaramati*, ed. Paraśurāma Lakshmaṇa Vaidya, Buddhist Sanskrit Texts 12 (Darbhanga: Mithila Institute, 1960), 161–62 vv. 8.111–116; Śāntideva, *A Guide to the Bodhisattva Way of Life: = (Bodhicaryāvatāra)*, trans. Vesna A. Wallace and B. Alan Wallace (Ithaca, NY: Snow Lion Publications, 1997), 103–04 vv. 8.111–16.
18. Here, I borrow from Linda Zagzebeski's notion of "omnisubjectivity," a rich theory of how an omniscient God would cognize each of our individual subjectivities. Linda Trinkaus Zagzebski, "The Attribute of Omnisubjectivity," in *God, Knowledge, and the Good*, 1st ed. (New York: Oxford University Press, 2022), 187–210, https://doi.org/10.1093/oso/9780197612385.003.0012. Still, my position is more radical. Unlike Christian traditions that (largely) describe God's experience as unattainable, Buddhists (largely) argue that our *lack* of omniscience is adventitious: we will all, someday, become buddhas, as guaranteed by our inherent buddha nature. Thus, read phenomenologically, Buddhist theories of omniscience describe *our* most fundamental experience. I also contend that this has consequences for how we understand subjectivity, as, perhaps, not fundamentally individuated, but distributed.
19. Mark Gifford, "Aristotle on Platonic Recollection and the Paradox of Knowing Universals: Prior Analytics B.21 67a8-30," *Phronesis* 44, no. 1 (February 1999): 4–7, https://doi.org/10.1163/156852899762447610.
20. Of course, Kant argues that synthetic a priori judgements about the properties of triangles are not developed empirically in this fashion, but I will not waylay us with that debate here. Kant, *Critique of Pure Reason*, B145–6.
21. Though Śāntarakṣita does not use the term "yogic perception" in this section, its reference is clear from the topic of *atīndriya-darśin*, that is, those who have supersensible sight. For a discussion of how this position links to Kamalaśīla's understanding of yogic perception as mental cognition, see Toru Funayama, "Kamalaśīla's View on Yogic Perception and the Bodhisattva Path," in *Religion and Logic in Buddhist Philosophical Analysis: Proceedings of the Fourth International Dharmakirti Conference, Vienna, August 23-27, 2005*, ed. Helmut Krasser et al. (Vienna: Verlag der Österreichischen Akademie der Wissenschaften, 2011), 105, especially n30.
22. For details on this progression, see Kamalaśīla, *Bhāvanākramaḥ of Ācārya Kamalaśīla*, ed. Gyaktsen Namdol (Varanasi: Central Institute of Higher Tibetan Studies, 1984), 245.13 ff.
23. Śāntarakṣita and Kamalaśīla, *Tattvasaṅgraha of Ācārya Śāntarakṣita with the "Pañjika" Commentary of Ācārya Śrī Kamalaśīla*, 2:750–51 vv. 3380–88.
24. Śāntarakṣita and Kamalaśīla, *Tattvasaṅgraha of Ācārya Śāntarakṣita*, 2:750 v. 3380.
25. Śāntarakṣita's position thus resembles Bhāsarvajña's, who (unlike his predecessors) argued that absorbed yogic perception perceives discrete objects in addition to their metaphysical subtleties without fourfold contact.

26. This "culmination of intense practice" (*abhyāsa-karṣa-paryanta*) echoes Dharmakīrti's analysis of meditation's role in cultivating yogic perception in his *Drop of Logic* (*Nyāyabindu*) (*bhāvanā-prakarṣa-paryanta*). Dharmakīrti, Dharmottara, and Durvekamiśra, *Paṇḍita Durveka Miśra's Dharmottarapradīpa: Being a Subcommentary on Dharmottara's Nyāyabinduṭīkā, a Commentary on Dharmakīrti's Nyāyabindu*, ed. Dalasukha Bhāī Mālavaṇiyā (Patna: Kashi Prasad Jayaswal Research Institute, 1971), 67 v. 1.11.
27. Śāntarakṣita and Kamalaśīla, *Tattvasaṅgraha of Ācārya Śāntarakṣita*, 2:751.7–9.
28. Śāntarakṣita's discussion of emptiness (*śūnyatā*) is indicative of his Middle Way (*madhyamaka*) philosophy. The theory of emptiness extends the insights of selflessness, arguing that not only does the person not have identity, but that all phenomena lack identity. Śāntarakṣita and Kamalaśīla, *Tattvasaṅgraha of Ācārya Śāntarakṣita*, 2:442 v. 1851.
29. Śāntarakṣita and Kamalaśīla, *Tattvasaṅgraha of Ācārya Śāntarakṣita*, 2:759 vv. 3442–44.
30. Śāntarakṣita and Kamalaśīla, *Tattvasaṅgraha of Ācārya Śāntarakṣita*, 2:759 v. 3448.
31. Sara L. McClintock, "Knowing All Through Knowing One: Mystical Communion or Logical Trick in the Tattvasaṃgraha and Tattvasaṃgrahapañjikā," *Journal of the International Association of Buddhist Studies* 23, no. 2 (2000).
32. Secondary scholarship confirms that Vācaspatimiśra is presenting the views of Kamalaśīla in this section. Sara L. McClintock, *Omniscience and the Rhetoric of Reason: Śāntarakṣita and Kamalaśīla on Rationality, Argumentation, and Religious Authority* (Boston: Wisdom, 2010), 229; Monkia Pemwieser, "Materialien Zur Theorie Der Yogischen Erkenntnis Im Buddhismus" (Masters thesis, Vienna, University of Vienna, 1991), 114.
33. Maṇḍanamiśra and Vācaspatimiśra, *Vidhiviveka of Śrī Maṇḍana Miśra: With the Commentary Nyāyakaṇikā of Vāchaspati Miśra*, ed. Mahāprabhu Lāla Gosvāmī (Varanasi: Tara Publications, 1978), 106.7–9.
34. Maṇḍanamiśra and Vācaspatimiśra, *Vidhiviveka of Śrī Maṇḍana Miśra*, 104.26–29.
35. Dharmakīrti, *The Pramanavarttikam of Dharmakīrti: The First Chapter with the Autocommentary*, ed. Raniero Gnoli (Roma: Instituto Italiano per il Medio ed Estremo Oriente, 1960), 42.12–22.
36. One possible answer to this question is a trope theory of properties. Each particular carries a certain trope that is individual but guarantees that the object bearing this trope is a member of the set defined by this property. But this merely passes the buck on the problem. What is it that unites all these individual tropes in a common set? To say they are all the same begs the question. Thus, tropes do not explain how universal, repeatable properties inhere in separate instantiations.
37. Maṇḍanamiśra and Vācaspatimiśra, *Vidhiviveka of Śrī Maṇḍana Miśra: With the Commentary Nyāyakaṇikā of Vāchaspati Miśra*, 105.3–5.
38. Jñānaśrīmitra, "Yoginirṇayaprakaraṇa," in *Jñānaśrīmitranibandhavāli: Buddhist Philosophical Works of Jñānaśrīmitra*, ed. Anantalāla Ṭhakkura, 2nd. ed. (Patna: Kashi Prasad Jayaswal Research Institute, 1987), 330.7–9.
39. Dharmakīrti, however, switches between this register and Yogācāra, which comes close to idealism, but qualified, since Asaṅga (its founder) argues that the mind is not ultimately real. Catherine Prueitt, "Shifting Concepts: The Realignment of

Dharmakīrti on Concepts and the Error of Subject/Object Duality in Pratyabhijñā Śaiva Thought," *Journal of Indian Philosophy* 45, no. 1 (2017): 21–47. As discussed, however, Yogācāra's view on the mind is highly debated. For one accessible presentation, along with a rendering of the entire Buddhist doxography, see Lhun-grub-bsod-pa and Jeffrey Hopkins, *Cutting through Appearances: The Practice and Theory of Tibetan Buddhism*, 2nd. ed. (Ithaca, NY: Snow Lion Publications, 1989), pt. 2.

40. Indeed, this motivates Dharmakīrti's quip about vultures. From the perspective of the *Commentary*, omniscience concerns the insight needed for liberation, not literal knowledge of everything, analogized to glorified vultures with overdeveloped remote seeing. Dharmakīrti, *Pramāṇavarttika-kārikā: (Sanskrit and Tibetan)*, vol. 2., ed. Yūshō Miyasaka (Acta Indologica. Narita: Naritasan Shinshōji, 1972), v. 2.33; Dharmakīrti, "*Pramāṇavārttikakārikā, Tshad ma rnam 'grel gyi tshig le'ur byas pa," in *Sde dge bstan 'gyur*, Ed. Tshul khrims rin chen, Toh. no. 4210., Tshad ma, ce:94a–151b (Delhi: Delhi Karmapae Choedhey, Gyalwae Sungrab Partun Khang, 1744), fol. 108b6–7.
41. The portion in brackets is supplied by Ratnakīrti, Jñānaśrīmitra's student, who cites this passage verbatim. Ratnakīrti, "Sarvajñasiddhiḥ," in *Ratnakīrtinibandhavāli: Buddhist Philosophical Works of Ratnakīrti*, ed. Anantalāla Ṭhakkura, 2nd ed. (Patna: Kashi Prasad Jayaswal Research Institute, 1975), 21.26–27.
42. Jñānaśrīmitra, "Yoginirṇayaprakaraṇa," 330.14–17.
43. Jñānaśrīmitra, "Yoginirṇayaprakaraṇa," 330.12; Prajñākaragupta, *Pramāṇavārtikabhāshyam or Vārtikālaṅkaraḥ of Prajñākaragupta (Being a Commentary on Dharmakīrti's Pramāṇavārtikam)*, ed. Rāhula Sāṅkṛtyāyana (Patna, India: Kashi Prasad Jayaswal Research Institute, 1943), 52 v. 375.
44. Dharmakīrti, *Pramāṇavarttika-kārikā: (Sanskrit and Tibetan)*, vol. 2, v. 3.532bcd.
45. Prajñākaragupta, *Pramāṇavārtikabhāshyam or Vārtikālaṅkaraḥ of Prajñākaragupta (Being a Commentary on Dharmakīrti's Pramāṇavārtikam)*, 460.16–17; Prajñākaragupta, "*Pramāṇavārttikālaṅkāra, Tshad ma rnam 'grel gyi rgyan," in *Sde dge bstan 'gyur*, ed. 'Phags pa shes rab, trans. Paṇḍita skal ldan rgyal po, Blo ldan shes rab, and Paṇḍita Kumāraśrī, Toh. no. 4221., Tshad ma, the:1a–282b (Delhi: Delhi Karmapae Choedhey, Gyalwae Sungrab Partun Khang, 1744), fol. 120a4.
46. Jñānaśrīmitra, "Yoginirṇayaprakaraṇa," 343.8–10.
47. McClintock, *Omniscience and the Rhetoric of Reason*, 85–91. Different levels of analysis also stem from Dharmakīrti's commentators', including Prajñākaragupta and Jñānaśrīmitra, attempt to differentiate conventional criteria for epistemic warrant concerning our everyday experience from the unique, ultimate epistemic warrant of a Buddha's omniscience. Motoi Ono, "Prajñākaragupta's Interpretation of Dharmakīrti's Two Definitions of Pramāṇa: A Reconsideration Based on the Newly Discovered Sanskrit Manuscript of Yamāri's Commentary," in *To the Heart of Truth: Felicitation Volume for Eli Franco on the Occasion of His Seventieth Birthday*, ed. Hiroko Matsuoka, Shinya Moriyama, and Tyler Neill, vol. 1, Wiener Studien Zur Tibetologie Und Buddhismuskunde, Heft 104 (Wien: Arbeitskreis für Tibetische und Buddhistische Studien Universität Wien, 2023), 591–617. Also see Shinya Moriyama, "The Reliability of Yogic Perception for Dharmakīrti, Prajñākaragupta and Jñānaśrīmitra," in *To the Heart of Truth: Felicitation Volume for Eli Franco on the Occasion of His Seventieth Birthday*, ed. Hiroko

Matsuoka, Shinya Moriyama, and Tyler Neill, vol. 1, Wiener Studien Zur Tibetologie Und Buddhismuskunde, Heft 104 (Wien: Arbeitskreis für Tibetische und Buddhistische Studien Universität Wien, 2023), 565–89.

48. Lawrence J. McCrea and Parimal G. Patil, *Buddhist Philosophy of Language in India: Jñānaśrīmitra on Exclusion* (New York: Columbia University Press, 2010), 3; Malcolm David Eckel, *Bhāviveka and His Buddhist Opponents*. Harvard Oriental Series, vol. 70 (Cambridge, MA: Harvard University Department of Sanskrit and Indian Studies, 2008), 213–300.
49. Haribhadrasūri similarly criticizes the Buddhist appeal to inconceivability on this point. Haribhadrasūri and Municandrasūri, *Anekāntajayapatākā by Haribhadra Sūri with His Own Commentary and Municandra Sūri's Supercommentary*, vol. 2, ed. H. R. Kapadia (Baroda: Oriental Institute, 1947), 57.8–58.4.
50. In response to an interlocutor who questions how universals and particulars connect, Dharmakīrti seems ultimately to efface the distinction, claiming they are merely conventions (*vyavahāra*).

    > [Objection:] *How is it to be understood that the particular is identical to a universal that is different from it? You might say it is otherwise, but what else could it be? If the universal is a particular, then how could it be a conceptual object? And if not, then how could the universal have pragmatic efficacy? And because there would be no recognition of impermanence, etc., with regard to particulars, there would be no identity relationship [between particulars and impermanence]; these would be properties of unreal things.*
    >
    > [Reply:] This poses no problem. Universals and their co-referentiality [with particulars], as well as properties and their bearers, are conventional [distinctions] with regard to the object that appears to consciousness.

    Dharmakīrti, *The Pramanavarttikam of Dharmakīrti: The First Chapter with the Autocommentary*, 42.8–13; Dharmakīrti, "*Pramāṇavārttikavṛtti, Tshad ma rnam 'grel gyi 'grel pa," in *Sde dge bstan 'gyur*, ed. Tshul khrims rin chen, Toh. no. 4216, vol. Tshad ma, ce (Delhi: Delhi Karmapae Choedhey, Gyalwae Sungrab Partun Khang, 1744), 284b3–4.
51. For Dignāga's theory to this effect, see Zhihua Yao, *The Buddhist Theory of Self-Cognition* (New York: Routledge, 2005), 141–45, https://doi.org/10.4324/9780203445280. Interestingly, Dignāga's conclusion opposes Kant's based on the same apperceptive premise. While Dignāga argues that apperception leads to an illusory *duality* between subject and object, Kant argues that apperception is necessary for a transcendental *unity* of consciousness. Kant, *Critique of Pure Reason*, A107–8.
52. Yao, *The Buddhist Theory of Self-Cognition*, 141–45.
53. As reconstructed from "*gnas ma gyur ba'i phyir*" in the Sanskrit version by the Central Institute for Higher Studies. Dharmakīrti and Vinītadeva, *Santānāntarasiddhiḥ of Ācārya Dharmakīrti and Santānāntarasiddhiḥ Ṭīkā of Ācārya Vinītadeva: Restored and Ed. J. S. Negi*, ed. J. S. Negi, Bibliotheca Indo Tibetica Series 37 (Varanasi: Central Institute of Higher Tibetan Studies, 1997), ll. 87–93, http://gretil.sub.uni-goettingen.de/gretil/1_sanskr/6_sastra/3_phil/buddh/bsa059_u.htm. Dharmakīrti often uses this term, "transformation of the basis"

(*āśrayaparivṛtti*) to denote the mental transformation that occurs through spiritual practice. Eli Franco, *Dharmakīrti on Compassion and Rebirth* (Vienna: Arbeitskreis für Tibetische und Buddhistische Studien, Universität Wien, 1997), 82 ff.

54. Dharmakīrti, "*Saṃtānāntarasiddhi, Rgyud gzhan grub pa zhes bya ba'i rab tu byed pa," ed. Tshul khrims rin chen, Toh. no. 4219., Tshad ma, ce:355b–59 (Delhi: Delhi Karmapae Choedhey, Gyalwae Sungrab Partun Khang, 1744), fol. 359a3–5.
55. Dharmakīrti, "*Saṃtānāntarasiddhi, Rgyud gzhan grub pa zhes bya ba'i rab tu byed pa," fol. 359a5–6; Dharmakīrti and Vinītadeva, *Santānāntarasiddhiḥ of Ācārya Dharmakīrti and Santānāntarasiddhiḥ Ṭīkā of Ācārya Vinītadeva*, ll. 87–93.
56. Dharmakīrti, "*Saṃtānāntarasiddhi, Rgyud gzhan grub pa zhes bya ba'i rab tu byed pa," fol. 359a6–7; Dharmakīrti and Vinītadeva, *Santānāntarasiddhiḥ of Ācārya Dharmakīrti and Santānāntarasiddhiḥ Ṭīkā of Ācārya Vinītadeva*, ll. 87–93.
57. It is worth noting that Dharmakīrti's description of telepathy here as both being vivid and informative closely matches his description of yogic perception in the *Exegesis on Epistemology* (*Pramāṇaviniścaya*). Compare "*mngon sum du ni de'i rnam pa'i rjes su byed pa gsal bar snang ba'i phyir dang/ mi slu pa'i tshad ma zhes bya bar 'dod do/*" with "*gsal bar snang zhing rnam par rtog pa med pa phyin ci ma log pa'i yul can gang yin pa de yang mngon sum gyi tshad ma yin no/*." Dharmakīrti, "*Saṃtānāntarasiddhi, Rgyud gzhan grub pa zhes bya ba'i rab tu byed pa," fol. 359a6; Dharmakīrti, "*Pramāṇaviniścaya, Tshad ma rnam par nges pa," fols. 161a7–161b1. This similarity is also attested by Shinya Moriyama, "On Self-Awareness in the Sautrāntika Epistemology," *Journal of Indian Philosophy* 38, no. 3 (2010): 272.
58. Dharmakīrti, *Pramāṇavarttika-kārikā: (Sanskrit and Tibetan)*, vol. 2, v. 3.532d.
59. Prajñākaragupta, *Pramāṇavārtikabhāshyam or Vārtikālaṅkaraḥ of Prajñākaragupta (Being a Commentary on Dharmakīrti's Pramāṇavārtikam)*, 460.18–23; Prajñākaragupta, "*Pramāṇavārttikālaṅkāra, Tshad ma rnam 'grel gyi rgyan," in *Sde dge bstan 'gyur*, ed. 'Phags pa shes rab, trans. Paṇḍita skal ldan rgyal po, Blo ldan shes rab, and Paṇḍita Kumāraśrī, Toh. no. 4221., Tshad ma, the:1a–282b (Delhi: Delhi Karmapae Choedhey, Gyalwae Sungrab Partun Khang), 1744, fol. 120a5–7. My translation of this passage and subsequent interpretation relies on two commentaries. Jina, "*Pramāṇavārttikālaṃkāraṭīkā, Tshad ma rnam 'grel gyi rgyan gyi 'grel bshad," in *Sde 'dge bstan 'gyur*, ed. Tshul khrims rin chen, trans. Sridipamkarararakṣita and Man hor byang chub shes rab, Toh. 4222, vol. Tshad ma, de (Delhi: Delhi Karmapae Choedhey, Gyalwae Sungrab Partun Khang, 1982), fols. 304a6–b3. Yamāri, "*Pramāṇavārttikālaṃkāraṭīkāsupariśuddhā, Tshad ma rnam 'grel rgyan gyi 'grel bshad shin tu yongs su dag pa zhes bya ba," in *Sde 'dge bstan 'gyur*, ed. Tshul khrims rin chen, trans. Rngog blo ldan shes rab, Toh. 4226, vol. Tshad ma, be (Delhi: Delhi Karmapae Choedhey, Gyalwae Sungrab Partun Khang, 1982), fols. 164b3–166a3.
60. Bhāsarvajña, *Nyāyabhūṣaṇam*, ed. Śvāmī Yogīndrānanda (Varanasi: Ṣaḍdarśana Prakāśana Pratiṣṭhānam, 1968), 172.9.
61. Bhāsarvajña, *Nyāyabhūṣaṇam*, 172.13–15.
62. Jñānaśrīmitra, "Yoginirṇayaprakaraṇa," 341.16–17.
63. Jñānaśrīmitra, "Yoginirṇayaprakaraṇa," 341.20–22.
64. Ratnakīrti, "Sarvajñasiddhiḥ," 21.23–25.

65. Jñānaśrīmitra, "Yoginirṇayaprakaraṇa," 330.14–17.
66. Ratnakīrti, "Sarvajñasiddhiḥ," 21.26–31.
67. While Ratnakīrti's citation of Dharmakīrti reads "subject and object" (*grāhya-grāhaka*), Miyasaka's edition has "the characteristic of an object" (*grāhya-lakṣaṇa*). Dharmakīrti, *Pramāṇavarttika-kārikā: (Sanskrit and Tibetan)*, vol. 2, v. 3.532bcd.
68. Ratnakīrti, "Sarvajñasiddhiḥ," 21.31–22.4.
69. The logical positivists, however, would be unlikely to assent to the epistemic warrant of prophetic dreams, though we might press them on the issue and ask whether their position has the resources to deny them outright.
70. Ratnakīrti, "Sarvajñasiddhiḥ," 22.6–8.
71. Ratnakīrti goes on to elaborate his point about precognition and dreams by drawing on Prajñākaragupta. See this discussed in detail in my forthcoming chapter, Forman, "Timeless Visions: Prajñākaragupta on Futureless Precognition and Temporal Intuitions."
72. Jill Bolte Taylor, *My Stroke of Insight: A Brain Scientist's Personal Journey* (New York: Viking, 2006), 3.
73. Taylor, *My Stroke of Insight*, 42.
74. Taylor, *My Stroke of Insight*, 3.
75. Heidegger, *Being and Time*, 343 and 417.
76. Taylor, *My Stroke of Insight*, 49.
77. Taylor, *My Stroke of Insight*, 35.
78. Alan Lightman, *Searching for Stars on an Island in Maine* (New York: Knopf Doubleday, 2018), 6.
79. Also worth exploring is Ann Taves's detailed analysis of Judith Skutch's similar experience. Ann Taves, *Revelatory Events: Three Case Studies of the Emergence of New Spiritual Paths* (Princeton, NJ: Princeton University Press, 2016), 207 ff.
80. Colette Cornubert, "Freud et Romain Rolland: Essai sur la découverte de la pensée psychanalytique par quelques écrivains français" (Diss., Faculté de médecine de Paris, 1966), 25.
81. Rebekah Richert, Justin L. Barrett, and Roxanne Moore Newman, "When Seeing Is Not Believing: Children's Understanding of Humans' and Non-Humans' Use of Background Knowledge in Interpreting Visual Displays," *Journal of Cognition and Culture* 3, no. 1 (2003): 91–108, https://doi.org/10.1163/156853703321598590; Henry M. Wellman, David Cross, and Julianne Watson, "Meta-Analysis of Theory-of-Mind Development: The Truth about False Belief," *Sage Family Studies Abstracts* 23, no. 4 (2001): 411–568; Jonathan D. Lane, Henry M. Wellman and E. Margaret Evans, "Sociocultural Input Facilitates Children's Developing Understanding of Extraordinary Minds," *Child Development* 83, no. 3 (2012): 1007–21, https://doi.org/10.1111/j.1467-8624.2012.01741.x.
82. Justin L. Barrett, "Coding and Quantifying Counterintuitiveness in Religious Concepts: Theoretical and Methodological Reflections," *Method & Theory in the Study of Religion* 20, no. 4 (2008): 328.
83. Calvin L. Warren, *Ontological Terror: Blackness, Nihilism, and Emancipation* (Durham, NC: Duke University Press, 2018), 1–25, https://doi.org/10.1215/9780822371847.
84. Warren, *Ontological Terror*, 28.

85. Warren, *Ontological Terror*, 145. Although Trish Glazebrook's project is to recover a genderless Dasein in Heidegger, her remarks can be interpreted to make a similar point about Dasein and gender: "Dasein is first and foremost being-in-a-world. This world is *very much informed* by gender. To think transcendently, then, in a gender-neutral way, would be precisely to transcend the world, to be worldless. This is, in Heidegger's own terms from *Being and Time*, impossible." Trish Glazebrook, "Heidegger and Ecofeminism," in *Feminist Interpretations of Martin Heidegger*, ed. Nancy J. Holland and Patricia J. Huntington, Re-Reading the Canon (University Park: Pennsylvania State University Press, 2001), 233. If to have Dasein is to be in the world, and that world oppresses a woman's freedom to have their being to be, then is not Dasein inscribed in a certain male mode of being?
86. I am thinking specifically of Heidegger's description of thrownness as individuating and circumscribing the bounds of Dasein's freedom. Heidegger, *Being and Time*, 343 and 417.
87. For an interesting comparison of collectivist versus individualistic modalities between African and Western cultures, see H. J. Pietersen, "Western Humanism, African Humanism and Work Organisations," *SA Journal of Industrial Psychology* 31, no. 3 (October 29, 2005), https://doi.org/10.4102/sajip.v31i3.209.
88. Heidegger, *Being and Time*, 167.
89. Heidegger, *Being and Time*, 463.
90. I see my proposal here as similar to Warren's understanding of the role of postmetaphysics. Warren, *Ontological Terror*, 7–9. He argues that postmetaphysics is a process of destruction that ungrounds the harmful metaphysical structures that perpetuate suffering. I argue that an omniphenomenology is also destructive, destroying the conceit of there being innate structures that belie phenomenology. But as Warren notes, postmetaphysics is insufficient. We still need to build a metaphysics that can rehabilitate black being. So too, I argue, with that ground upended by omniphenomenology, can new structures be built that are more equitable.
91. Those familiar with Heidegger will counter that I have omitted the importance of "care" and "solicitude" in his analysis. In other words, Dasein's Being-in-the-world is primordially Being-alongside, including Others. Heidegger, *Being and Time*, sec. 41. According to Heidegger, then, our ability to be with others compassionately is *predicated* on Dasein, our ability to recognize that Others have their own Being to be. Heidegger, *Being and Time*, sec. 26. But, although Heidegger gives an avenue for care within his system, the primacy of the individual over its relation to others leaves him open to the criticism that I (and others like Levinas) have leveled here. For example, Heidegger concedes, "The expression 'Dasein,' however, shows plainly that 'in the first instance' this entity is unrelated to Others, and that of course it can still be 'with' Others afterwards" (156).
92. This is also a goal of Zagzebski's "omnisubjectivity." Zagzebski, "The Attribute of Omnisubjectivity." By democratizing phenomenology via omniphenomenology, we develop a higher-order respect for differing ways of being in the world.
93. For a similar view, see Christian Coseru, *Perceiving Reality: Consciousness, Intentionality, and Cognition in Buddhist Philosophy* (New York: Oxford University Press, 2012), passim.

5. Gelug Representationalism

1. Again, I am reading Asaṅga under the "progressive model" of Yogācāra rather than the "pivot model." Sponberg, "The Trisvabhāva Doctrine in India & China;" Brennan, "The Three Natures and the Path to Liberation in Yogācāra-Vijñānavāda Thought," 621–48.
2. Avrum Stroll, Twentieth-Century Analytic Philosophy (New York: Columbia University Press, 2000), 50.
3. Bertrand Russell, "Letter on Sense-Data [1915]," in *The Philosophy of Logical Atomism and Other Essays, 1914–19*, ed. John Greer Slater, The McMaster University edition, The Collected Papers of Bertrand Russell (London: George Allen & Unwin, 1986), 87–88.
4. Unless, of course, we say that concepts correspond with appearances. But I mean "correspondence" here in a realist sense, meaning a "real" object as something extramental, such that it could adjudicate discrepancies between individual, idiosyncratic mental appearances. So, for correspondence to serve as an epistemic criterion, a concept's referent must be beyond what merely appears, since some mental appearance will categorically "correspond" with every concept, even those that are fictitious.
5. The three Middle Way figures here are Śāntarakṣita, Kamalaśīla, and Jñānagarbha (ca. eighth century). For a brief introduction to this text, see Pascale Hugon, "Proving Emptiness: The Epistemological Background for the 'Neither One Nor Many' Argument and the Nature of Its Probandum in Phya pa Chos kyi seng ge's Works," *Journal of Buddhist Philosophy* 1, no. 1 (2015): 58 ff., https://doi.org/10.1353/jbp.2015.0006.
6. Phya pa chos kyi seng ge, *Dbu ma shar gsum gyi stong thun*, ed. Helmut Tauscher (Vienna: Arbeitskreis für Tibetische und Buddhistische Studien, Universität Wien, 1999), 21.2–4.
7. Phya pa chos kyi seng ge, *Dbu ma shar gsum gyi stong thun*, 21.5–8.
8. Phya pa chos kyi seng ge, *Dbu ma shar gsum gyi stong thun*, 21.9–12. This assessment informs Chapa's sophisticated differentiation between absolute negation (*med dgag*) and nonexhaustive negation (*ma yin dgag*). Indeed, these terms are used by Chapa in a much different sense than by his Gelug successors. He is largely in line with later Gelugpas about the former: absolute negations are total absences. But per the latter, in the place of an "implicative" negation—that is, a negation that implies something *else* that is positive—Chapa means a negation that does not completely vitiate the thing to which it is applied. This is important for Chapa's theory of inference, for he argues even in the case of negative inferences, which negate some property, the probandum must be a nonexhaustive negation, since that negation is always about some positive entity. Pascale Hugon, "Proving Emptiness," 62–67. Hence, Chapa's view that it is impossible to make arguments about pure absences per se, since inferences by nature are predicative.
9. Phya pa chos kyi seng ge, *Dbu ma shar gsum gyi stong thun*, 21.20–21.
10. Mi pham rgya mtsho, *The Wisdom Chapter: Jamgön Mipham's Commentary on the Ninth Chapter of "The Way of the Bodhisattva,"* trans. Padmakara Translation Group, 1st ed. (Boulder: Shambhala, 2017), 8–9.

11. Georges B. J. Dreyfus, *Recognizing Reality: Dharmakīrti's Philosophy and Its Tibetan Interpretations*, SUNY Series in Buddhist Studies (Albany: State University of New York Press, 1997), 30–33; Thupten Jinpa, "Tsongkhapa's Qualms about Early Tibetan Interpretations of Madhyamaka Philosophy," *The Tibet Journal* 24, no. 2 (1999): 4.
12. Georges Dreyfus similarly calls the Gelug position "moderate realism." He argues that, unlike Dignāga, Gelugpas argue universals are moderately real, impossible to disentangle from the objects which instantiate them. They are thus not robust enough to have some ontological status independent of particulars, but still have some real instantiation in particulars. Universals are thus moderately real. Dreyfus, *Recognizing Reality*, 179–82. I agree with Dreyfus that Gelugpas solve the correspondence problem by arguing universals and particulars are ultimately indistinguishable. I disagree, however, that this position is tantamount to a type of realism afforded to universals. While it is true that on the Gelug position there has to be something real with which conceptual universals correspond, this is not tantamount to the claim that universals themselves are real. Jed Forman, "Tsongkhapa's Difficult Point: Saying What Cannot be Said about Particulars, Universals, and Relations" (Paper presentation presented at the American Philosophical Association Pacific Conference, Portland, OR, March 22, 2024).
13. Blo bzang grags pa, "Bstan bcos chen po dbu ma la 'jug pa'i rnam bshad dgongs pa rab gsal," in *Rje tsong kha pa chen po'i gsung 'bum*, BDRC W3PD188, vol. 16 (Beijing: Krung go'i bod rig pa'i dpe skrun khang, 2012), 262.5–13.
14. Although Tsongkhapa does not make the point exactly like this, it is articulated by one of his most important commentators, Purchok Ngawang Jampa (1682–1762). Purchok Ngawang Jampa, "Diamond Slivers: A Rejoinder to Taktsang Lotsawa," in *Knowing Illusion Volume: Bringing a Tibetan Debate into Contemporary Discourse*, trans. Ryan Conlon et al., vol. 2 (New York: Oxford University Press, 2021), 386–87.
15. Specifically, Taktsang makes his criticism in the context of the Gelug argument that the human's and hungry ghost's differing and contradictory perceptions of liquid as water or pus are both epistemically warranted. Shes rab rin chen, "Grub mtha' kun shes kyi rnam par bshad pa legs bshad kyi rgya mtsho," in *Stag tshang lo tsā ba shes rab rin chen gyi gsung 'bum*, BDRC W2DB4577, vol. 1 (Beijing: Krung go'i bod rig pa dpe skrun khang, 2007), 281.16–82.8; also see Forman, "What Is the World? Neckties, Ghosts, Falling Hairs, and Celestial Cities in a Coherentist Epistemology," 914–15.
16. Shes rab rin chen, "Grub mtha' kun shes kyi rnam par bshad pa legs bshad kyi rgya mtsho," 281.16–82.8; also see Forman, "What Is the World? Neckties, Ghosts, Falling Hairs, and Celestial Cities in a Coherentist Epistemology," 914–15.
17. Blo bzang grags pa, "Mngon sum le'u'i brjed byang," in *Rje tsong kha pa chen po'i gsung 'bum*, ed. Dar ma rin chen, BDRC W20510, vol. 10 (Zi ling: Mtsho sngon mi rigs dpe skrun khang, 1999), 346.22–26.
18. Blo bzang grags pa, "Mngon sum le'u'i brjed byang," 347.3–6.
19. For a discussion of the Tibetan advent of these categories, see Dreyfus, *Recognizing Reality*, 384–85.

20. For a more detailed discussion of Gelug thought on this point, see Jonathan Stoltz, "Sakya Pandita and the Status of Concepts," *Philosophy East and West* 56, no. 4 (2006): 567–82, https://doi.org/10.1353/pew.2006.0064.
21. To reiterate from chapter 3, however, this is a strawman of Yogācārin views, some of which do not reify the mind either. Sponberg, "The Trisvabhāva Doctrine in India & China"; Brennan, "The Three Natures and the Path to Liberation in Yogācāra-Vijñānavāda Thought."
22. This is emptiness of the coarse person and the subtle person. For details, see a helpful chart in Jampa Tegchok, and Steve Carlier, *Insight into Emptiness*, ed. Thubten Chodron (Boston: Wisdom Publications, 2012), 100.
23. Blo bzang grags pa, "Mngon sum le'u'i brjed byang," 346.3–10.
24. For details, see a helpful chart in Jampa Tegchok and Carlier, *Insight into Emptiness*, 100.
25. Tom Tillemans goes as far to say that, according to Tsongkhapa, this is not just an epistemological requirement, but an ontological one as well. In other words, Tsongkhapa's representationalism also commits him to the existence of real universals, not merely as representations but also as inherent in reality. See Tom J. F. Tillemans, *Scripture, Logic, Language: Essays on Dharmakirti and His Tibetan Successors*, Studies in Indian and Tibetan Buddhism (Boston: Wisdom, 1999), 215–16. I argue, however, that Tsongkhapa's epistemological view does not entail such ontological commitments. Forman, "Tsongkhapa's Difficult Point: Saying What Cannot be Said about Particulars, Universals, and Relations."
26. As Ethan Mills demonstrates, Candrakīrti argues that this is impossible on the assumption that inference and perception have distinct objects. Mills, "On the Coherence of Dignāga's Epistemology," *Asian Philosophy* 25, no. 4 (October 2, 2015): 339–57, https://doi.org/10.1080/09552367.2015.1102694.
27. Tsongkhapa here subscribes the "pivot model" interpretation of the three natures. Sponberg, "The Trisvabhāva Doctrine in India & China."
28. Tsongkhapa uses the term "Vijñāptimātrin" (*rnam rig pa*), but it is synonymous with Mind Only (**cittamātrin, sems tsam pa*).
29. Blo bzang grags pa, "Mngon sum le'u'i brjed byang," 346.10–12.
30. I am grateful to Geshe Lobsang Tsultrim at the Central Institute for Higher Tibetan Studies who explained this unique feature in Tsongkhapa's understanding of the Mind Only school (personal communication, December 12, 2019).
31. Dignāga, *Dignāga's Pramāṇasamuccaya, Chapter 1: A Hypothetical Reconstruction of the Sanskrit Text with the Help of the Two Tibetan Translations on the Basis of the Hitherto Known Sanskrit Fragments and the Linguistic Materials Gained from Jinendrabuddhi's Ṭīkā*, ed. Ernst Steinkellner (Vienna: Österreichische Akademie der Wissenschaften, 2005), 3.10; Dignāga, "*Pramāṇasamuccaya, Tshad ma kun las btus pa zhes bya ba'i rab tu byed pa," in *Sde dge bstan 'gyur*, ed. Tshul khrims rin chen, Toh. no. 4203, Tshad ma, ce: fols. 1a–13b (Delhi: Delhi Karmapae Choedhey, Gyalwae Sungrab Partun Khang, 1744), fol. 2a1.
32. Blo bzang grags pa, "Mngon sum le'u'i brjed byang," 346.17–19.
33. For a lucid explanation of how Gelugpas use the notion of implicit cognition to explain how perception perceives conceptual entities, see Dreyfus, *Recognizing Reality*, 370–73.

34. Rongtön Sheja Kunrig (Rong ston shes bya kun rig, 1367–1449), following Sakya Paṇḍita (Sa skya paṇ ḍi ta, 1182–1251), understands the notion of implicit cognition as a Tibetan invention. Rong ston, "Rigs gter rnam bshad nyi ma'i snying po," in *The Collection of the Eighteen Renowned Scriptures: Root Texts and Commentaries*, ed. Sachen International (Kathmandu: Sachen International, 2011), 202.12 ff. I admittedly agree that I find it difficult to see how the notion of implicit cognition could square with Dharmakīrti's formulation.
35. Peter A. Schwabland, "Direct and Indirect Cognition and the Definition of Pramāna in Early Tibetan Epistemology," *Asiatische Studien: Zeitschrift Der Schweizerischen Asiengesellschaft* 49, no. 4 (1995): 796, https://doi.org/10.5169/seals-147199.
36. Gendün Drubpa (1391–1474), one of Tsongkhapa's primary students, discusses this point in some detail. Dge 'dun grub, "Tshad ma'i bstan bcos chen mo rigs pa'i rgyan las mngon sum le'u," in *Dge 'dun grub kyi gsung 'bum*, BDRC W1KG14505, vol. 7 (Lhasa: Ser gtsug nang bstan dpe rnying 'tshol bsdu phyogs sgrig khang, 2011), 93.5–94.5.
37. Blo bzang grags pa, "Mngon sum le'u'i brjed byang," 346.19–21.
38. Thakchoe, "Candrakīrti's Theory of Perception: A Case for Non-Foundationalist Epistemology in Madhyamaka," *Acta Orientalia Vilnensia* 11, no. 1 (2010): 105–11.
39. Unlike Tsongkhapa, other Tibetan exegetes argue that Middle Way analysis undermines epistemic warrant entirely, as well as representationalism a fortiori. For a discussion, see Jay L. Garfield and Georges B. J. Dreyfus, "The Madhyamaka Contribution to Skepticism" (Unpublished manuscript, 2017).
40. The Gelug school in general is known (and criticized) for adopting a view of Middle Way that is highly reliant on the epistemological view of Dharmakīrti. Taktsang Lotsāwa (1405–1477) thus dubbed Gelugpas as those who advocate that the traditions of Dharmakīrti and Candrakīrti are like "two lions with their necks intertwined." Shes rab rin chen, "Grub mtha' kun shes kyi rnam par bshad pa legs bshad kyi rgya mtsho," in *Stag tshang lo tsā ba shes rab rin chen gyi gsung 'bum*, BDRC W2DB4577, 1:121–361 (Beijing: Krung go'i bod rig pa dpe skrun khang, 2007), 273.13–15. The famed Gelug scholar Lobsang Chökyi Gyeltsen (Blo bzang chos kyi rgyal mtshan, 1570–1662) proudly adopts the slogan. Blo bzang chos kyi rgyal mtshan, "Sgra pa shes rab rin chen pa'i rtsod lan lung rigs seng ge'i nga ro," in *Collected Works (gsun 'bum) of Blo-bzan-chos-kyi-rgyal-mtshan*, BDRC W23430., 4:559–648 (New Delhi: Mongolian Lama Gurudeva, 1973), 618.2–3. The question is whether these two intertwined necks protect or choke each other.
41. Tillemans, *Scripture, Logic, Language*, 215–16.
42. Note that this parallels Vincent Eltschinger's position, who also cites the benefit of meditation on unreal objects for the sake of spiritual ends but argues this is not a form of yogic perception. Eltschinger, "On the Career and the Cognition of Yogins," 194.
43. Nor was it lost on Indian Buddhist Tantric commentators, who also recruit Dharmakīrti's views on yogic perception to explain the Creation Stage. Davey K. Tomlinson, "Yogic Perception, Tantric Vision Practice, and the Norms of Attention," presentation at the American Academy of Religion, San Antonio, 2023.

44. This is a technical point about the argument for the existence of yogis. In order for such an argument to be conclusive, there needs to be an example (*dṛṣṭānta*) that exemplifies the pervasion between the reason (*hetu*) and the probandum (*sādhya*). Because the opponent does not accept the existence of veritable yogis, they reject any example that exemplifies the quality of developing yogic perception and thus that could serve as a locus for both the reason and the probandum.
45. Blo bzang grags pa, "Rgyal ba khyab bdag rdo rje 'chang chen po'i lam gyi rim pa gsang ba kun gyi gnad rnam par phye ba," in *Rje tsong kha pa chen po'i gsung 'bum*, BDRC W3PD188, vol. 3 (Beijing: Krung go'i bod rig pa'i dpe skrun khang, 2012), 548.6–15.
46. Blo bzang grags pa, "Rgyal ba khyab bdag rdo rje 'chan chen po'i lam gyi rim pa gsang ba kun gyi gnad rnam par phye ba," 582.20–83.5.
47. Blo bzang grags pa, "Rgyal ba khyab bdag rdo rje 'chang chen po'i lam gyi rim pa gsang ba kun gyi gnad rnam par phye ba," 574.22–75.4.
48. Blo bzang grags pa, "Rgyal ba khyab bdag rdo rje 'chang chen po'i lam gyi rim pa gsang ba kun gyi gnad rnam par phye ba," 575.4–5; Dharmakīrti, *Pramāṇavarttika-kārikā: (Sanskrit and Tibetan)*, vol. 2, v. 2.112cd; Dharmakīrti, "*Pra māṇavārttikakārikā, Tshad ma rnam 'grel gyi tshig le'ur byas pa," fol. 111b6.
49. Blo bzang grags pa, "Rgyal ba khyab bdag rdo rje 'chang chen po'i lam gyi rim pa gsang ba kun gyi gnad rnam par phye ba," 575.5–8.
50. Blo bzang grags pa, "Rgyal ba khyab bdag rdo rje 'chan chen po'i lam gyi rim pa gsang ba kun gyi gnad rnam par phye ba," 582.17–22.
51. By the contrapositive, I am not presenting Tsongkhapa as arguing that *someone else* can tell who is a buddha empirically through the senses. See Jed Forman, "Double Hiddenness: Governmentality and Subjectivization in Gelug Buddhism," *Critical Research on Religion*, 2021, 1–15, https://doi.org/10.1177/2050303220986985. Nonetheless, he does seem to suggest that a buddha sees *themself* as a buddha with *all* of their enlightened senses, not just the mental sense.
52. But Tsongkhapa does make clear that these vivid appearances in deity yoga are epistemic warrants (*tshad ma*) because they undo self-grasping. This speaks to a certain pragmatist reading. Still, he contends these appearances are mistaken (*phyin ci log pa*). Blo bzang grags pa, "Rgyal ba khyab bdag rdo rje 'chang chen po'i lam gyi rim pa gsang ba kun gyi gnad rnam par phye ba," 608.16–10.4. Tsongkhapa thus appears to define deity yoga's epistemic warrant to be like that of inferences, which are also pragmatically informative but mistaken. But this would preclude these meditative appearances from being authentic *perceptions*, which must be unmistaken. Tsongkhapa's position here counters that of Mipham (1846–1912), who maintains that mediative appearances during the Creation Stage are not just effective but "pure" and therefore *not* mistaken. Douglas S. Duckworth, *Mipam on Buddha-Nature: The Ground of the Nyingma Tradition* (Albany: State University of New York Press, 2008), 124–31.
53. This is an inherent ambiguity in Dharmakīrti that is reflected both in these primary sources as well in secondary-literature debates. Again, see Dunne and Eltschinger. Dunne, "Realizing the Unreal: Dharmakīrti's Theory of Yogic Perception," *Journal of Indian Philosophy* 34, no. 6 (2007): 497–519. https://doi.org/10

.1007/s10781-006-9008-y; Eltschinger, "On the Career and the Cognition of Yogins," 169n1.

54. Compare *"rnam shes don gzhan chags pa yis/ /nus med don gzhan mi 'dzin phyir/ /"* with *"anya-artha-āsakti-viguṇe jñāne anartha-antara-grahāt."* Dharmakīrti, "*Pramāṇavārttikakārikā, Tshad ma rnam 'grel gyi tshig le'ur byas pa," fol. 111b6; Dharmakīrti, *Pramāṇavarttika-kārikā: (Sanskrit and Tibetan)*, vol. 2, v. 2.112cd. The discrepancy with the Tibetan is somewhat bewildering. *Āsakti* may have been mis-rendered as *aśakti* in the Tibetan *nus med,* but does seem correctly translated as *chags pa*. If so, then *nus med* may be *viguṇa*, which is a slightly strange translation choice, since *yon tan med pa* or some variant would be more standard. The Tibetan phrase *don gzhan mi 'dzin phyir* would be more appropriately *artha-antara-agrahāt* in Sanskrit, as in, "it does not grasp another object," but the Sanskrit recension, *anartha-antara-grahāt*, more felicitously means "it grasps something which is not another object." Finally, the Tibetan trades the locative *jñāne*, which denotes a conditional, for an instrumental, also significantly changing the meaning. It is also possible that the Tibetan was translated from another recession of the Sanskrit than that currently available.
55. Prajñākaragupta, *Pramāṇavārtikabhāshyam or Vārtikālaṅkaraḥ of Prajñākaragupta (Being a Commentary on Dharmakīrti's Pramāṇavārtikam)*, ed. Rāhula Sāṅkṛtyāyana (Patna, India: Kashi Prasad Jayaswal Research Institute, 1943), 102.8–9.
56. G. E. Moore, "Visual Sense-Data," in *British Philosophy in the Mid-Century*, ed. J. H. Muirhead (George Allen and Unwin, 1957), 130–37, https://doi.org/10.1525/9780520315167-008.
57. Moore, "Visual Sense-Data," 136–37.
58. Of course, this distortion is different according to each theorist. On Tsongkhapa's position, this distortion is global, since representations always depict impermanent entities as permanent, empty entities as nonempty, and so forth. Representations, on this view, have some *inherent* error. Moore, on the other hand, does not subscribe to a global error theory. The distortion occurs as a product of physical limits, since the multiple surfaces of an object cannot simultaneously present themselves to a singular observer.

6. Sakya Antirepresentationalism

1. Sonam Thakchoe, "Candrakīrti's Theory of Perception: A Case for Non-Foundationalist Epistemology in Madhyamaka," *Acta Orientalia Vilnensia* 11, no. 1 (2010): 107.
2. Candrakīrti, "*Madhyamakāvatārabhāṣya, Dbu ma la 'jug pa'i bshad pa," in *Sde dge bstan 'gyur*, ed. Tshul khrims rin chen, Toh. no. 3862. Dbu ma, 'a:220b–348a (Delhi: Delhi Karmapae Choedhey, Gyalwae Sungrab Partun Khang, 1744), fol. 254a3–7.
3. Ludwig Wittgenstein, *Preliminary Studies for the "Philosophical Investigations:" Generally Known as the Blue and Brown Books* (Oxford: Blackwell, 1960), 108–10.

4. Ludwig Wittgenstein, *Philosophische Untersuchungen = Philosophical Investigations*, ed. Peter Michael Stephan Hacker, trans. Gertrude Elizabeth Margaret Anscombe and Joachim Schulte, rev. 4th ed. (Chichester, West Sussex, UK: Wiley-Blackwell, 2009), 53; also see Avrum Stroll, *Twentieth-Century Analytic Philosophy* (New York: Columbia University Press, 2000), 128–29.
5. Robert Thurman wrote the seminal paper noting the affinities between Candrakīrti and Wittgenstein. Robert A. F. Thurman, "Philosophical Nonegocentrism in Wittgenstein and Candrakirti in Their Treatment of the Private Language Problem," Philosophy East and West 30, no. 3 (1980): 321–337, https://doi .org/10.2307/1399191.
6. Ludwig Wittgenstein, "Tractatus Logico-Philosophicus," in *Major Works: Selected Philosophical Writings*, trans. C. K. Ogden, 1st ed. (New York: HarperPerennial, 2009), sec. 6.522.
7. Wittgenstein, "Tractatus Logico-Philosophicus," sec. 6.52–6.52.1.
8. Wittgenstein, "Tractatus Logico-Philosophicus," sec. 6.54.
9. Majjhima Nikāya MN 22, *Alagaddūpamasuttaṃ*, 134.30–35.25. Trenckner, V., Robert Chalmers, and T. W. Rhys Davids, eds, *The Majjhima Nikaya*, vol. 1 (Oxford: Pali Text Society, 1991).
10. Interestingly, Sangpu and Sakya monasteries were founded in the same year: 1073.
11. Bsod nams rtse mo, "Byang chub sems dpa'i spyod pa la 'jug pa'i 'grel pa," in *'Phags yul rgyan drug mchog gnyis kyi zhal lung*, BDRC W3CN3408, vol. 68 (Lhasa: Bod ljongs bod yig dpe rnying dpe skrun khang, 2015), 114.16–115.1.
12. Bsod nams rtse mo, "Byang chub sems dpa'i spyod pa la 'jug pa'i 'grel pa," 115.1–2.
13. Bsod nams rtse mo, "Byang chub sems dpa'i spyod pa la 'jug pa'i 'grel pa," 115.3–13.
14. Asaṅga, "*Mahāyānasaṃgraha, Theg pa chen po bsdus pa," in *Sde dge bstan 'gyur*, ed. Tshul khrims rin chen, Toh. no. 4048, Sems tsam, ri:1a–43b (Delhi: Delhi Karmapae Choedhey, Gyalwae Sungrab Partun Khang, 1744), fols. 15b6–16a4.
15. Bsod nams rtse mo, "Byang chub sems dpa'i spyod pa la 'jug pa'i 'grel pa," 115.13–14.
16. Bsod nams rtse mo, "Byang chub sems dpa'i spyod pa la 'jug pa'i 'grel pa," 116.16–17.4.
17. The only place I have found this distinction in the works of Tsongkhapa, Kedrub Gelek Pelzang, and Gyaltsab Darma Rinchen—considered the three foundational philosophers of the Gelug tradition—is in Gyaltab's commentary on the *Treasury of Reasoning and Epistemology* (*Tshad ma rigs gter*). Dar ma rin chen, "Tshad ma rigs pa'i gter gyi rnam bshad," in *Rgyal tshab thams cad mkhyen pa dar ma rin chen gyi gsung 'bum*, vol. 28 (Mundgod, India: Rje yab sras gsum gyi gsung 'bum sdud sgrig khang, 2019), 158.14 ff. This commentary is accepted by Sakyapas themselves and so may reflect Gyaltsab's views as a Sakyapa before becoming a disciple of Tsongkhapa.
18. Kun dga' rgyal mtshan, "Tshad ma rigs pa'i gter gyi rang 'grel," in *Tshad ma'i 'grel pa phyogs bsgrigs*, vol. 7 (Rdzong sar khams bye: Rdzong sar khams bye'i slob gling thub bstan dar rgyas gling, 2009), 280.2–5.

19. Kun dga' rgyal mtshan, "Tshad ma rigs pa'i gter gyi rang 'grel," 303.6–304.1.
20. This is made clear by Sapen's reference to "inconceivable wisdom with its basis transformed (*āsraya-parivṛtti)." Dharmakīrti, "*Saṃtānāntarasiddhi, Rgyud gzhan grub pa zhes bya ba'i rab tu byed pa," ed. Tshul khrims rin chen, Toh. no. 4219., Tshad ma, ce:355b–59 (Delhi: Delhi Karmapae Choedhey, Gyalwae Sungrab Partun Khang, 1744), fol. 359a3–7.
21. Kun dga' rgyal mtshan, "Tshad ma rigs pa'i gter gyi rang 'grel," 303.1–4.
22. Dharmakīrti, *Pramāṇavarttika-kārikā: (Sanskrit and Tibetan)*, ed. Yūshō Miyasaka (Acta Indologica. Narita: Naritasan Shinshōji, 1972), vol. 2, v. 3.281d; Dharmakīrti, "*Pramāṇavārttikakārikā, Tshad ma rnam 'grel gyi tshig le'ur byas pa," in *Sde dge bstan 'gyur*, ed. Tshul khrims rin chen, Toh. no. 4210, vol. Tshad ma, ce (Delhi: Delhi Karmapae Choedhey, Gyalwae Sungrab Partun Khang, 1744), fol. 129a4–5.
23. At the level of Middle Way, however, Gelugpas do indeed argue that yogic perception of emptiness initially does *not* involve appearances, exactly because it is a mere absence (*med dgag*). But this is not a product of ultimate reality itself being bereft of appearances, such as argued by Sönam Tsemo and subsequent Sakyapas. Rather, it is merely because before buddhahood, the yogi is unable to cognize this emptiness simultaneously with appearances. The lack of appearances is a product of spiritual incompleteness, not an ontological fact about ultimate reality. Thus, the yogi oscillates between their cognition of emptiness and appearances until they can be seen simultaneously in the final stage. Blo bzang grags pa, "Dbu ma la 'jug pa'i rnam bshad," in *'Jam mgon bla ma tsong kha pa chen po'i gsung 'bum*, vol. 16 (Mundgod, India: Rje yab sras gsum gyi gsung 'bum sdud sgrig khang, 2019), 161.12–17. In other words, the object of yogic perception (emptiness) is not beyond appearances inherently; it only seems that way due to a lack in the yogi's meditative skill. We saw Tsongkhapa make a similar point in chapter 5, where the appearance of the deity in deity yoga does not appear alongside sensorial appearances merely because the mind does not have the capacity to grasp both simultaneously; but this fact does not vitiate the validity of sensory appearances.
24. Dar ma rin chen, "Rnam nges ṭika chen dgongs pa rab gsal," in *Rgyal tshab thams cad mkhyen pa dar ma rin chen gyi gsung 'bum*, vol. 26 (Mundgod, India: Rje yab sras gsum gyi gsung 'bum sdud sgrig khang, 2019), 133.12–15.
25. Kun dga' rgyal mtshan, "Tshad ma rigs pa'i gter gyi rang 'grel," 283.6–84.2. Rongtön Sheja Kunrig (Rong ston Shes bya Kun rig, 1367–1449) also deals with this issue extensively. Rong ston, "Rigs gter rnam bshad nyi ma'i snying po," in *The Collection of the Eighteen Renowned Scriptures: Root Texts and Commentaries*, ed. Sachen International (Kathmandu: Sachen International, 2011), 202.12 ff.
26. Schwabland, "Direct and Indirect Cognition and the Definition of Pramāna in Early Tibetan Epistemology," *Asiatische Studien: Zeitschrift Der Schweizerische-nAsiengesellschaft* 49, no. 4 (1995): 803, https://doi.org/10.5169/seals-147199.
27. Go bo rab 'byams pa, *Freedom from Extremes: Gorampa's "Distinguishing the Views" and The Polemics of Emptiness*, trans. José Ignacio Cabezón and Lobsang Dargyay, Studies in Indian and Tibetan Buddhism (Boston: Wisdom, 2007); Sonam Thakchoe, *The Two Truths Debate: Tsongkhapa and Gorampa on the Middle Way* (Boston: Wisdom, 2007).

28. Go bo rab 'byams pa, "Tshad ma rigs pa'i gter gyi don gsal," in *The Collection of the Eighteen Renowned Scriptures: Root Texts and Commentaries*, ed. Sachen International (Kathmandu: Sachen International, 2011), 99.9–12.
29. Again, this is one of Dharmakīrti's requirements for epistemic warrant. Dharmakīrti, *Pramāṇavarttika-kārikā: (Sanskrit and Tibetan)*, vol. 2, v. 2.3.
30. Go bo rab 'byams pa, "Tshad ma rigs pa'i gter gyi don gsal," 99.12–14.
31. Go bo rab 'byams pa, "Tshad ma rigs pa'i gter gyi don gsal," 99.14–18.
32. Kun dga' rgyal mtshan, "Tshad ma rigs pa'i gter gyi rang 'grel," 284.6–85.1; Go bo rab 'byams pa, "Tshad ma rigs pa'i gter gyi don gsal," 100.4.
33. Kun dga' rgyal mtshan, "Tshad ma rigs pa'i gter gyi rang 'grel," 284.5–6.
34. Go bo rab 'byams pa, "Tshad ma rigs pa'i gter gyi don gsal," 99.12–14.
35. Kun dga' rgyal mtshan, "Tshad ma rigs pa'i gter gyi rang 'grel," 284.6–85.2.
36. Go bo rab 'byams pa, "Rgyas pa'i bstan bcos tshad ma rnam 'grel gyi rnam par bshad pa kun tu bzang po'i 'od zer: Mngon sum le'u," in *The Collection of the Eighteen Renowned Scriptures: Root Texts and Commentaries*, ed. Sachen International (Kathmandu: Sachen International, 2011), 92.6–10.
37. Mkhas grub dge legs dpal bzang po, "Tshad ma rnam 'grel gyi mngon sum le'u rgya cher bshad pa," in *Mkhas grub thams cad mkhyen pa dge legs dpal bzang gi gsung 'bum*, vol. 33 (Mundgod, India: Rje yab sras gsum gyi gsung 'bum sdud sgrig khang, 2019), 152.13–17.
38. It is unlikely that this is typo, since it is found in at least three recensions of the text: Go bo rab 'byams pa, "Rgyas pa'i bstan bcos tshad ma rnam 'grel gyi rnam par bshad pa kun tu bzang po'i 'od zer: Mngon sum le'u," 2011, 92.10; Go bo rab 'byams pa, "Rgyas pa'i bstan bcos tshad ma rnam 'grel gyi rnam par bshad pa kun tu bzang po'i 'od zer," in *Kun mkhyen go rams pa bsod nams seng+ge'i gsung 'bum*, BDRC W1KG16651, vol. 1 (Beijing: Krung go'i bod rig pa dpe skrun khang, 2013), 385.21–22; Go bo rab 'byams pa, "Rgyas pa'i bstan bcos tshad ma rnam 'grel gyi rnam par bshad pa kun tu bzang po'i 'od zer: Mngon sum le'u," in *Kun mkhyen go rams pa bsod nams seng+ge'i gsung 'bum*, BDRC W1PD1725, vol. 1 (Derge: Dzong sar khams bye'i slob gling, 2014), 635.4.
39. Dr. Venerable Tashi Tsering, a modern-day authority of the Sakya school, argues that instead of "seeing those appearances with an epistemic instrument," Gorampa may mean something like "the fact that those appearances are seen is established with an authentic epistemic instrument" (personal communication, January 19, 2021). This would resolve the issue, since it is not that those objects themselves are epistemically warranted, but it is the fact of their being seen by some people that is so warranted. On the other hand, this assertion would seem more felicitously rendered in Tibetan as "*mthong ba tshad mas grub*," as in their being seen is epistemically warranted. But, as it is, "*tshad mas mthong*" suggests that *tshad ma* is the instrument of the seeing itself, not the warrant of the fact of their being seen seeing. There are also philosophical reasons that may preclude such a reading. To say that *the fact* that people see those objects is true, even though those objects themselves are not, would be tantamount to saying that there is a real appearance of those objects even though they are referentless. But Sakyapas in general deny that appearances can be epistemically warranted qua appearances despite failing to be so qua referent object. The Sakya point is

deflationary: it is not true that someone sees false appearances, it is just false that they see an appearance. Gorampa corroborates this position elsewhere when discussing the notion of the "appearing object" (*snang yul*): "In mistaken, nonconceptual cognition (*rtog med log shes*), all that actually 'appears' is the absence of an appearing object. . . . Although this is the 'appearing object' of this cognition, generally speaking, it is not an appearing object." Go bo rab 'byams pa, "Tshad ma rigs pa'i gter gyi don gsal," 2.17–19. Thus, illusions entail no appearing object. There is not some appearance the mind authentically grasps despite that appearance's failure to refer. Gorampa therefore is in general agreement with the Sakya rejection of the Gelug distinction between appearance qua referent and an appearance qua appearance. Given this deflationary position, it does not seem that Gorampa would assent to the *fact* of something being seen as true independent of whether that visual appearance refers to a real object.

40. Go bo rab 'byams pa, "Rgyas pa'i bstan bcos tshad ma rnam 'grel gyi rnam par bshad pa kun tu bzang po'i 'od zer: Mngon sum le'u," 2011, 4.20–5.7.
41. For all its paradox, "false truth" is also another felicitous translation of both the Tibetan, "*kun rdzob bden pa*," as is "deceptive reality."
42. Sonam Thakchoe, "How Many Truths? Are There Two Truths or One in the Tibetan Prāsaṅgika Madhyamaka?," *Contemporary Buddhism* 5, no. 2 (2004): 121–41, https://doi.org/10.1080/1463994042000291547.
43. Dharmakīrti, *Pramāṇavarttika-kārikā: (Sanskrit and Tibetan)*, ed. Yūshō Miyasaka, (Acta Indologica. Narita: Naritasan Shinshōji, 1972), vol. 2, v. 3.286abc.
44. Go bo rab 'byams pa, "Rgyas pa'i bstan bcos tshad ma rnam 'grel gyi rnam par bshad pa kun tu bzang po'i 'od zer: Mngon sum le'u," 2011, 92.14–18.
45. Vincent Eltschinger, "On the Career and the Cognition of Yogins," in *Yogic Perception, Meditation and Altered States of Consciousness*, ed. Eli Franco and Dagmar Eigner (Vienna: Verlag der Österreichischen Akademie der Wissenschaften, 2009), sec. 3.1 and 5.2.
46. Mkhas grub dge legs dpal bzang po, "Tshad ma rnam 'grel gyi mngon sum le'u rgya cher bshad pa," 153.2–6.
47. It is also of note, however, that here Gorampa defines yogic perception as an "authentic epistemic instrument" in contrast to his earlier assessment that *unreal* meditative appearances are "seen by an authentic epistemic instrument." He thus appears to contradict himself. He may be bound by the root text here, since the former claim is Dharmakīrti's while the latter is his own addition. There is also another possibility. In the first case, the apparition is seen with an authentic epistemic instrument, while in the latter, yogic perception is said to be an authentic *perceptual* epistemic instrument. Gorampa, then, may elevate perceptual epistemic instruments above what we see on a day-to-day basis, which is not truly perceptual, given that it is ensconced in appearances.
48. Bsod nams rtse mo, "Byang chub sems dpa'i spyod pa la 'jug pa'i 'grel pa," 114.12–14.
49. Go bo rab 'byams pa, "Rgyas pa'i bstan bcos tshad ma rnam 'grel gyi rnam par bshad pa kun tu bzang po'i 'od zer: Mngon sum le'u," 2011, 92.18–19.
50. Mkhas grub dge legs dpal bzang po, "Tshad ma rnam 'grel gyi mngon sum le'u rgya cher bshad pa," 153.6–8.

51. We saw Tsongkhapa make a similar point when he argued that a falling hair is neither an epistemically warranted universal nor a particular because it does not exist.
52. Thakchoe, *The Two Truths Debate*; Go bo rab 'byams pa, *Freedom from Extremes*, 115–202.
53. Go bo rab 'byams pa, *Freedom from Extremes*, 196.
54. Blo bzang grags pa, "Dbu ma la 'jug pa'i rnam bshad," 161.12–17.
55. Dignāga, *Dignāga's Pramāṇasamuccaya, Chapter 1: A Hypothetical Reconstruction of the Sanskrit Text with the Help of the Two Tibetan Translations on the Basis of the Hitherto Known Sanskrit Fragments and the Linguistic Materials Gained from Jinendrabuddhi's Ṭīkā*, ed. Ernst Steinkellner (Vienna: Österreichische Akademie der Wissenschaften, 2005), 3.10; Dignāga, "*Pramāṇasamuccaya, Tshad ma kun las btus pa zhes bya ba'i rab tu byed pa," in *Sde dge bstan 'gyur*, ed. Tshul khrims rin chen, Toh. no. 4203. Tshad ma, ce:1a–13b (Delhi: Delhi Karmapae Choedhey, Gyalwae Sungrab Partun Khang, 1744), fol. 2a1.
56. Like Tsongkhapa, Śākya Chokden uses the term "Vijñāptimātra" (*rnam par rig pa tsam*). But again, it is synonymous with "Cittamātra."
57. Śākya mchog ldan, "Tshad ma rigs pa'i gter gyi dgongs rgyan lung dang rigs pa'i 'khor los lugs ngan pham," in *The Collection of the Eighteen Renowned Scriptures: Root Texts and Commentaries*, ed. Sachen International (Kathmandu: Sachen International, 2011), 488.2–9.
58. Tsongkhapa also understands emptiness to be a non-implicative negation. But he means this in a completely different sense than Śākya Chokden. On his position, this negation does not vitiate objects entirely, merely their impossible ways of existing. Blo bzang grags pa, *The Great Treatise on the Stages of the Path to Enlightenment*, trans. Joshua W. C. Cutler, Guy Newland, and Lamrim Chenmo Translation Committee, vol. 3 (Ithaca, NY: Snow Lion Publications, 2015), chap. 15. Although he uses the terminology differently from Chapa, Tsongkhapa still means this total negation of impossible ways of existing is predictable of existing objects that are not so vitiated.
59. Wittgenstein, "Tractatus Logico-Philosophicus," sec. 7.
60. Wittgenstein, "Tractatus Logico-Philosophicus," sec. 1.1.
61. John Ó Maoilearca, *All Thoughts Are Equal: Laruelle and Nonhuman Philosophy* (Minneapolis: University of Minnesota Press, 2015), 7–12.
62. François Laruelle, *Dictionary of Non-Philosophy*, trans. Taylor Adkins, 1st. ed, Univocal (Minneapolis, MN: Univocal, 2013), 129.
63. François Laruelle, *Principles of Non-Philosophy*, trans. Nicola Rubczak and Anthony Paul Smith (London: Bloomsbury, 2013), 56.
64. Laruelle, *Principles of Non-Philosophy*, 56.
65. Laruelle, *Principles of Non-Philosophy*, 56.
66. Laruelle, *Principles of Non-Philosophy*, passim.
67. Laruelle, *Dictionary of Non-Philosophy*, 131.
68. François Laruelle and Philippe Petit, *Intellectuals and Power: The Insurrection of the Victim*, trans. Anthony Paul Smith (Wiley, Polity Press, 2015), 8.
69. Laruelle and Petit, *Intellectuals and Power*, 122.

70. Ó Maoilearca, *All Thoughts Are Equal*, 17.
71. François Laruelle, *Une biographie de l'homme ordinaire: Des autorités et des minorités*, Collection Analyse et raisons (Paris: Aubier, 1985), 105 and 111.
72. *dmigs med brtse ba'i gter chen spyan ras gzigs*
73. There are parallels here between (reconstructed) Sakya nonrepresentationalism and the omniphenomenology explored in chapter 4. Both are destructive and thus accommodative in ways that promote inclusion, tolerance, and empathy.

Conclusion

1. Hans-Georg Gadamer, *Truth and Method*, trans. Joel Weinsheimer and Donald G. Marshall, 2nd. rev. ed. Continuum Impacts (New York: Continuum, 2004), 301–5.
2. Reading Gadamer as a relativist, however, misses the nuance of his position. John McDowell, "Gadamer and Davidson on Understanding and Relativism," in *Gadamer's Century: Essays in Honor of Hans-Georg Gadamer*, ed. Hans-Georg Gadamer et al., Studies in Contemporary German Social Thought (Cambridge, MA: MIT Press, 2002), 173–94.
3. Also see my work on this in Forman, "Subtle, Hidden, and Far-Off: The Intertextuality of the Yogasūtras," *The Journal of Hindu Studies*, April 10, 2023, 1–24. https://doi.org/10.1093/jhs/hiad013.
4. Federico Squarcini's intertextual analysis of the *Yogasūtras*, for example, is a great example of this kind of burgeoning scholarship. Federico Squarcini, *Patañjali: Yogasūtra: A Cura di Federico Squarcini*, Et Classici (Turin, Italy: Giulio Einaudi Editore, 2019).
5. Martin Heidegger, *Being and Time*, trans. John Macquarrie and Edward Robinson (Cambridge, MA: Blackwell, 2001), 105.
6. As cited in Frederick C. Beiser, "The Concept of Bildung in Early German Romanticism," in *Philosophers on Education: Historical Perspectives*, ed. Amélie Rorty (London: Routledge, 1998), 294; also see Novalis, "Fragments from the Notebooks," in *The Early Political Writings of The German Romantics*, ed. and trans. Frederick C. Beiser, repr. Cambridge Texts in the History of Political Thought (Cambridge: Cambridge University Press, 1999), 85.
7. Benjamin Grant Purzycki and Richard Sosis, *Religion Evolving: Cultural, Cognitive, and Ecological Dynamics*. Advances in the Cognitive Science of Religion (Sheffield, UK: Equinox Publishing Ltd, 2022), 96–99.
8. Wayne Proudfoot, *Religious Experience* (Berkeley: University of California Press, 1985), 196–99.
9. My concluding sentiments here reflect the insights of Jason Ānanda Josephson Storm, who considers social kinds like "philosophy," as an academic discipline, to be processes rather than static entities with ossified demarcations and closed canons. Jason Ānanda Josephson Storm, *Metamodernism: The Future of Theory* (Chicago: University of Chicago Press, 2021), chaps. 3–4. As a social, diachronic category, philosophy is (and must) evolve to be more capacious.

References

Abe, Hiroshi. "Haidegā no tasharon." *Kinsei tetsugaku kenkyū* 5 (February 10, 1999): 47–63. https://doi.org/10.14989/189800.

Abhinavagupta and Utpaladeva. *Īśvara-Pratyabhijñā-Vimarśinī of Abhinavagupta: Doctrine of Divine Recognition*. Ed. K.A. Subramania Iyer, K. C. Pandey, and Rāma Candra Dvivedī. Vol. 2. Delhi: Motilal Banarsidass, 1986.

Abou-Khalil, Rima, and Lealani Mae Y Acosta. "A Case Report of Acquired Synesthesia and Heightened Creativity in a Musician after Traumatic Brain Injury." *Neurocase*, 2023, 1–4. https://doi.org/10.1080/13554794.2023.2208271.

Adams, Reginald B., Heather L. Gordon, Abigail A. Baird, Nalini Ambady, and Robert E. Kleck. "Effects of Gaze on Amygdala Sensitivity to Anger and Fear Faces." *Science* 300, no. 5625 (2003): 1536.

Agniveśa and Cakrapāṇidatta. *The Charakasaṃhitā by Agniveśa, Revised by Charaka and Dṛidhabala, with the Āyurveda-Dīpikā Commentary of Chakrapāṇidatta. Ed. Vaidya Jādavaji Trikamji Āchārya*. Ed. Jādavaji Trikamji. Bombay: Satyabhāmābāi Pāndurang, 1941.

Akalaṅka and Anantavīrya. *Siddhiviniścaya With the Commentaries Siddhiviniścayavṛtti, Siddhiviniścayaṭīkā*. Ed. Liudmila Olalde. SARIT: Enriching Digital Text Collections in Indology. Baden-Württemberg, Germany: University of Heidelberg, 2018. https://sarit.indology.info/siddhiviniscayatika.

Akṣapāda Gautama and Uddyotakara. *Nyāyabhāṣyavārttikam of Bhāradvāja Uddyotakara*. Ed. Anantalāla Ṭhakkura. New Delhi: Bhāratīyadārśanikānusandhānapari ṣatprakaśitam, 1997.

Akṣapāda Gautama and Vācaspatimiśra. *Nyāyavārttikatātparyaṭīkā*. Ed. Anantalāla Ṭhakkura. New Delhi: Bhāratīyadārśnikanusandhāna Pariṣatprakāśitā, 1996.

Akṣapāda Gautama and Vātsyāyana. *Savātsyāyanabhāṣyaṃ Gautamīyaṃ Nyāyadarśanam with Bhāṣya of Vātsyāyana*. Ed. Anantalāla Ṭhakkura. New Delhi: Bhāratīyadārśa nikānusandhānapariṣatprakāśitam, 1997.

Arnold, Dan. *Buddhists, Brahmins, and Belief: Epistemology in South Asian Philosophy of Religion*. New York: Columbia University Press, 2005.

——. "Candrakīrti on Dignāga on Svalakṣaṇas." *Journal of the International Association of Buddhist Studies* 26, no. 1 (2003).

——. "Givenness as a Corollary to Non-Conceptual Awareness: Thinking About Thought in Buddhist Philosophy." In *Wilfrid Sellars and Buddhist Philosophy: Freedom from Foundations*, Google Play Edition, 214–56. New York: Routledge, 2019.

——. "The Philosophical Works and Influence of Dignāga and Dharmakīrti." *Oxford Research Encyclopedia of Religion*, July 27, 2017. https://doi.org/10.1093/acrefore/9780199340378.013.198.

Āryadeva, Dharmapāla, and Candrakīrti. *Materials for the Study of Āryadeva, Dharmapāla, and Candrakīrti: The Catuḥśataka of Āryadeva, Chapters XII and XIII With the Commentaries of Dharmapāla and Candrakīrti: Introduction, Translation, Sanskrit, Tibetan, and Chinese Texts, Notes*. Trans. Tom J. F. Tillemans. Wiener Studien Zur Tibetologie Und Buddhismuskunde ; Heft 24. Wien: Arbeitskreis für Tibetische und Buddhistische Studien, Universität Wien, 1990.

Asaṅga. "*Mahāyānasaṃgraha, Theg pa chen po bsdus pa." In *Sde dge bstan 'gyur*. Ed. Tshul khrims rin chen, Toh. no. 4048, Sems tsam, ri:1a–43b. Delhi: Delhi Karmapae Choedhey, Gyalwae Sungrab Partun Khang, 1744.

Audi, Robert. "Philosophy: A Brief Guide for Undergraduates." The American Philosophical Association, 2017. https://www.apaonline.org/page/undergraduates.

——. *The Place of Testimony in the Fabric of Knowledge and Justification. Rational Belief.* Oxford University Press, 2015.

Ayer, A. J. "Has Austin Refuted the Sense-Datum Theory?" *Synthese* 17, no. 2 (1967): 117–40.

Babb, Lawrence A. "Glancing: Visual Interaction in Hinduism." *Journal of Anthropological Research* 37 (1981): 387–401.

Balakrishna, Narayana Godabole, and Kāśīnātha Pāṇḍuraṅga Paraba, eds. *Hitopadeśa*. 5th rev. ed. Bombay: Tukârâm Jâvajî, 1904.

Balcerowicz, Piotr. "Extrasensory Perception (Yogi-Pratyakṣa) in Jainism, Proofs of Its Existence and Its Soteriological Implications." In *Yoga in Jainism*. Ed. Christopher Key Chapple, 48–108. London: Routledge, 2016.

Barrett, Justin L. "Coding and Quantifying Counterintuitiveness in Religious Concepts: Theoretical and Methodological Reflections." *Method & Theory in the Study of Religion* 20, no. 4 (2008): 308–38.

Beiser, Frederick C. "The Concept of Bildung in Early German Romanticism." In *Philosophers on Education: Historical Perspectives*. Ed. Amélie Rorty, 284–99. London: Routledge, 1998.

Bellah, Robert N. "Rousseau on Society and the Individual." In *The Social Contract: And, The First and Second Discourses*. Ed. Susan Dunn and Gita May, 266–87. Rethinking the Western Tradition. New Haven, CT: Yale University Press, 2002.

Bhartṛhari. *Versuch Einer Vollständigen Deutschen Erstübersetzung Nach Der Kritischen Edition Der Mūla-Kārikās*. Ed. and trans. Wilhelm Rau. Mainz: Steiner, 2000.

Bhāsarvajña. *Nyāyabhūṣaṇam*. Ed. Śvāmī Yogīndrānanda. Varanasi: Ṣaḍdarśana Prakāśana Pratiṣṭhānam, 1968.

Blo bzang chos kyi rgyal mtshan. "Sgra pa shes rab rin chen pa'i rtsod lan lung rigs seng ge'i nga ro." In *Collected Works (gsun 'bum) of Blo-bzan-chos-kyi-rgyal-mtshan*, BDRC W23430. 4:559–648. New Delhi: Mongolian Lama Gurudeva, 1973.

Blo bzang grags pa. "Bstan bcos chen po dbu ma la 'jug pa'i rnam bshad dgongs pa rab gsal." In *Rje tsong kha pa chen po'i gsung 'bum*, BDRC W3PD188. 16:1–460. Beijing: Krung go'i bod rig pa'i dpe skrun khang, 2012.

——. "Dbu ma la 'jug pa'i rnam bshad." In *'Jam mgon bla ma tsong kha pa chen po'i gsung 'bum*, 16:49–227. Mundgod, India: Rje yab sras gsum gyi gsung 'bum sdud sgrig khang, 2019.

——. "Mngon sum le'u'i brjed byang." In *Rje tsong kha pa chen po'i gsung 'bum*. Ed. Dar ma rin chen, BDRC W20510. 10:342–95. Zi ling: Mtsho sngon mi rigs dpe skrun khang, 1999.

——. "Rgyal ba khyab bdag rdo rje 'chang chen po'i lam gyi rim pa gsang ba kun gyi gnad rnam par phye ba." In *Rje tsong kha pa chen po'i gsung 'bum*, BDRC W3PD188. 3:1–770. Beijing: Krung go'i bod rig pa'i dpe skrun khang, 2012.

——. *The Great Treatise on the Stages of the Path to Enlightenment*. Trans. Joshua W. C. Cutler, Guy Newland, and Lamrim Chenmo Translation Committee. 3 vols. Ithaca, NY: Snow Lion Publications, 2015.

Bråten, Ivar, Helge I. Strømsø, and Marit S. Samuelstuen. "Are Sophisticated Students Always Better? The Role of Topic-Specific Personal Epistemology in the Understanding of Multiple Expository Texts." *Contemporary Educational Psychology* 33, no. 4 (2008): 814–40. https://doi.org/10.1016/j.cedpsych.2008.02.001.

Brennan, Joy Cecile. "The Three Natures and the Path to Liberation in Yogācāra-Vijñānavāda Thought." *Journal of Indian Philosophy* 46, no. 4 (September 2018): 621–48. https://doi.org/10.1007/s10781-018-9356-4.

Bsod nams rtse mo. "Byang chub sems dpa'i spyod pa la 'jug pa'i 'grel pa." In *'Phags yul rgyan drug mchog gnyis kyi zhal lung*, BDRC W3CN3408. 68:1–190. Lhasa: Bod ljongs bod yig dpe rnying dpe skrun khang, 2015.

Buddhaghoṣa. *The Path of Purification*. Trans. Ñāṇamoli Thera. 4th ed. Kandy, Sri Lanka: Buddhist Publication Society, 2010.

——. *The Visuddhi-magga of Buddhaghosa*. 2 vols. Ed. Caroline A. F. Rhys Davids. London: Pali Text Society, 1920.

Buswell, Robert E., ed. *Encyclopedia of Buddhism*. 2 vols. New York: Macmillan Library Reference, 2003.

Campbell, George. *A Dissertation on Miracles*. Edinburgh: Bell & Bradfute, 1797.

Candrakīrti. *In Clear Words: The Prasannapadā, Chapter One 1: Introduction, Manuscript Description, Sanskrit Text*. Ed. Anne MacDonald. 2 vols. Vienna: Verlag der Österreichischen Akademie der Wissenschaften, 2015.

——. "*Madhyamakāvatārabhāṣya, Dbu ma la 'jug pa'i bshad pa." In *Sde dge bstan 'gyur*. Ed. Tshul khrims rin chen, Toh. no. 3862. Dbu ma, 'a:220b–348a. Delhi: Delhi Karmapae Choedhey, Gyalwae Sungrab Partun Khang, 1744.

——. "'Madhyamakāvatāra-Kārikā' Chapter 6." Ed. Li Xuezhu. *Journal of Indian Philosophy* 43, no. 1 (2015): 1–30.

——. "*Mūlamadhyamakavṛttiprasannapadā, Dbu ma rtsa ba'i 'grel pa tshig gsal ba." In *Sde dge bstan 'gyur*. Ed. Kanakavarman and Pa tshab lo tsā ba nyi ma grags,

Trans. Mahāsumati and Pa tshab lo tsā ba nyi ma grags, Toh. no. 3860. Dbu ma, 'a:1b–200a. Delhi: Delhi Karmapae Choedhey, Gyalwae Sungrab Partun Khang, 1744.

Candrakīrti and Jayānanda. "*Madhyamakāvatāraṭīkā, Dbu ma la 'jug pa'i 'grel pa." In *Sde dge bstan 'gyur*. Ed. Tshul khrims rin chen, Toh. no. 3870., Dbu ma, ra:1b–365a. Delhi: Delhi Karmapae Choedhey, Gyalwae Sungrab Partun Khang, 1744.

Caspar, Émilie A., and Régine Kolinsky. "Review of an Unusual Phenomenon: Synesthesia." *L'Année psychologique* 113, no. 4 (2013): 629. https://doi.org/10.3917/anpsy.134.0629.

Castelnovo, A., S. Cavallotti, O. Gambini, and A. D'Agostino. "Post-Bereavement Hallucinatory Experiences: A Critical Overview of Population and Clinical Studies." *Journal of Affective Disorders* 186 (2015): 266–74. https://doi.org/10.1016/j.jad.2015.07.032.

Chanter, Tina. *Time, Death, and the Feminine: Levinas with Heidegger*. Stanford, CA: Stanford University Press, 2001.

Chen, Yi-Chia, and Su-Ling Yeh. "Look into My Eyes and I Will Wee You: Unconscious Processing of Human Gaze." *Consciousness and Cognition* 21, no. 4 (2012): 1703–10. https://doi.org/10.1016/j.concog.2012.10.001.

Clough, Bradley S. "The Cultivation of Yogic Powers in the Pāli Path Manuals of Theravāda Buddhism." In *Yoga Powers: Extraordinary Capacities Attained Through Meditation and Concentration*. Ed. Knut A. Jacobsen, 77–95. Leiden: Brill, 2012.

Coady, C. A. J. *Testimony: A Philosophical Study*. New York: Clarendon Press, 1992.

Code, Lorraine. *Epistemic Responsibility*. 2nd ed. Albany: State University of New York Press, 2020.

Collerton, Daniel, Elaine Perry, and Ian McKeith. "Why People See Things That Are Not There: A Novel Perception and Attention Deficit Model for Recurrent Complex Visual Hallucinations." *Behavioral and Brain Sciences* 28, no. 6 (December 2005): 737–57. https://doi.org/10.1017/S0140525X05000130.

Cornubert, Colette. "Freud et Romain Rolland: Essai sur la découverte de la pensée psychanalytique par quelques écrivains française." Diss., Faculté de médecine de Paris, 1966.

Coseru, Christian. "Buddhist 'Foundationalism' and the Phenomenology of Perception." *Philosophy East and West* 59, no. 4 (2009): 409–39.

——. *Perceiving Reality: Consciousness, Intentionality, and Cognition in Buddhist Philosophy*. New York: Oxford University Press, 2012.

Cottrell, Jane E., and Gerald A. Winer. "Development in the Understanding of Perception: The Decline of Extramission Perception Beliefs." *Developmental Psychology* 30, no. 2 (1994): 218–28.

Coward, Harold G., and K. Kunjunni Raja. *The Philosophy of the Grammarians*. Princeton, NJ: Princeton University Press, 1990. https://doi.org/10.1515/9781400872701.

Cuevas, Joshua. "Is Learning Styles-Based Instruction Effective? A Comprehensive Analysis of Recent Research on Learning Styles." *Theory and Research in Education* 13, no. 3 (November 1, 2015): 308–33. https://doi.org/10.1177/1477878515606621.

Dar ma rin chen. "Rnam nges ṭika chen dgongs pa rab gsal." In *Rgyal tshab thams cad mkhyen pa dar ma rin chen gyi gsung 'bum*, 26:1–443. Mundgod, India: Rje yab sras gsum gyi gsung 'bum sdud sgrig khang, 2019.

——. "Tshad ma rigs pa'i gter gyi rnam bshad." In *Rgyal tshab thams cad mkhyen pa dar ma rin chen gyi gsung 'bum*, 28:49–227. Mundgod, India: Rje yab sras gsum gyi gsung 'bum sdud sgrig khang, 2019.

Davids, Caroline A. F. Rhys, and Estlin Carpenter, eds. *The Dīgha Nikāya*. London: Pali Text Society, 1890.

Dennett, Daniel C. "Quining Qualia." In *Consciousness in Contemporary Science*. Ed. A. J. Marcel and E. Bisiach, 42–77. New York: Oxford University Press, 1992. https://doi.org/10.1093/acprof:oso/9780198522379.003.0003.

Devendrabuddhi. "*Pramāṇavārttikapañjikā, Tshad ma rnam 'grel kyi dka' 'grel." In *Sde dge bstan 'gyur*. Ed. Tshul khrims rin chen, Trans. Subhutiśrī and Dge ba'i blo gros, Toh. no. 4217., Tshad ma, che:1b–326b. Delhi: Delhi Karmapae Choedhey, Gyalwae Sungrab Partun Khang, 1744.

Dge 'dun grub. "Tshad ma'i bstan bcos chen mo rigs pa'i rgyan las mngon sum le'u." In *Dge 'dun grub kyi gsung 'bum*, BDRC W1KG14505. 7:1–503. Lhasa: Ser gtsug nang bstan dpe rnying 'tshol bsdu phyogs sgrig khang, 2011.

Dhammajoti, Kuala Lumpur. *Abhidharma Doctrines and Controversies on Perception*. 3rd ed. Hong Kong: Centre of Buddhist Studies, University of Hong Kong, 2007.

Dharmakīrti. *Pramāṇavārttika of Acharya Dharmakirtti: With the Commentary "Vritti" of Acharya Manorathanandin*. Ed. Dvārikādāsa Śāstrī. Bauddha Bharati Series 3. Varanasi: Bauddha Bharati, 1968.

——. *Pramāṇavarttika-kārikā: (Sanskrit and Tibetan)*. Ed. Yūshō Miyasaka. Vol. 2. Acta Indologica. Narita: Naritasan Shinshōji, 1972.

——. "*Pramāṇavārttikakārikā, Tshad ma rnam 'grel gyi tshig le'ur byas pa." In *Sde dge bstan 'gyur*. Ed. Tshul khrims rin chen, Toh. no. 4210., Tshad ma, ce:94a–151b. Delhi: Delhi Karmapae Choedhey, Gyalwae Sungrab Partun Khang, 1744.

——. "*Pramāṇavārttikavṛtti, Tshad ma rnam 'grel gyi 'grel pa." In *Sde dge bstan 'gyur*. Ed. Tshul khrims rin chen, Toh. no. 4216., Tshad ma, ce:261b–365a. Delhi: Delhi Karmapae Choedhey, Gyalwae Sungrab Partun Khang, 1744.

——. "*Pramāṇaviniścaya, Tshad ma rnam par nges pa." In *Sde dge bstan 'gyur*. Ed. Tshul khrims rin chen, Toh. no. 4211, Tshad ma, ce:152a–230b. Delhi: Delhi Karmapae Choedhey, Gyalwae Sungrab Partun Khang, 1744.

——. "*Saṃtānāntarasiddhi, Rgyud gzhan grub pa zhes bya ba'i rab tu byed pa." In *Sde dge bstan 'gyur*. Ed. Tshul khrims rin chen, Toh. no. 4219., Tshad ma, ce:355b–59. Delhi: Delhi Karmapae Choedhey, Gyalwae Sungrab Partun Khang, 1744. http://gretil.sub.uni-goettingen.de/gretil/1_sanskr/6_sastra/3_phil/buddh/bsa059_u.htm.

——. *The Pramanavarttikam of Dharmakīrti: The First Chapter with the Autocommentary*. Ed. Raniero Gnoli. Roma: Instituto Italiano per il Medio ed Estremo Oriente, 1960.

Dharmakīrti, Dharmottara, and Durvekamiśra. *Paṇḍita Durveka Miśra's Dharmottarapradīpa: Being a Subcommentary on Dharmottara's Nyāyabinduṭīkā, a Commentary on Dharmakīrti's Nyāyabindu*. Ed. Dalasukha Bhāī Mālavaṇiyā. Patna: Kashi Prasad Jayaswal Research Institute, 1971.

Dharmakīrti and Vinītadeva. *Santānāntarasiddhiḥ of Ācārya Dharmakīrti and Santānāntarasiddhiḥ Ṭīkā of Ācārya Vinītadeva: Restored and Ed. J. S. Negi*. Ed. J. S. Negi. Bibliotheca Indo Tibetica Series 37. Varanasi: Central Institute of Higher Tibetan Studies, 1997.

Dignāga. *Dignaga: On Perception, Being the Pratyakṣapariccheda of Dignaga's Pramāṇasamuccaya from the Sanskrit Fragments and the Tibetan Versions*. Ed. and trans. Masaaki Hattori. Harvard Oriental Series 47. Cambridge, MA: Harvard University Press, 1968.

——. *Dignāga's Pramāṇasamuccaya, Chapter 1: A Hypothetical Reconstruction of the Sanskrit Text with the Help of the Two Tibetan Translations on the Basis of the Hitherto Known Sanskrit Fragments and the Linguistic Materials Gained from Jinendrabuddhi's Ṭīkā*. Ed. Ernst Steinkellner. Vienna: Österreichische Akademie der Wissenschaften, 2005.

——. "*Pramāṇasamuccaya, Tshad ma kun las btus pa zhes bya ba'i rab tu byed pa." In *Sde dge bstan 'gyur*. Ed. Tshul khrims rin chen, Toh. no. 4203. Tshad ma, ce:1a–13b. Delhi: Delhi Karmapae Choedhey, Gyalwae Sungrab Partun Khang, 1744.

——. "*Pramāṇasamuccayavṛtti, Tshad ma kun las btus pa'i 'grel pa." In *Sde dge bstan 'gyur*. Ed. Tshul khrims rin chen, Trans. Vasudhararakṣita and Zha ma seng rgyal, Toh. no. 4204. Tshad ma, ce:14a–85a. Delhi: Delhi Karmapae Choedhey, Gyalwae Sungrab Partun Khang, 1744.

Dreyfus, Georges B. J. *Recognizing Reality: Dharmakīrti's Philosophy and Its Tibetan Interpretations*. SUNY Series in Buddhist Studies. Albany: State University of New York Press, 1997.

Duckworth, Douglas S. *Mipam on Buddha-Nature: The Ground of the Nyingma Tradition*. Albany: State University of New York Press, 2008.

Dundas, Paul. "Haribhadra." *Brill's Encyclopedia of Jainism Online*, February 14, 2020. https://referenceworks.brillonline.com/entries/brill-s-encyclopedia-of-jainism-online/haribhadra-COM_034908.

Dunne, John D. *Foundations of Dharmakīrti's Philosophy*. 1st ed. Boston: Wisdom, 2004.

——. "Key Features of Dharmakīrti's Apoha Theory." In *Apoha: Buddhist Nominalism and Human Cognition*. Ed. Mark Siderits, Tom Tillemans, and Arindam Chakrabarti, 84–108. Columbia University Press, 2011.

——. "Pac-Man to the Rescue? Conceptuality and Non-Conceptuality in the Dharmakīrtian Theory of Pseudo-Perception." *Philosophy East & West* 70, no. 3 (2020): 571–93. https://doi.org/10.1353/pew.2020.0045.

——. "Realizing the Unreal: Dharmakīrti's Theory of Yogic Perception." *Journal of Indian Philosophy* 34, no. 6 (2007): 497–519. https://doi.org/10.1007/s10781-006-9008-y.

Eck, Diana L. *Darśan: Seeing the Divine Image in India*. 3rd ed. New York: Columbia University Press, 1998.

Eckel, Malcolm David. *Bhāviveka and His Buddhist Opponents*. Harvard Oriental Series, vol. 70. Cambridge, MA: Harvard University Department of Sanskrit and Indian Studies, 2008.

Eltschinger, Vincent. *Can the Veda Speak? Dharmakīrti Against Mīmāṃsā Exegetics and Vedic Authority: An Annotated Translation of PVSV 164,24–176,16*. Ed. Helmut Krasser and John Taber. Vienna: Verlag der Österreichischen Akademie der Wissenschaften, 2012.

——. "On the Career and the Cognition of Yogins." In *Yogic Perception, Meditation and Altered States of Consciousness*. Ed. Eli Franco and Dagmar Eigner, 169–213. Vienna: Verlag der Österreichischen Akademie der Wissenschaften, 2009.

Ferrante, Marco. "On Ṛṣis and Yogins: Immediate and Mediate Extraordinary Cognitions in Early Brahmanical Thought." *Proceedings of the Meeting of the Italian Association of Sanskrit Studies* 89 (2016): 41–62.

Forer, Bertram R. "The Fallacy of Personal Validation: A Classroom Demonstration of Gullibility." *The Journal of Abnormal and Social Psychology* 44, no. 1 (1949): 118–23. https://doi.org/10.1037/h0059240.

Forman, Jed. "Believing Is Seeing: A Buddhist Theory of Creditions." *Frontiers in Psychology* 13 (August 3, 2022): 938731. https://doi.org/10.3389/fpsyg.2022.938731.

——. "Developing Good Taste: Jñānaśrīmitra's Theory of Imagination and Aesthetic Epistemology." In *The Imagination and Imaginal Worlds in the Mirror of Buddhism*. Eds. Karin Meyers and Hugh Joswick, eds. Berkeley: Mangalam Press, forthcoming.

——. "Double Hiddenness: Governmentality and Subjectivization in Gelug Buddhism." *Critical Research on Religion*, 2021, 1–15. https://doi.org/10.1177/2050303220986985.

——. "Subtle, Hidden, and Far-Off: The Intertextuality of the Yogasūtras." *The Journal of Hindu Studies*, April 10, 2023, 1–24. https://doi.org/10.1093/jhs/hiad013.

——. "Timeless Visions: Prajñākaragupta on Futureless Precognition and Temporal Intuitions." In *The Handbook of Intuitions*. Logic, Epistemology, and the Unity of Sciences. New York: Springer, forthcoming.

——. "Tsongkhapa's Difficult Point: Saying What Cannot be Said about Particulars, Universals, and Relations." Paper presented at the American Philosophical Association Pacific Conference, Portland, OR, March 22, 2024.

——. "What Is the World? Neckties, Ghosts, Falling Hairs, and Celestial Cities in a Coherentist Epistemology." *Philosophy East and West* 70, no. 4 (2020): 906–31. https://doi.org/10.1353/pew.2020.0066.

Franco, Eli. *Dharmakīrti on Compassion and Rebirth*. Vienna: Arbeitskreis für Tibetische und Buddhistische Studien, Universität Wien, 1997.

——. "Did Dignāga Accept Four Types of Perception?" *Journal of Indian Philosophy* 21, no. 3 (1993): 295–99.

——. "Once Again on Dharmakīrti's Deviation from Dignāga on 'Pratyakṣâbhāsa.'" *Journal of Indian Philosophy* 14, no. 1 (1986): 79–97.

——. "Variant Readings from Tucci's Photographs of the Yoginirṇayaprakaraṇa Manuscript." In *Sanskrit Texts from Giuseppe Tucci's Collection*, 157–86. Rome: Istituto italiano per l'Africa e l'Oriente, 2008.

Feer, Léon, and Caroline A. F. Rhys Davids, eds. *Saṃyutta-nikāya*. 5 vols. London: Pali Text Society, 1960.

Fricker, Elizabeth. "Against Gullibility." In *Knowing from Words: Western and Indian Philosophical Analysis of Understanding and Testimony*. Ed. Bimal Krishna Matilal and Arindam Chakrabarti, 125–61. Dordrecht: Kluwer Academic, 1994.

——. "Trusting Others in the Sciences: A Priori or Empirical Warrant." *Studies in History and Philosophy of Science* 33, no. 2 (2002): 373–83. https://doi.org/10.1016/S0039-3681(02)00006-7.

Funayama, Toru. "Kamalaśīla's View on Yogic Perception and the Bodhisattva Path." In *Religion and Logic in Buddhist Philosophical Analysis: Proceedings of the Fourth International Dharmakirti Conference, Vienna, August 23-27, 2005*. Ed. Helmut Krasser, Horst

Lasic, Eli Franco, and Birgit Kellner, 99–111. Vienna: Verlag der Österreichischen Akademie der Wissenschaften, 2011.
Gadamer, Hans-Georg. *Truth and Method*. Trans. Joel Weinsheimer and Donald G. Marshall. 2nd, rev. ed ed. Continuum Impacts. New York: Continuum, 2004.
Garfield, Jay L. "Practicing Without a License and Making Trouble Along the Way: My Life in Buddhist Studies." 2018. https://jaygarfield.files.wordpress.com/2018/10/practicing-without-a-license.pdf.
——. *The Concealed Influence of Custom: Hume's Treatise From the Inside Out*. New York: Oxford University Press, 2019.
Garfield, Jay L., and Georges B. J. Dreyfus. "The Madhyamaka Contribution to Skepticism." Unpublished manuscript, 2017.
Gašpar, Veronika Nela. "Le apparizioni mariane nel nostro tempo. Il significato e i criteri del discernimento nella teologia." *IKON* 6 (2013): 17–26.
Gelfert, Axel. "Hume on Testimony Revisited." *History of Philosophy & Logical Analysis* 13, no. 1 (April 5, 2010): 60–75. https://doi.org/10.30965/26664275-01301004.
George, Alexander. *The Everlasting Check: Hume on Miracles*. Cambridge, MA: Harvard University Press, 2016.
Gethin, Rupert. *The Foundations of Buddhism*. Oxford: Oxford University Press, 1998.
Gifford, Mark. "Aristotle on Platonic Recollection and the Paradox of Knowing Universals: Prior Analytics B.21 67a8-30." *Phronesis* 44, no. 1 (February 1999): 1–29. https://doi.org/10.1163/156852899762447610.
Glazebrook, Trish. "Heidegger and Ecofeminism." In *Feminist Interpretations of Martin Heidegger*. Ed. Nancy J. Holland and Patricia J. Huntington, 221–51. Re-Reading the Canon. University Park: Pennsylvania State University Press, 2001.
Go bo rab 'byams pa. *Freedom from Extremes: Gorampa's "Distinguishing the Views" and The Polemics of Emptiness*. Trans. José Ignacio Cabezón and Lobsang Dargyay. Studies in Indian and Tibetan Buddhism. Boston: Wisdom, 2007.
——. "Rgyas pa'i bstan bcos tshad ma rnam 'grel gyi rnam par bshad pa kun tu bzang po'i 'od zer." In *Kun mkhyen go rams pa bsod nams seng+ge'i gsung 'bum*, BDRC W1KG16651. 1:68–568. Beijing: Krung go'i bod rig pa dpe skrun khang, 2013.
——. "Rgyas pa'i bstan bcos tshad ma rnam 'grel gyi rnam par bshad pa kun tu bzang po'i 'od zer: Mngon sum le'u." In *The Collection of the Eighteen Renowned Scriptures: Root Texts and Commentaries*. Ed. Sachen International. Kathmandu: Sachen International, 2011.
——. "Rgyas pa'i bstan bcos tshad ma rnam 'grel gyi rnam par bshad pa kun tu bzang po'i 'od zer: Mngon sum le'u." In *Kun mkhyen go rams pa bsod nams seng+ge'i gsung 'bum*, BDRC W1PD1725. 1:479–759. Derge: Dzong sar khams bye'i slob gling, 2014.
——. "Tshad ma rigs pa'i gter gyi don gsal." In *The Collection of the Eighteen Renowned Scriptures: Root Texts and Commentaries*. Ed. Sachen International. Kathmandu: Sachen International, 2011.
Gokhale, Pradeep P. *The Yogasutra of Patañjali: A New Introduction to the Buddhist Roots of the Yoga System*. London: Routledge, 2020.
Goldberg, Robert F., and Sharon L. Thompson-Schill. "Developmental 'Roots' in Mature Biological Knowledge." *Psychological Science* 20, no. 4 (April 1, 2009): 480–87. https://doi.org/10.1111/j.1467-9280.2009.02320.x.

Goldman, Alvin I. "Experts: Which Ones Should You Trust?" *Philosophy and Phenomenological Research* 63, no. 1 (July 2001): 85–110. https://doi.org/10.1111/j.1933-1592.2001.tb00093.x.

——. *Pathways to Knowledge: Private and Public*. Oxford: Oxford University Press, 2002.

Gonda, Jan. *Eye and Gaze in the Veda*. Amsterdam: North Holland Publishing Company, 1969.

Grimby, A. "Bereavement Among Elderly People: Grief Reactions, Post-Bereavement Hallucinations and Quality of Life." *Acta Psychiatrica Scandinavica* 87, no. 1 (1993): 72–80.

Guterstam, Arvid, Hope H Kean, Taylor W Webb, Faith S Kean, and Michael S. A Graziano. "Implicit Model of Other People's Visual Attention as an Invisible, Force-Carrying Beam Projecting From the Eyes." *Proceedings of the National Academy of Sciences—PNAS* 116, no. 1 (2019): 328–33. https://doi.org/10.1073/pnas.1816581115.

Haack, Susan. *Evidence and Inquiry: Towards Reconstruction in Epistemology*. Cambridge, MA: Blackwell, 1993.

Hadjikhani, Nouchine, Rick Hoge, Josh Snyder, and Beatrice de Gelder. "Pointing with the Eyes: The Role of Gaze in Communicating Danger." *Brain and Cognition* 68, no. 1 (2008): 1–8. https://doi.org/10.1016/j.bandc.2008.01.008.

Hall, Harrison. "The Other Minds Problem in Early Heidegger." *Human Studies : A Journal for Philosophy and the Social Sciences* 3, no. 1 (1980): 247–54. https://doi.org/10.1007/BF02331812.

Haribhadrasūri. *The Śāstravārtāsamuccaya: With Hindi Translation, Notes and Introduction*. Ed. Jitendra B. Shah. Trans. Krsna Kumara Diksita. Lalbhai Dalpatbhai Series 22. Ahmedabad: Lalbhai Dalpatbhai Bharatiya Sanskriti Vidyamandira, 1969.

Haribhadrasūri and Municandrasūri. *Anekāntajayapatākā by Haribhadra Sūri with His Own Commentary and Municandra Sūri's Supercommentary*. Ed. H. R. Kapadia. 2 vols. Baroda: Oriental Institute, 1947.

Hartle, James B. *Gravity: An Introduction to Einstein's General Relativity*. 1st ed. Harlow, UK: Pearson, 2014.

Haugeland, John, and Joseph Rouse. *Dasein Disclosed: John Haugeland's Heidegger*. Cambridge, MA: Harvard University Press, 2013.

Heidegger, Martin. *Being and Time*. Trans. John Macquarrie and Edward Robinson. Cambridge, MA: Blackwell, 2001.

Hellwig, Oliver, ed. *Matsyapurāṇa, 1-176*. Göttingen: Göttingen Register of Electronic Texts in Indian Languages (GRETIL), 2020. http://gretil.sub.uni-goettingen.de/gretil/corpustei/transformations/html/sa_matsyapurANa1-176.htm.

Hemacandra. *Pramāṇamīmāṃsā: With the Commentary Pramāṇamīmāṃsāvṛtti*. Ed. Sukhlalji Saṅghavi. Ahmedabad: The Sañcālaka-Siṅghī Jaina Granthamālā, 2016.

Ho, Chien-Hsing. "Saying the Unsayable." *Philosophy East and West* 56, no. 3 (2006): 409–27.

Hota, K. N. "Is Sense-Organ Prāpyakārin in Perception?" *Bulletin of the Deccan College Research Institute* 75 (2015): 255–62.

Hugon, Pascale. "Proving Emptiness: The Epistemological Background for the 'Neither One Nor Many' Argument and the Nature of Its Probandum in Phya Pa Chos Kyi Seng Ge's Works." *Journal of Buddhist Philosophy* 1, no. 1 (2015): 58–94. https://doi.org/10.1353/jbp.2015.0006.

Hume, David. *An Enquiry Concerning Human Understanding*. Ed. Tom L. Beauchamp. Oxford Philosophical Texts. Oxford: Oxford University Press, 1999.

——. *Essays, Moral, Political, and Literary*. Ed. Eugene F. Miller. Rev. ed. Indianapolis: LibertyClassics, 1987.

Husserl, Edmund. *The Crisis of European Sciences and Transcendental Phenomenology: An Introduction to Phenomenological Philosophy*. Trans. David Carr. 6th printing. Studies in Phenomenology & Existential Philosophy. Evanston, IL: Northwestern University Press, 1984.

Jaimini and Śabarasvāmī. *The Aphorisms of the Mīmāmsa with the Commentary of Sāvarasvāmin*. Ed. Maheśacandra Bhaṭṭācārya. Bibliotheca Indica 45. Calcutta: Asiatic Society of Bengal, 1873.

Jampa Tegchok and Steve Carlier. *Insight into Emptiness*. Edited by Thubten Chodron. Boston: Wisdom Publications, 2012.

James, William. "The Will to Believe." In *William James: Writings 1878–1899: Psychology: Briefer Course, The Will to Believe, Talks to Teachers and Students, and Essays*, 457–79. New York: Library of America, 1992.

Jayanta Bhaṭṭa. *Nyāyamañjarī of Jayanta Bhaṭṭa with the Commentary of Granthibhaṅga by Cakradhara*. 2 vols. Ed. Gaurinath Sastri. Varanasi: Sampurnanand Sanskrit Vishvavidyalaya, 1982.

Jena, Siddheswar, ed. *[Śrīnarasiṃhapurāṇam] = The Narasiṃha Purāṇam: Text with English Translation and Notes*. Delhi: Nag Publishers, 1987.

Jina. "*Pramāṇavārttikālaṃkāraṭīkā, Tshad ma rnam 'grel gyi rgyan gyi 'grel bshad." In *Sde 'dge bstan 'gyur*. Ed. Tshul khrims rin chen, Trans. Sridipamkararakṣita and Man hor byang chub shes rab, Toh. 4222, Tshad ma, de:1b–365a. Delhi: Delhi Karmapae Choedhey, Gyalwae Sungrab Partun Khang, 1982.

Jinpa, Thupten. "Tsongkhapa's Qualms about Early Tibetan Interpretations of Madhyamaka Philosophy." *The Tibet Journal* 24, no. 2 (1999): 3–28.

Jñānaśrīmitra. "Yoginirṇayaprakaraṇa." In *Jñānaśrīmitranibandhavāli: Buddhist Philosophical Works of Jñānaśrīmitra*. Ed. Anantalāla Ṭhakkura, 2nd. ed., 324–43. Patna: Kashi Prasad Jayaswal Research Institute, 1987.

Jones, Karen. "The Politics of Credibility." In *A Mind of One's Own: Feminist Essays on Reason and Objectivity*. Ed. Louise M. Antony and Charlotte Witt, 2nd ed., 154–76. Feminist Theory and Politics. Boulder, CO: Westview Press, 2001.

Jong, J. W. de. "Book Review: Outline of Indian Philosophy." *Indo-Iranian Journal* 16, no. 2 (1974): 147–49.

Kajiyama, Yūichi. "Controversy between the Sākāra- and Nirākāra-Vādins of the Yogācāra School—Some Materials." *Journal of Indian and Buddhist Studies (Indogaku Bukkyogaku Kenkyu)* 14, no. 1 (1965): 429–418. https://doi.org/10.4259/ibk.14.429.

Kamalaśīla. *Bhāvanākramaḥ of Ācārya Kamalaśīla*. Ed. Gyaktsen Namdol. Varanasi: Central Institute of Higher Tibetan Studies, 1984.

Kambala. *A Garland of Light: Kambala's Ālokamālā*. Trans. Christian Lindtner. Fremont, CA: Asian Humanities Press, 2003.

Kaṇāda, Praśastapāda, and Udayana. *The Aphorisms of the Vaiśeshika Philosophy by Kaṇâda, with the Commentary of Praśastapâda, and the Gloss of Udayanâchârya*. Ed. Vindhyeśvarīprasāda Dvivedī. Varanasi: Braj Bhushan Das, 1919.

Kanai, Ryota, Yutaka Komura, Stewart Shipp, and Karl Friston. "Cerebral Hierarchies: Predictive Processing, Precision and the Pulvinar." *Philosophical Transactions of the Royal Society B: Biological Sciences* 370, no. 1668 (May 19, 2015): 20140169. https://doi.org/10.1098/rstb.2014.0169.

Kant, Immanuel. *Critique of Pure Reason*. Trans. Paul Guyer and Allen W Wood. Cambridge: Cambridge University Press, 1998.

Keller, Pierre. *Husserl and Heidegger on Human Experience*. Cambridge: Cambridge University Press, 1999.

Kerwer, Martin, and Tom Rosman. "Epistemic Change and Diverging Information: How Do Prior Epistemic Beliefs Affect the Efficacy of Short-Term Interventions?" *Learning and Individual Differences* 80 (2020). https://doi.org/10.1016/j.lindif.2020.101886.

King, Richard. *Indian Philosophy: An Introduction to Hindu and Buddhist Thought*. Washington, DC: Georgetown University Press, 1999.

Klaczynski, Paul A, and Kristen L Lavallee. "Domain-Specific Identity, Epistemic Regulation, and Intellectual Ability as Predictors of Belief-Biased Reasoning: A Dual-Process Perspective." *Journal of Experimental Child Psychology* 92, no. 1 (2005): 1–24. https://doi.org/10.1016/j.jecp.2005.05.001.

Kumāra, Śaśiprabhā. *Categories, Creation and Cognition in Vaisesika Philosophy*. New York: Springer Berlin Heidelberg, 2018.

Kumārila Bhaṭṭa and Sucaritamiśra. *The Mîmâmsāślokavârtika with the Commentary Kāśikā of Sucaritamiśra*. Ed. K. Sambasiva Sastri. Trivandrum Sanskrit Series 99. Trivandrum: Superintendent, Gov. Press, 1929.

Kundakunda, Amrṛtacandra, and Jayasena. *Srī Kundakundācārya's Pravacanasāra (Pavayaṇasāra): A Pro-canonical Text of the Jainas*. Ed. and trans. A. N. Upādhye. Agas: Srimad Rajachandra Ashrama, 1964.

Kun dga' rgyal mtshan. "Tshad ma rigs pa'i gter gyi rang 'grel." In *Tshad ma'i 'grel pa phyogs bsgrigs*, 7:3–481. Rdzong sar khams bye: Rdzong sar khams bye'i slob gling thub bstan dar rgyas gling, 2009.

Lackey, Jennifer. *Learning From Words: Testimony as a Source of Knowledge*. Oxford: Oxford University Press, 2008.

Lakoff, George. *Women, Fire, and Dangerous Things: What Categories Reveal About the Mind*. Chicago: University of Chicago Press, 1990.

Lakoff, George, and Mark Johnson. *Metaphors We Live By*. Chicago: University of Chicago Press, 2003.

Lane, Jonathan D., Henry M. Wellman, and E. Margaret Evans. "Sociocultural Input Facilitates Children's Developing Understanding of Extraordinary Minds." *Child Development* 83, no. 3 (2012): 1007–21. https://doi.org/10.1111/j.1467-8624.2012.01741.x.

Laruelle, François. *Dictionary of Non-Philosophy*. Trans. Taylor Adkins. First edition. Univocal. Minneapolis, MN: Univocal, 2013.

——. *Principles of Non-Philosophy*. Trans. Nicola Rubczak and Anthony Paul Smith. London: Bloomsbury, 2013.

——. *Une biographie de l'homme ordinaire: Des autorités et des minorités*. Collection Analyse et raisons. Paris: Aubier, 1985.

Laruelle, François, and Philippe Petit. *Intellectuals and Power: The Insurrection of the Victim*. Trans. Anthony Paul Smith. Wiley, Polity Press, 2015.

Levinas, Emmanuel. *Totality and Infinity: An Essay on Exteriority*. Martinus Nijhoff Philosophy Texts, vol. 1. The Hague: Martinus Nijhoff Publishers, 1979.

Lhun-grub-bsod-pa, and Jeffrey Hopkins. *Cutting through Appearances: The Practice and Theory of Tibetan Buddhism*. 2nd. ed. Ithaca, NY: Snow Lion Publications, 1989.

Lightman, Alan. *Searching for Stars on an Island in Maine*. New York: Knopf Doubleday, 2018.

Lingis, Alphonso. "The First Person Singular: Missteps on Heidegger's Path." *Philosophy Today* 61, no. 1 (2017): 85–97. https://doi.org/10.5840/philtoday2017320148.

Livingston, Paul M. *The Politics of Logic: Badiou, Wittgenstein, and the Consequences of Formalism*. Routledge Studies in Contemporary Philosophy 27. New York: Routledge, 2012.

Locke, John. *An Essay Concerning Humane Understanding, Volume 2MDCXC, Based on the 2nd Edition, Books 3 and 4*. Ed. Steve Harris and David Widger. Chapel Hill, NC: Project Gutenberg, 2004.

Lorenzen, David N. "Who Invented Hinduism?" *Comparative Studies in Society and History* 41, no. 4 (1999): 630–59.

Lusthaus, Dan. "A Pre-Dharmakīrti Indian Discussion of Dignāga Preserved in Chinese Translation: The Buddhabhūmy-Upadeśa." *Journal of Buddhist Studies* 6 (2009): 19–81.

MacDonald, Anne. "Knowing Nothing: Candrakīrti and Yogic Perception." In *Yogic Perception, Meditation and Altered States of Consciousness*. Ed. Eli Franco and Dagmar Eigner, 133–68. Vienna: Verlag der Österreichischen Akademie der Wissenschaften, 2009.

Maṇḍanamiśra and Vācaspatimiśra. *Vidhiviveka of Śrī Maṇḍana Miśra: With the Commentary Nyāyakaṇikā of Vāchaspati Miśra*. Ed. Mahāprabhu Lāla Gosvāmī. Varanasi: Tara Publications, 1978.

McClintock, Sara L. "Knowing All Through Knowing One: Mystical Communion or Logical Trick in the Tattvasaṃgraha and Tattvasaṃgrahapañjikā." *Journal of the International Association of Buddhist Studies* 23, no. 2 (2000).

——. *Omniscience and the Rhetoric of Reason: Śāntarakṣita and Kamalaśīla on Rationality, Argumentation, and Religious Authority*. Boston: Wisdom, 2010.

McCrea, Lawrence J., and Parimal G. Patil. *Buddhist Philosophy of Language in India: Jñānaśrīmitra on Exclusion*. New York: Columbia University Press, 2010.

McCullin, Irene. *Time and the Shared World: Heidegger on Social Relations*. Northwestern University Studies in Phenomenology and Existential Philosophy. Evanston, IL: Northwestern University Press, 2013.

McDowell, John. "Gadamer and Davidson on Understanding and Relativism." In *Gadamer's Century: Essays in Honor of Hans-Georg Gadamer*. Ed. Hans-Georg Gadamer, Jeff Malpas, Ulrich Arnswald, and Jens Kertscher, 173–94. Studies in Contemporary German Social Thought. Cambridge, Mass: MIT Press, 2002.

McMyler, Benjamin. *Testimony, Trust, and Authority*. Oxford: Oxford University Press, 2011.

Mealor, Andy D, Julia Simner, and Jamie Ward. "Does Synaesthesia Protect against Age-Related Memory Loss?" *Journal of Neuropsychology* 14, no. 2 (2020): 197–212. https://doi.org/10.1111/jnp.12182.

Merleau-Ponty, Maurice. *Phenomenology of Perception*. Trans. Colin Smith. Routledge Classics. London: Routledge, 2002.

Mi pham rgya mtsho. *The Wisdom Chapter: Jamgön Mipham's Commentary on the Ninth Chapter of "The Way of the Bodhisattva."* Trans. Padmakara Translation Group. 1st ed. Boulder, CO: Shambhala, 2017.

Middleton, Chad A., and Michael Langston. "Circular Orbits on a Warped Spandex Fabric." *American Journal of Physics* 82, no. 4 (April 2014): 287–94. https://doi.org/10.1119/1.4848635.

Mikogami, Esho. "Some Remarks on the Concept of Arthakriyā." *Journal of Indian Philosophy* 7, no. 1 (1979): 79–94.

Mill, John Stuart. *A System of Logic, Ratiocinative and Inductive; Being a Connected View of the Principles of Evidence, and the Methods of Scientific Investigation*. Ed. J. M. Robson. 2 vols. Toronto: University of Toronto Press, 1973.

Mills, Ethan. "On the Coherence of Dignāga's Epistemology: Evaluating the Critiques of Candrakīrti and Jayarāśi." *Asian Philosophy* 25, no. 4 (October 2, 2015): 339–57. https://doi.org/10.1080/09552367.2015.1102694.

Mishra, Jwala Prasad, ed. *Śiva Māhapurāṇa*. Vol. 1. Mumbai: Sri Venkateswar Steam Press, 1920.

Mkhas grub dge legs dpal bzang po. "Tshad ma rnam 'grel gyi mngon sum le'u rgya cher bshad pa." In *Mkhas grub thams cad mkhyen pa dge legs dpal bzang gi gsung 'bum*, 33:1–298. Mundgod, India: Rje yab sras gsum gyi gsung 'bum sdud sgrig khang, 2019.

Mookerjee, Satkari. *The Buddhist Philosophy of Universal Flux. An Exposition of the Philosophy of Critical Realism as Expounded by the School of Dignāga*. Calcutta: University of Calcutta, 1935.

Moore, G. E. "Visual Sense-Data." In *British Philosophy in the Mid-Century*. Ed. J. H. Muirhead, 130–37. George Allen and Unwin, 1957. https://doi.org/10.1525/9780520315167-008.

Moriyama, Shinya. "On Self-Awareness in the Sautrāntika Epistemology." *Journal of Indian Philosophy* 38, no. 3 (2010): 261–77.

——. "Pramāṇapariśuddhasakalatattvajña, Sarvajña and Sarvasarvajña." In *Religion and Logic in Buddhist Philosophical Analysis Proceedings of the Fourth International Dharmakīrti Conference Vienna, August 23–27, 2005*. Ed. Helmut Krasser, Horst Lasic, Eli Franco, and Birgit Kellner, 329–39. Vienna: Verlag der Österreichischen Akademie der Wissenschaften, 2011.

——. "The Reliability of Yogic Perception for Dharmakīrti, Prajñākaragupta and Jñānaśrīmitra." In *To the Heart of Truth: Felicitation Volume for Eli Franco on the Occasion of His Seventieth Birthday*. Ed. Hiroko Matsuoka, Shinya Moriyama, and Tyler Neill, 1:565–89. Wiener Studien Zur Tibetologie Und Buddhismuskunde, Heft 104. Wien: Arbeitskreis für Tibetische und Buddhistische Studien Universität Wien, 2023.

Muis, Krista R., Lisa D. Bendixen, and Florian C. Haerle. "Domain-Generality and Domain-Specificity in Personal Epistemology Research: Philosophical and

Empirical Reflections in the Development of a Theoretical Framework." *Educational Psychology Review* 18, no. 1 (2006): 3–54.

Mulvey, Laura. "Visual Pleasure and Narrative Cinema." *Screen* 16, no. 3 (September 1, 1975): 6–18. https://doi.org/10.1093/screen/16.3.6.

Mundra, Anil. "Engaging Religious Difference: The Case of Haribhadrasūri." Santa Barbara: University of California, Santa Barbara, 2023.

Nāgārjuna and Candrakīrti. *Madhyamakasāstra of Nāgārjuna with the Commentary: Prasannapadā by Candrakīrti*. Ed. Paraśurāma Lakshmaṇa Vaidya. Buddhist Sanskrit Texts 10. Darbhanga: Mithila Institute, 1960.

——. *Mūlamadhyamakakārikās (Mādhyamikasūtras) de Nāgārjuna Avec Le Prasannapadā Commentaire de Candrakīrti*. Ed. Louis de la Valle Poussin. Bibliotheca Buddhica IV. Saint Petersburg: l'Académie Imperiale des sciences, 1903.

Ñāṇamoli Thera and Bodhi Bhikkhu, eds. *The Middle Length Discourses of the Buddha: A [New] Translation of the Majjhima Nikāya*. 4. ed. Boston: Wisdom, 2009.

Novalis. "Fragments from the Notebooks." In *The Early Political Writings of The German Romantics*. Ed. and trans. Frederick C. Beiser, 81–92. Repr. Cambridge Texts in the History of Political Thought. Cambridge: Cambridge University Press, 1999.

Ó Maoilearca, John. *All Thoughts Are Equal: Laruelle and Nonhuman Philosophy*. Minneapolis: University of Minnesota Press, 2015.

O'Brien, Dan. *Hume on Testimony*. 1st ed. New York: Routledge, 2023.

Ono, Motoi. "Prajñākaragupta's Interpretation of Dharmakīrti's Two Definitions of Pramāṇa: A Reconsideration Based on the Newly Discovered Sanskrit Manuscript of Yamāri's Commentary." In *To the Heart of Truth: Felicitation Volume for Eli Franco on the Occasion of His Seventieth Birthday*. Ed. Hiroko Matsuoka, Shinya Moriyama, and Tyler Neill, 1:591–617. Wiener Studien Zur Tibetologie Und Buddhismuskunde, Heft 104. Wien: Arbeitskreis für Tibetische und Buddhistische Studien Universität Wien, 2023.

Pantañjali. *Pantañjali's Yoga-Sūtras with the Yoga-Bhāṣya Attributed to Veda-Vyāsa and the Explanation Entitled Tattva-Vāiçāradī of Vacaspati-Miçra and the Brief Explanation of Bālarāma*. Ed. Svāmi Bālarāma of Saṁvat. Varanasi: Svāmi Bālarāma of Saṁvat, 1908.

——. *Patañjali's Yoga Sūtra*. Trans. Shyam Ranganathan. London: Penguin, 2009.

——. *Pātañjali's Yoga Sūtras: With the Commentary of Vyāsa and the Gloss of Vāchaspati Miśra*. Trans. Rāma Prasāda. New Delhi: Munshiram Manoharlal, 1998.

——. *The Complete Commentary by Śaṅkara on the Yoga Sūtras: A Full Translation of the Newly Discovered Text*. Trans. Trevor Leggett. London: Kegan Paul International, 1990.

Peirce, Charles Sanders. *Philosophical Writings of Peirce*. Ed. Justus Buchler. New York: Dover Publications, 1955.

Pemwieser, Monkia. "Materialien Zur Theorie Der Yogischen Erkenntnis Im Buddhismus." Masters thesis, University of Vienna, 1991.

Phya pa chos kyi seng ge. *Dbu ma shar gsum gyi stong thun*. Ed. Helmut Tauscher. Vienna: Arbeitskreis für Tibetische und Buddhistische Studien, Universität Wien, 1999.

Piaget, Jean. *The Child's Conception of the World*. Trans. Joan Tomlinson and Andrew Tomlinson. London: Routledge & Kegan Paul Ltd., 1971.

Picascia, Rosanna. "Our Epistemic Dependence on Others: Nyāya and Buddhist Accounts of Testimony as a Source of Knowledge." *Journal of Hindu Studies*, April 18, 2023, hiad003. https://doi.org/10.1093/jhs/hiad003.

Pietersen, H. J. "Western Humanism, African Humanism and Work Organisations." *SA Journal of Industrial Psychology* 31, no. 3 (October 29, 2005). https://doi.org/10.4102/sajip.v31i3.209.

Pilasse, Chandaratana. "Divergent Doctrinal Interpretations on the Nature of Mind and Matter in Theravāda Abhidhamma: A Study Mainly Based on the Pāli and Siṃhala Buddhist Exegetical Literature." Diss., University of Hong Kong, 2011.

Poleshchuk, Irina. "Heidegger and Levinas: Metaphysics, Ontology and the Horizon of the Other." *Indo-Pacific Journal of Phenomenology* 10, no. 2 (October 2010): 1–10. https://doi.org/10.2989/IPJP.2010.10.2.4.1085.

Powers, John, trans. *Wisdom of Buddha: The Saṁdhinirmocana Sūtra*. Tibetan Translation Series 16. Berkeley, CA: Dharma Publications, 1995.

Prajñākaragupta. *Pramāṇavārtikabhāshyam or Vārtikālaṅkaraḥ of Prajñākaragupta (Being a Commentary on Dharmakīrti's Pramāṇavārtikam)*. Ed. Rāhula Sāṅkṛtyāyana. Patna, India: Kashi Prasad Jayaswal Research Institute, 1943.

——. "*Pramāṇavārttikālaṅkāra, Tshad ma rnam 'grel gyi rgyan." In *Sde dge bstan 'gyur*. Ed. 'Phags pa shes rab, Trans. Paṇḍita skal ldan rgyal po, Blo ldan shes rab, and Paṇḍita Kumāraśrī, Toh. no. 4221., Tshad ma, te:1b–308a. Delhi: Delhi Karmapae Choedhey, Gyalwae Sungrab Partun Khang, 1744.

——. "*Pramāṇavārttikālaṅkāra, Tshad ma rnam 'grel gyi rgyan." In *Sde dge bstan 'gyur*. Ed. 'Phags pa shes rab, Trans. Paṇḍita skal ldan rgyal po, Blo ldan shes rab, and Paṇḍita Kumāraśrī, Toh. no. 4221., Tshad ma, the:1a–282b. Delhi: Delhi Karmapae Choedhey, Gyalwae Sungrab Partun Khang, 1744.

Praśastapāda and Śrīdhara. *Nyāyakandalī: Being a Commentary on Prasastapadabhasya with Three Sub-Commentaries*. Ed. J. S. Jetly and Vasant G. Parikh. Vadodara: Oriental Institute, 1991.

——. *The Praśastapāda Bhāshya, With the Commentary Nyāyakandali of Sridhara*. Ed. Vindhyeśvarīprasāda Dvivedī. 2nd ed. Delhi: Sri Satguru Publications, 1984.

Proudfoot, Wayne. *Religious Experience*. Berkeley: University of California Press, 1985.

Prueitt, Catherine. "Shifting Concepts: The Realignment of Dharmakīrti on Concepts and the Error of Subject/Object Duality in Pratyabhijñā Śaiva Thought." *Journal of Indian Philosophy* 45, no. 1 (2017): 21–47.

Purchok Ngawang Jampa. "Diamond Slivers: A Rejoinder to Taktsang Lotsawa." In *Knowing Illusion Volume: Bringing a Tibetan Debate into Contemporary Discourse*, Trans. Ryan Conlon, Thomas Doctor, Jay L. Garfield, and John Powers, 2:340–406. New York: Oxford University Press, 2021.

Purzycki, Benjamin Grant, and Richard Sosis. *Religion Evolving: Cultural, Cognitive, and Ecological Dynamics*. Advances in the Cognitive Science of Religion. Sheffield, UK: Equinox Publishing Ltd, 2022.

Raffoul, François. "The Question of Responsibility Between Levinas and Heidegger." In *Between Levinas and Heidegger*. Ed. John E. Drabinski and Eric S. Nelson, 175–206. SUNY Series in Contemporary Continental Philosophy. Albany: State University of New York Press, 2014.

Ram-Prasad, C. "Knowledge and Action I: Means to the Human End in Bhāṭṭa Mīmāṃsā and Advaita Vedānta." *Journal of Indian Philosophy* 28, no. 1 (2000): 1–24.

Ratié, Isabelle. *Le soi et l'autre: identité, différence et altérité dans la philosophie de la Pratyabhijñā*. Jerusalem studies in religion and culture, vol. 13. Leiden: Brill, 2011.

Ratnakīrti. "Sarvajñasiddhiḥ." In *Ratnakīrtinibandhavāli: Buddhist Philosophical Works of Ratnakīrti*. Ed. Anantalāla Ṭhakkura, 2nd ed., 1–31. Patna: Kashi Prasad Jayaswal Research Institute, 1975.

Raynaud, Dominique. "Les normes de la rationalité dans une controverse scientifique: le cas de l'optique médiévale." *L'Année sociologique* 48, no. 2 (1998): 447–66.

Richert, Rebekah, Justin L. Barrett, and Roxanne Moore Newman. "When Seeing Is Not Believing: Children's Understanding of Humans' and Non-Humans' Use of Background Knowledge in Interpreting Visual Displays." *Journal of Cognition and Culture* 3, no. 1 (2003): 91–108. https://doi.org/10.1163/156853703321598590.

Ridder, Jeroen de. "How to Trust a Scientist." *Studies in History and Philosophy of Science* 93 (June 2022): 11–20. https://doi.org/10.1016/j.shpsa.2022.02.003.

Rolin, Kristina. "Trust in Science." In *The Routledge Handbook of Trust and Philosophy*. Ed. Judith Simon, 354–66. Routledge Handbooks in Philosophy. London: Routledge, 2020.

Rong ston. "Rigs gter rnam bshad nyi ma'i snying po." In *The Collection of the Eighteen Renowned Scriptures: Root Texts and Commentaries*. Ed. Sachen International. Kathmandu: Sachen International, 2011.

Rosu, Arion. *Les conceptions psychologuqes dans les texts médicaux indiens*. Paris: De Boccard, 1978.

Russell, Bertrand. *Human Knowledge: Its Scope and Limits*. Routledge, 2009. https://doi.org/10.4324/9780203875353.

——. "Letter on Sense-Data [1915]." In *The Philosophy of Logical Atomism and Other Essays, 1914–19*. Ed. John Greer Slater, The McMaster University edition, 87–88. The Collected Papers of Bertrand Russell. London: George Allen & Unwin, 1986.

——. *The Problems of Philosophy*. London: Oxford University Press, 2001.

Saccone, Margherita Serena. "Of Authoritativeness and Perception: The Establishment of an Omniscient Person (Against the Mīmāṃsakas)." In *Wind Horses: Tibetan, Himalayan and Mongolian Studies*. Ed. Giacomella Orofino, 455–83. Napoli: Università degli studi di Napoli "L'Orientale," 2019.

Sacks, Oliver W. *Hallucinations*. New York: Vintage Books, 2013.

Śākya mchog ldan. "Tshad ma rigs pa'i gter gyi dgongs rgyan lung dang rigs pa'i 'khor los lugs ngan pham." In *The Collection of the Eighteen Renowned Scriptures: Root Texts and Commentaries*. Ed. Sachen International. Kathmandu: Sachen International, 2011.

Salvini, Mattia. "Etymologies of What Can(Not) Be Said: Candrakīrti on Conventions and Elaborations." *Journal of Indian Philosophy* 47, no. 4 (September 2019): 661–95. https://doi.org/10.1007/s10781-019-09402-4.

Śaṅkara. *The Bṛhadāraṇyaka Upaniṣad: With the Commentary of Śaṅkarācārya*. Trans. Madhavananda Swami. 3rd ed. Mayavati, Almora: Advaita Ashrama, 1950.

Śāntarakṣita and Kamalaśīla. *Tattvasaṅgraha of Ācārya Śāntarakṣita with the "Pañjika" Commentary of Ācārya Śrī Kamalaśīla*. Ed. Dvārikādāsa Śāstrī. Vol. 2. Varanasi: Baudha, 1981.

Śāntideva. *A Guide to the Bodhisattva Way of Life: = (Bodhicaryāvatāra).* Trans. Vesna A. Wallace and B. Alan Wallace. Ithaca, NY: Snow Lion Publications, 1997.

Śāntideva and Prajñākaramati. *Bodhicaryāvatāra of Śāntideva with the Commentary Pañjika of Prajñākaramati.* Ed. Paraśurāma Lakshmaṇa Vaidya. Buddhist Sanskrit Texts 12. Darbhanga: Mithila Institute, 1960.

Sartre, Jean-Paul. *Being and Nothingness: A Phenomenological Essay on Ontology.* Trans. Hazel E. Barnes. New York: Washington Square Press, 1978.

Schmitt, Frederick F. "Justification, Sociality, and Autonomy." *Synthese* 73, no. 1 (1987): 43–85.

Schwabland, Peter A. "Direct and Indirect Cognition and the Definition of Pramāna in Early Tibetan Epistemology." *Asiatische Studien: Zeitschrift Der Schweizerischen Asiengesellschaft* 49, no. 4 (1995): 793–816. https://doi.org/10.5169/seals-147199.

Sellars, Wilfrid. "Empiricism and The Philosophy of Mind." In *Knowledge, Mind, and the Given: Reading Wilfrid Sellars's "Empiricism and the Philosophy of Mind," Including the Complete Text of Sellars's Essay.* Ed. Willem A. DeVries and Timm Triplett, 205–76. Indianapolis, IN: Hackett Pub, 2000.

Sharf, Robert H. "Knowing Blue: Early Buddhist Accounts of Non-Conceptual Sense." *Philosophy East & West* 68, no. 3 (2018): 826–70. https://doi.org/10.1353/pew.2018.0075.

Shes rab rin chen. "Grub mtha' kun shes kyi rnam par bshad pa legs bshad kyi rgya mtsho." In *Stag tshang lo tsā ba shes rab rin chen gyi gsung 'bum*, BDRC W2DB4577. 1:121–361. Beijing: Krung go'i bod rig pa dpe skrun khang, 2007.

Shieber, Joseph. "Locke on Testimony: A Reexamination." *History of Philosophy Quarterly* 26, no. 1 (2009): 21–41.

Shirazibeheshti, Amirali, Jennifer Cooke, Srivas Chennu, Ram Adapa, David K Menon, Seyed Ali Hojjatoleslami, Adrien Witon, Ling Li, Tristan Bekinschtein, and Howard Bowman. "Placing Meta-Stable States of Consciousness within the Predictive Coding Hierarchy: The Deceleration of the Accelerated Prediction Error." *Consciousness and Cognition* 63 (2018): 123–42. https://doi.org/10.1016/j.concog.2018.06.010.

Singleton, Mark, and James Mallinson. *Roots of Yoga.* Penguin Classics. London: Penguin, 2017.

Sinha, Jadunath. *Indian Psychology: Perception.* London: Kegan Paul, Trench, Trubner and Co., 1934.

Sjödin, Anna-Pya. "The Girl Who Knew Her Brother Would Be Coming Home: Ārṣajñāna in Praśastapādabhāṣya, Nyāyakandalī and Vyomavatī." *Journal of Indian Philosophy* 40, no. 4 (2012): 469–88.

Sperber, Dan. *Explaining Culture: A Naturalistic Approach.* Malden, MA: Blackwell, 1996.

Sponberg, Alan. "The Trisvabhāva Doctrine in India & China: A Study of Three Exegetical Models." *Bulletin of Buddhist Cultural Institute, Ryukoku University* 21 (November 30, 1982): 97–119.

Squarcini, Federico. *Patañjali: Yogasūtra: A Cura Di Federico Squarcini.* Et Classici. Turin, Italy: Giulio Einaudi Editore, 2019.

Stambaugh, Joan. *Thoughts on Heidegger.* Current Continental Research 217. Washington, DC: Center for Advanced Research in Phenomenology and University Press of America, 1991.

Stern, Robert. *Hegelian Metaphysics.* New York: Oxford University Press, 2009.
Stoltz, Jonathan. "Sakya Pandita and the Status of Concepts." *Philosophy East and West* 56, no. 4 (2006): 567–82. https://doi.org/10.1353/pew.2006.0064.
Storm, Jason Ānanda Josephson. *Metamodernism: The Future of Theory.* Chicago: University of Chicago Press, 2021.
Stroll, Avrum. *Twentieth-Century Analytic Philosophy.* New York: Columbia University Press, 2000.
Taber, John. "Yoga and Our Epistemic Predicament." In *Yogic Perception, Meditation and Altered States of Consciousness.* Ed. Eli Franco and Dagmar Eigner, 71–92. Vienna: Verlag der Österreichischen Akademie der Wissenschaften, 2009.
Talmy, Leonard. "Fictive Motion in Language and 'Ception." In *Speech, Language, and Communication.* Ed. Joanne L. Miller and Peter D. Eimas, 211–76. San Diego, CA: Academic Press, 1995.
Tanabe, Hajime. *Philosophy as Metanoetics.* Trans. Takeuchi Yoshinori, Valdo Viglielmo, and James W. Heisig. Nanzan Studies in Religion and Culture. Berkeley: University of California Press, 1986.
Taves, Ann. *Revelatory Events: Three Case Studies of the Emergence of New Spiritual Paths.* Princeton, NJ: Princeton University Press, 2016.
Taylor, Charles. *Sources of the Self: The Making of the Modern Identity.* Cambridge, MA: Harvard University Press, 1989.
Taylor, Jill Bolte. *My Stroke of Insight: A Brain Scientist's Personal Journey.* New York: Viking, 2006.
Thakchoe, Sonam. "Candrakīrti's Theory of Perception: A Case for Non-Foundationalist Epistemology in Madhyamaka." *Acta Orientalia Vilnensia* 11, no. 1 (2010): 93–124.
——. "How Many Truths? Are There Two Truths or One in the Tibetan Prāsaṅgika Madhyamaka?" *Contemporary Buddhism* 5, no. 2 (2004): 121–41. https://doi.org/10.1080/1463994042000291547.
——. *The Two Truths Debate: Tsongkhapa and Gorampa on the Middle Way.* Boston: Wisdom, 2007.
Thompson, Evan. *Why I Am Not a Buddhist.* New Haven, CT: Yale University Press, 2020. https://doi.org/10.2307/j.ctvt1sgfz.
Thurman, Robert A. F. "Philosophical Nonegocentrism in Wittgenstein and Candrakirti in Their Treatment of the Private Language Problem." *Philosophy East and West* 30, no. 3 (1980): 321–337. https://doi.org/10.2307/1399191.
Tillemans, Tom J. F. "Metaphysics for Madhyamikas." In *The Svātantrika-Prāsaṅgika Distinction: What Difference Does a Difference Make?* Ed. Georges B. J. Dreyfus and Sara L. McClintock, 93–123. Studies in Indian and Tibetan Buddhism. Boston: Wisdom, 2002.
——. *Scripture, Logic, Language: Essays on Dharmakirti and His Tibetan Successors.* Studies in Indian and Tibetan Buddhism. Boston: Wisdom, 1999.
Tomlinson, Davey K. "A Buddhist's Guide to Self-Destruction: Jñānaśrīmitra on the Structure of Yogic Perception." *Religious Studies* 60, no. 2 (2023): 1–16. https://doi.org/10.1017/S003441252300032X.
——. "Yogic Perception, Tantric Vision Practice, and the Norms of Attention." Presentation at the American Academy of Religion, San Antonio, 2023.

Torella, Raffaele. "Observations on Yogipratyakṣa." In *Saṁskṛta-Sādhutā: Goodness of Sanskrit. Studies in Honour of Professor Ashok N. Aklujkar.* Ed. Chikafumi Watanabe, Michele Desmarais, and Yoshichika Honda, 470–87. Delhi: D.K. Printworld, 2012.

Townley, Cynthia. *A Defense of Ignorance: Its Value for Knowers and Roles in Feminist and Social Epistemologies.* Lanham, MD: Lexington Books, 2011.

Trenckner, V., Robert Chalmers, and T. W. Rhys Davids, eds. *The Majjhima Nikaya.* Vol. 1. Oxford: Pali Text Society, 1991.

Tripāṭhī, Rāmaśaṅkara, ed. *Prajñāpāramitopadeśaśāstre Abhisamayālaṅkāravṛttiḥ Sphuṭārthā.* Varanasi: Central Institute of Higher Tibetan Studies, 1977.

Tryon Edwards. *A Dictionary of Thoughts, Being a Cyclopedia of Laconic Quotations from the Best Authors, Both Ancient and Modern.* New York: Cassell publishing company, 1893.

"Unidentified Anomalous Phenomena: Implications on National Security, Public Safety, and Government Transparency." 2154 Rayburn House Office Building, Washington, DC, July 26, 2023.

Vālmīki. *Rāmāyaṇa.* Ed. Muneo Tokunaga. Göttingen: Göttingen Register of Electronic Texts in Indian Languages, 2020. http://gretil.sub.uni-goettingen.de/gretil/corpustei/transformations/html/sa_rAmAyaNa.htm.

Van Den Bossche, Frank. "God, the Soul and the Creatrix: Haribhadra Sūri on Nyāya and Sāṃkhya." *International Journal of Jaina Studies* 6, no. 6 (2010): 1–49.

Vasubandhu. "*Abhidharmakośabhāṣya, Chos mngon pa'i mdzod kyi bshad pa." In *Sde dge bstan 'gyur.* Ed. Tshul khrims rin chen, Toh. no. 4090., Mngon pa, khu:1b–95a. Delhi: Delhi Karmapae Choedhey, Gyalwae Sungrab Partun Khang, 1744.

——. *Abhidharmakośabhāṣyam.* Ed. Prahlad Pradhan. Patna: K. P. Jayaswal Research Institute, 1975.

Veṅkaṭanātha and Nivāsa. *Nayâyaparishuddhi by Venkatnath Vedântâchârya: Nyāyapariśuddhiḥ. With a Commentary Called Nyayasar(a) by Niwâsachârya [Nivāsa Ācārya]. Edited with Notes by Vidyabhushan Laksńmanàchàrya.* Ed. Vidyabhuṣana Lakṣmanācārya. Varanasi: Chowkhambâ Sanskrit Series Office, 1918.

Voltaire. *Dictionnaire philosophique.* Vol. 8. Paris: Chez l'Editeur, 1822.

Walser, Joseph. "Buddhism without Buddhists? Academia & Learning to See Buddhism Like a State." *Pacific World*, 4, no. 3 (2022): 103–70.

Walsh, Kevin S., David P. McGovern, Andy Clark, and Redmond G. O'Connell. "Evaluating the Neurophysiological Evidence for Predictive Processing as a Model of Perception." *Annals of the New York Academy of Sciences* 1464, no. 1 (March 2020): 242–68. https://doi.org/10.1111/nyas.14321.

Ward, Jamie. "Synaesthesia: A Distinct Entity That Is an Emergent Feature of Adaptive Neurocognitive Differences." *Philosophical Transactions of the Royal Society of London. Series B, Biological Sciences* 374, no. 1787 (2019): 20180351. https://doi.org/10.1098/rstb.2018.0351.

Warren, Calvin L. *Ontological Terror Blackness, Nihilism, and Emancipation.* Durham, NC: Duke University Press, 2018. https://doi.org/10.1215/9780822371847.

Watson, Alex. "Light as an Analogy for Cognition in Buddhist Idealism (Vijñānavāda)." *Journal of Indian Philosophy* 42, no. 2–3 (2014): 401–21.

Webb, Mark Owen. "Why I Know About as Much as You: A Reply to Hardwig." *The Journal of Philosophy* 90, no. 5 (1993): 260–70.

Wellman, Henry M., David Cross, and Julianne Watson. "Meta-Analysis of Theory-of-Mind Development: The Truth about False Belief." *Sage Family Studies Abstracts* 23, no. 4 (2001): 411–568.

White, David Gordon. "How Big Can Yogis Get? How Much Can Yogis See?" In *Yoga Powers: Extraordinary Capacities Attained Through Meditation and Concentration*. Ed. Knut A. Jacobsen, 61–76. Leiden: Brill, 2012.

——. *Sinister Yogis*. Chicago: The University of Chicago Press, 2009.

Williams, Paul. *Yogācāra, The Epistemological Tradition and Tathāgatagarbha*. Vol. 5. Buddhism: Critical Concepts in Religious Studies. London: Routledge, 2005.

Winer, Gerald A., Jane E. Cottrell, Virginia Gregg, Jody S. Fournier, and Lori A. Bica. "Fundamentally Misunderstanding Visual Perception." *American Psychologist* 57, no. 6/7 (2002).

Winer, Gerald A., Aaron W. Rader, and Jane E. Cottrell. "Testing Different Interpretations for the Mistaken Belief That Rays Exit the Eyes During Vision." *The Journal of Psychology* 137, no. 3 (2003): 243–61. https://doi.org/10.1080/00223980309600612.

Wittgenstein, Ludwig. *Philosophische Untersuchungen = Philosophical Investigations*. Ed. Peter Michael Stephan Hacker. Trans. Gertrude Elizabeth Margaret Anscombe and Joachim Schulte. Rev. 4th ed. Chichester, West Sussex, UK: Wiley-Blackwell, 2009.

——. *Preliminary Studies for the "Philosophical Investigations:" Generally Known as the Blue and Brown Books*. Oxford: Blackwell, 1960.

——. "Tractatus Logico-Philosophicus." In *Major Works: Selected Philosophical Writings*, Trans. C. K. Ogden, 1st ed., 1–82. New York: HarperPerennial, 2009.

Wollstonecraft, Mary, and Janet Todd. *A Vindication of the Rights of Men A Vindication of the Rights of Woman Historical and Moral View of the French Revolution*. Oxford World's Classics. Oxford: Oxford University Press, 1999.

Woo, Jeson. "Kamalaśīla on 'Yogipratyakṣa.'" *Indo-Iranian Journal* 48, no. 1–2 (2005): 111–21.

Wynn, April N., Irvin L. Pan, Elizabeth E. Rueschhoff, Maryann A. B. Herman, and E. Kathleen Archer. "Student Misconceptions about Plants—A First Step in Building a Teaching Resource." *Journal of Microbiology & Biology Education*, April 2017. https://doi.org/10.1128/jmbe.v18i1.1253.

Yamāri. "*Pramāṇavārttikālaṃkāraṭīkāsupariśuddhā, Tshad ma rnam 'grel rgyan gyi 'grel bshad shin tu yongs su dag pa zhes bya ba." In *Sde 'dge bstan 'gyur*. Ed. Tshul khrims rin chen, Trans. Rngog blo ldan shes rab, Toh. 4226, Tshad ma, be:1b–261a. Delhi: Delhi Karmapae Choedhey, Gyalwae Sungrab Partun Khang, 1982.

Yāmunācārya and Dāmodara Prapanācārya. "Īśvarasiddhiḥ." In *Siddhitrayam: Ātma-Īśvara-Saṃvitsiddhayaḥ*, Prathama saṃskaraṇa, 246–341. Caukhambā surabhāratī granthamālā 587. Vārāṇasī: Caukhambā Surabhāratī Prakāśana, 2015..

Yao, Zhihua. *The Buddhist Theory of Self-Cognition*. New York: Routledge, 2005. https://doi.org/10.4324/9780203445280.

Zagzebski, Linda Trinkaus. "The Attribute of Omnisubjectivity." In *God, Knowledge, and the Good*, 187–210, 1st ed. New York: Oxford University Press, 2022. https://doi.org/10.1093/oso/9780197612385.003.0012.

Index

Figures are indicated by an italic *f* following the page number.

abductive inference, 79–80
Abhinavagupta, 66–68, 70
Absorbed (*yukta*) yogic perception, 19–21, 24–25, 29–30, 34, 36, 46, 60, 216n53, 232n27, 239n25
achieving desired ends (*arthakriyā*), 79, 94
Anti-Essentialist, 185–87, 193
antirealism, 5, 136, 142, 168, 172, 206
antirepresentationalism, 5, 136, 142. *See also* Sakya (Sa skya) antirepresentationalism
appearanceless wisdom, 174, 182
appearing *vs.* conceived objects, 155
argument from ignorance, 42, 48, 51, 53, 55, 57, 64, 69–70
Aristotle, 113, 117–18
Arnold, Dan, 78
Asaṅga, 83–88, 86*f*, 139, 169–71, 173–76, 182, 196, 204, 240–41n39
ascertainments, 177–81, 197
Audi, Robert, 6, 40–43, 58
authentic cognition, 23, 98, 178, 180
authentic perception, 179, 188–92
authentic testimony, 39, 57–58, 205
authority and testimony, 43, 46–47, 52–55, 60, 68. *See also* testimony in yogic perception
Ayer, Alfred J., 77–78

being there (Dasein), 108, 110–12, 135–36, 245n85, 245n91
beyond the senses (*atīndriya*), 44–45, 223n33
Bhartṛhari, 48–51, 56, 69, 75
Bhāsarvajña, 23–25, 29, 36, 126–28
black-box theory of perception, 80, 101, 107–8
Bouquet of Reasons (*Nyāyamañjarī*) (Jayanta Bhaṭṭa), 22–23
Bṛhadāraṇyaka Upaniṣad, 15, 34, 203
Buddha, as lord of yogis, 125
Buddhaghoṣa, 26–27, 30, 36, 43, 63, 203
Buddhist theory of yogic perception, 81–93
Buddhist tradition, 25–29

Campbell, George, 40
Candrakīrti, 63–68, 70, 148–52, 170–71

Chapa Chökyi Senge, 143–47, 172–75, 182, 190, 195, 197, 201
Clear Words (*Prasannapadā*) (Candrakīrti), 64–65
cognition: authentic, 23, 98, 178, 180; Candrakīrti on, 170; Dharmakīrti on, 103, 155, 184–86; dual-process theories of, 31, 33; elaborations and, 144; four components in, 19; Gorampa on, 189–90; mental, 115–16, 239n21; mistaken, 90; nonconceptual, 85, 89, 153, 185; as objectless, 63–64, 68; omniphenomenology and, 124–32; omniscient, 53; of past and future objects, 23–24; Peirce on, 78–80, 102; precognitions, 126, 128, 131, 244n71; Ratnakīrti on, 100; reflexive awareness and, 124–25; remote seeing and, 19, 23–25, 35; Sapen on, 178–80; seer cognition (*ārṣa*), 24, 46; sense cognition, 149, 214n28; subsequent, 178–80; Sucaritamiśra on, 98; supersensible, 53; Taktsang Lotsāwa on, 152–53; Tsongkhapa on, 157–59, 161–62; Vācaspatimiśra on, 94–95; yogic, 92, 131, 185
coherentism, 59–62, 65, 68, 70–71, 75–81, 101–6
Collection of Mahāyāna (*Mahāyānasaṃgraha*) (Asaṅga), 84
Commentary on the Compendium of Epistemology (Dharmakīrti), 54–55
communal knowledge, 65, 67
comparative philosophy, 1, 209
Compendium on Commentarial Doctrine (*Śāstravārtāsamuccaya*) (Haribhadrasūri), 51
conception, 76, 81, 89–92, 94, 103–9, 112–20, 178, 197, 203–4
consciousness, 16, 21–22, 25, 32–35, 64, 79, 84–85, 111, 116–17, 133, 150, 153, 161–64, 208
conventional knowledge, 65, 67, 171
conventional truth (*saṃvṛti-satya*), 65, 188, 192, 200–201
Creation Stage (*utpattikrama, bskyed rim*), 159–65
"credible-unless-otherwise-indicated," 41–42, 45, 58, 69

deceptive reality (*saṃvṛti-satya*), 173
delusions, 4, 89, 104
desired ends (*arthakriyā*), 79–80, 94, 97, 131, 164, 179, 186
dharma: Bhartṛhari on, 50; Dignāga on, 88; Jaimini on, 43–44, 55; Jñānaśrīmitra on, 116; Kūṭadanta on, 82–83; Praśastapāda on, 45–46; Ratnakīrti on, 100; Śabara on, 56; Sucaritamiśra on, 99; Uddyotakara on, 52
dharma eye, 82–83, 88, 216n53
Dharmakīrti: black-box theory of perception, 80, 101, 107–8; conception *vs.* perception, 76, 78–80; Gelug representationalism and, 152–59, 163–64, 204; Indian Buddhism and, 87–97, 102–6; omniphenomenology/omniscience and, 117–26; other minds, 123–24; remote seeing and, 28–29, 36; Sakya (Sa skya) antirepresentationalism and, 176–77, 180–81, 183–85, 188–89, 192–94, 196, 206; testimony, 54–56; Tsongkhapa's commentary on, 152–59, 163–64
Digest on Phenomena and Meanings (*Padārthadharmasaṃgraha*) (Praśastapāda), 19
Dignāga, 25–29, 49, 76, 78–80, 87–92, 170, 194–95
discrete objects, 25
divine eye, 26–27, 30, 43, 83, 216n48, 216n53
divine pride (*lha'i nga rgyal*), 159–62

Edwards, Tryon, 1, 2
elaborations, 143–46, 172–73, 190
emanation (*nirmāṇa*), 66–67
embodied gaze, 37, 111, 116, 220n92
enlightenment, 1, 16, 160, 193, 201, 232n32

enumerative knowledge, 3–5, 14–15, 24–25, 29, 43–44, 108, 113–16, 120, 129, 177
epistemic authenticity, 185, 193
epistemic instrument (*pramāṇa*), 22, 24, 44, 47, 51, 56, 66, 69–70, 75, 87, 92, 98–100, 115–16, 155–56, 159, 174–93, 195–98, 204–6, 254n39, 255n47
epistemic warrant (*pramāṇa*), 44, 51, 56, 68, 90–97, 102–6, 116, 124, 144, 152, 155, 163–68, 173, 178–80, 183–92, 200, 212n8, 243n69, 249n39, 250n52
epistemological chain, 6, 42, 46, 49–54, 57–58, 61–71, 75, 80
Essential Teachings of the Three Mādhyamikas from the East (*Dbu ma shar gsum gyi stong thun*) (Chapa), 144
Euro-American philosophy, 2, 206
extending light, 16, 26–27, 35
extramission, 6, 14–16, 25–26, 29–37, 220n85
extramissive intuitions, 29–34, 37

False Aspectarian position (*alīkākāra/ nirākāravāda*), 87, 139–40, 182
feminism, 2, 210
first-person perspective, 7, 109–14, 123, 126, 131–34, 206
forward direction, 75–76, 80–81, 91–92, 97, 101–4, 107, 113–14, 119
foundationalism, 6, 41, 50, 58–59, 61–62, 65, 69–71, 75, 91–92, 101–2, 205, 223n22
Four Noble Truths, 82–86, 90–105, 120–21, 129, 189–90, 204
freedom from elaborations, 144–46, 172–73, 190

gaze (*darśana*) of Śiva, 15–16
Gelug representationalism: Chapa Chökyi Senge and, 143–47; Creation Stage (*utpattikrama, bskyed rim*), 159–65; Dharmakīrti and, 152–59, 163–64, 204; introduction to, 7–8; Jñānaśrīmitra and, 139, 141, 147, 154, 164; Mind Only (*cittamātra*) and, 155–59; quasirepresentationalism and, 8, 165–69; Russell, Bertrand and, 139–41; Sutrist perspectives, 155–59; Tibetan Buddhism and, 141–43; Tsongkhapa Losang Drakpa and, 143, 147–67
global requirement in testimony, 40–41, 47–48, 58, 64–65, 69–70, 222n13
Gorampa Sonam Senge, 179–94, 192*f*
Great Treatise on the Stages of Mantra (*Sngags rim chen mo*) (Tsongkhapa), 160

hallucinations, 4, 63, 90–91, 104–5, 126, 152, 154, 159, 184–85
Haribhadrasūri, 51–55
Hegel, Georg Wilhelm Friedrich, 36–37
Heidegger, Martin, 107–12, 135
Hemacandra, 52–55, 70, 226n57
human intuition, 29–37
human rights, 2
Hume, David: global requirement, 40–41, 47–48, 58, 64–65, 69–70, 222n13; introduction to, 1, 6; mutual destruction of arguments, 39, 42, 51; reductionism and, 39–41, 206; testimony and, 38–42, 51, 65
Husserl, Edmund, 7, 107–12

ideal forms theory, 2
impermanence/impermanent things, 94–98, 101, 112, 116, 143, 153–57, 165, 177–79, 183, 187, 189, 195, 198, 234n56, 242n50, 251n58
inconceivable power, 34, 121
incongruity of yogic perception: Buddhist tradition and, 25–29; extramission, 6, 14–16, 25–26, 29–37, 220n85; introduction to, 13–15; intuitions, 6, 27, 29–35, 37–40, 205–9, 218n69, 231n19, 237n1; metaphors and, 32–33; *Nyāya* tradition and, 22–25; remote seeing, 14–15, 17–21, 23–30, 35–36, 55–57, 83, 197, 203–4; VARK model of learning, 13–14, 37
incredibility, 39

Indian Buddhism: analysis of, 1; Asaṅga and, 83–88, 86*f*, 139, 169–71, 173–76, 182, 196, 204, 240–41n39; coherentism and, 75–81, 101–6; critique from redundancy, 98–101; critique of concepts, 93–98; Dharmakīrti and, 87–97, 102–6; Dignāga and, 87–92; foundationalism and, 75, 91–92, 101–2, 205; inference and, 75–81; introduction into Tibet, 55; Jñānaśrīmitra and, 92–93, 95–101, 103–4; mental perception, 29, 34–35, 88; Peirce, Charles S. and, 7, 78–80, 103–5; pragmatism and, 79–80, 90–91, 94, 96–105; Ratnakīrti and, 99–101, 104; reflexive awareness, 88, 122–32; self-authenticating perception and, 61, 75, 91–92, 101–2; sense perception, 34, 44, 88, 133, 170; Sucaritamiśra and, 98–100; Vācaspatimiśra and, 93–95, 103; Vasubandhu and, 27, 63, 83–87, 232n28; waning of, 4
Indo-Tibetan philosophy, 2–3
inference, 75–81, 87–88, 102
inferential thinking, 102, 158, 174–75
informative (*saṃvāda*) knowledge, 52–53, 99
informative yogic perception, 90–92, 97, 99, 103, 116, 124, 129–31, 188–90, 243n57, 250n52
intellectual development of yogic perception, 4–5, 81, 203
intrinsic validity (*svataḥ prāmāṇya*), 45, 48
Introduction to the Way of the Bodhisattva (*Bodhisattvacaryāvatāra*) (Śāntideva), 172–76
intuitions, 6, 27, 29–35, 37–40, 205–9, 218n69, 231n19, 237n1
Investigation of Epistemology (*Pramāṇamīmāṃsā*) (Hemacandra), 52–53

Jaimini, 43–44, 55
Jayanta Bhaṭṭa, 22–23
Jñānaśrīmitra: domain-specific reasoning, 33–36; Gelug representationalism and, 139, 141, 147, 154, 164; Indian Buddhism and, 57–59, 69, 92–93, 95–101, 103–4; omniphenomenology/omniscience and, 115–16, 119–24, 127–32; pragmaticism and, 205; remote seeing and, 57–59, 204; Sakya (Sa skya) antirepresentationalism, 179, 204–6
Jones, Karen, 40
justification for believing, 40–41, 45, 50, 52, 58, 70

Kamalaśīla, 24, 55–57, 115–17, 120, 204
Kandala Flower of Logic (*Nyāyakandalī*) (Śrīdhara), 20
Kedrub Gelek Pelzang, 182–94, 192*f*
knowing all through one, 112–15
Kūṭadanta, 81–84

Laruelle, François, 199–202
Lightman, Alan, 134
Light on Reality (*Tattvapradīpika*), 21
literal knowledge, 28, 111, 115, 241n40
logic and epistemology, 176–79

Matsyapurāṇa, 16
McClintock, Sara, 117, 121
meditation (*saṃyama*), 18
meditative ability, 63, 84, 86, 86*f*
meditative fixation, 7, 154
meditative objects, 75, 84, 89–91, 152, 161, 167
meditative realization, 85–86, 86*f*, 177
mental cognition, 115–16, 239n21
mental (*manas*) light, 18
mental perception (*mānasa-pratyakṣa*), 29, 34–35, 88
Merleau-Ponty, Maurice, 111
metaphors, 32–33
metaphysical objects, 25, 43
Middle Way theory, 65, 148, 157–59, 165, 185, 187–88, 193–94, 197, 249nn39–40, 253n23

Migtsema Mantra (*Dmigs brtse ma*), 202
Mill, John Stuart, 40
Mīmāṃsakas, 7, 41–50, 53–57, 69, 160, 204, 223n22, 227n72
Mīmāṃsāsūtras (Jaimini), 43–44, 55
Mind Only (*cittamātra*), 155–59, 194–95
miracles, 38–40, 44, 222n13
mistaken cognition (*bhrānti-jñāna*), 90
Moore, G. E., 165–69
mutual destruction of arguments, 39, 42, 51
mysticism, 62

Naiyāyikas, 6, 16, 30–31, 46–48, 69, 204, 224n35
Noble One, 83–84, 160, 180
nonconceptual cognition, 85, 89, 153, 185
nonconceptual yogic perception, 85–91, 106, 108, 114–16, 122–23, 132–34, 153, 166, 180, 185, 189–91, 205
nonsensory *prāpyakārin*, 21
normal perception, 3, 43, 60, 68, 114
no self (*anātman*), 26, 216n54
Nyāya tradition, 22–25, 79

omniphenomenology/omniscience: Bhāsarvajña and, 24, 126–28; defined, 7; Dharmakīrti and, 117–26; Heidegger, Martin and, 107–12, 135; Husserl, Edmund and, 7, 107–12; introduction to, 7; Jñānaśrīmitra and, 119–24, 127–32; Kamalaśīla and, 115–17, 120; knowing all through one, 112–22; mental cognition and, 115–16, 239n21; phenomenalism and, 121–32; Prajñākaragupta and, 119–26; Ratnakīrti and, 127–32; reflexive awareness and, 122–32; Śāntarakṣita and, 115–17; selflessness and, 116–19; spiritual capacity for, 29; subject-object duality, 84–85, 109–10, 123–26, 131–33; Vācaspatimiśra and, 117–19
omniscient cognition (*kevala-jñāna*), 53
On Sentences and Words (*Vākyapadīya*) (Bhartṛhari), 49
On the Demonstrability of Yogis (*Yoginirṇayaprakaraṇa*) (Jñānaśrīmitra), 92, 95
Ontological Terror: Blackness, Nihilism, and Emancipation (Warren), 135
Ornament for Logic (*Nyāyabhūṣaṇa*) (Bhāsarvajña), 126
other minds, 123–24

Pāli *suttas*, 81–83, 88
Patañjali's *Yogasūtras*, 6, 17–19, 23, 25, 44, 55
Path of Purification (*Visuddhimagga*) (Buddhaghoṣa), 26
Peirce, Charles S., 7, 78–80, 103–5
phenomenalism, 121–32, 139–44, 162
Piaget, Jean, 31
Pith Instructions (*Pravacanasāra*), 21
Plato, 2
pragmatism, 5, 7–8, 75–81, 90–91, 94, 96–105
Prajñākaragupta, 28–30, 36, 119–26, 163
prāpyakārin: Buddhaghoṣa and, 26–27, 30, 36, 43, 63, 203; defined, 15–16, 18; extramissive thinking and, 29–31; nonsensory, 21; sensory, 34; yogic perception and, 20–21
Praśastapāda, 19–20, 204
precognitions, 126, 128, 131, 244n71
Proof of Other Minds (*Saṃtānāntarasiddhi*) (Dharmakīrti), 123–24
properties of objects (*vastu-dharma*), 96–97, 101, 116, 120
Pūrva Mīmāṃsā tradition, 6

quasirepresentationalism, 8, 165–69

rāj yog, 16
Rāmāyaṇa, 17, 57
Ratnakīrti, 99–101, 104, 127–32, 181–82
reductionism, 39–41, 206
referent objects, 63, 144, 151–54, 159, 165, 183, 195
reflexive awareness (*svasaṃvedanā*), 88, 122–32
reliable testimony, 46–47, 49, 55

religious testimony, 62
remote seeing, 14–15, 17–21, 23–30, 35–36, 55–57, 83, 197, 203–4
representationalism: introduction to, 5; Jñānasrīmitra's rejection of, 131, 164; limits of, 199–201; phenomenalism and, 121–32, 139–44, 162; quasirepresentationalism, 8, 165–69. *See also* Gelug representationalism
representative realism, 7, 77–78, 140, 164
Ṛg Veda, 15
Rousseau, Jean-Jacques, 2
Russell, Bertrand, 7, 77, 139–41

Śabara, 44–48, 56, 69, 203–4
Śākya Chokden, 194–96, 198, 203
Sakya Paṇḍita (Sapen), 176–82, 187, 194, 197, 200–201
Sakya (Sa skya) antirepresentationalism: Asaṅga and, 169–71, 173–76, 182, 196; ascertainments and, 177–81, 197; authentic perception and, 179, 188–92; Candrakīrti and, 170–71; Chapa Chökyi Senge and, 172–75, 182, 190, 195, 197, 201; Dharmakīrti and, 176–77, 180–81, 183–85, 188–89, 192–94, 196, 206; Dignāga and, 170, 194–95; epistemic instruments (*pramāṇa*) and, 183–93, 195–98; epistemic warrant (*pramāṇa*), 173, 178–80, 183–92, 200; Gorampa Sonam Senge, 179–94, 192*f*; impermanence and, 177–79, 183, 187, 189, 195, 198; introduction to, 5, 8, 169–72; Kedrub Gelek Pelzang, 182–94, 192*f*; Laruelle, François and, 199–202; limits of representationalism, 199–201; logic and epistemology, 176–79; Ratnakīrti and, 181–82; Śākya Chokden and, 194–96, 198; Sakya Paṇḍita (Sapen) and, 176–82, 187, 194, 197, 200–201; selflessness and, 176–79, 183, 187, 198; Sönam Tsemo and, 172–76, 178, 182–83, 190, 195, 197; subsequent cognition and, 178–80; Tsongkhapa and, 169, 173, 177, 179, 182–84, 187–88, 193–98, 202; Wittgenstein, Ludwig and, 169–75, 182–83, 185–86, 193–94, 198–99
Śāntarakṣita, 24, 55–57, 115–17, 204
Śāntideva, 172–76
Sapen. *See* Sakya Paṇḍita (Sapen)
Sartre, Jean-Paul, 111
scientist testimony and yogic perception, 68–71
scriptural authority, 6, 68, 75, 205
scriptural testimony, 42, 44, 52, 68–69, 75, 223n22. *See also* testimony in yogic perception
seeing without the teacher, 88–89
seer cognition (*ārṣa*), 24, 46
self-authenticating perception, 61, 75, 91–92, 101–2
selflessness, 116–19, 176–79, 183, 187, 198
sense cognition, 149, 214n28
sense objects, 35, 149–50, 217n58
sense perception (*indriya-pratyakṣa*), 34, 44, 88, 133, 170
sensory *prāpyakārin,* 34
Śiva Purāṇa, 15
social gaze, 37
solipsism, 109–11, 115, 123–26, 131–32, 139, 165
Sönam Tsemo, 172–76, 178, 182–83, 190, 195, 197
soul/self (*ātman*), 15, 19, 34
space-time, 62
spiritual insight, 6, 14–15, 25, 28, 70, 75, 83, 204, 216n53
spiritual knowledge, 4–5, 44, 160, 177
spiritual practice, 3, 59, 88–89
Śrīdhara, 20–21, 25–26, 30, 35–36, 121
Stream Entry, 82–86
subject-object duality, 7, 33, 84–85, 109–10, 123–26, 131–33, 156, 176–77, 182
subsequent cognition, 178–80
Sucaritamiśra, 98–100
supersensible (*atīndriya*) cognition, 53

supersensible objects, 45–48, 54–57, 68–69
supersensory abilities, 17, 34, 47, 56, 69, 83
superstition, 1–2, 105
Sutrist (*sautrāntika*) perspectives, 155–59

Taktsang Lotsāwa, 151–52
Tantric practice, 66, 159, 162–63, 165–66, 209
Taylor, Jill Bolte, 133–34
testimony in yogic perception: Abhinavagupta, 66–68, 70; argument from ignorance, 42, 48, 51, 53, 55, 57, 64, 69–70; Audi, Robert, 40–43, 58; authentic, 39, 57–58, 205; authority and, 43, 46–47, 52–55, 60, 68; Bhartṛhari, 48–51, 56, 69, 75; Candrakīrti, 63–68, 70; coherentism and, 59–62, 65, 68, 70–71; "credible-unless-otherwise-indicated," 41–42, 45, 58, 69; Dharmakīrti, 54–56; epistemological chain and, 6, 42, 46, 49–54, 57–58, 61–71, 75, 80; global requirement in, 40–41, 47–48, 58, 64–65, 69–70, 222n13; Haribhadrasūri, 51–55; Hemacandra, 52–55, 69, 226n57; Hume, David, 38–42, 65; introduction to, 38; Kamalaśīla, 55–57; Mīmāṃsā and, 43–45; Mīmāṃsakas and, 41–50, 53–57, 68–69; Naiyāyikas and, 46–48; perception as foundation of scripture, 48–59; reliable, 46–47, 49, 55; religious, 62; Śāntarakṣita, 55–57; scientists and, 68–71; scriptural, 42, 44, 52, 68–69, 75, 223n22; supersensible objects and, 45–48; Uddyotakara and, 47–53, 58, 79, 223n33; Utpaladeva, 66–68, 70; Vedic, 6–7, 44–45, 68, 223n22; Veṅkaṭanātha, 59–61, 65, 70–71, 75, 227n73; yogis and, 68–71
Tibetan Buddhism, 1, 4, 141–43, 147, 201, 208
transcendental idealism, 109
Treasury of Higher Knowledge (*Abhidharmakośa*) (Vasubandhu), 83–84
Treasury of Reasoning and Epistemology (*Tshad ma rigs gter*) (Sakya Paṇḍita), 176–82, 187, 194, 197, 200–201
True Aspectarian position (*sākāravādin*), 87, 139
Tsongkhapa Losang Drakpa, 143, 147–67, 169, 173, 177, 179, 182–84, 187–88, 193–98, 202
two truths (*dvaya-satya*), 65, 177, 197–98

Uddyotakara, 47–53, 58, 79, 223n33
ultimate reality, 142, 157, 171–73, 182–83, 186–87, 192–93, 197–98, 253n23
ultimate truth (*paramārtha-satya*), 65, 118, 156, 173–74, 176–77, 183, 186, 188, 190, 192–95, 201
unabsorbed (*viyukta*) yogic perception, 19–20, 23–25, 28–29, 36, 46, 60
Unchanging Absolute (*pariniṣpanna*), 156, 158, 161, 165, 194–95
uninterrupted transmission/succession, 50, 94
unmistaken yogic perception, 90, 97–98, 101, 176, 180, 195
Utpaladeva, 66–68, 70

Vācaspatimiśra, 93–95, 103, 117–19
Vaiśeṣikas, 6, 19–22, 24–25, 30, 45, 68–69
VARK model of learning, 13–14, 37
Vasubandhu, 27, 63, 83–87, 232n28
Vātsyāyana, Pakṣilasvāmin, 22
Vedic testimony, 6–7, 44–45, 68, 223n22
Veṅkaṭanātha, 59–61, 65, 70–71, 75, 227n73
vivid yogic perception, 63–64, 89–91, 95, 97, 120, 124
Voltaire, 1

Warren, Calvin, 135
Wittgenstein, Ludwig, 169–75, 182–83, 185–86, 193–94, 198–99
Wollstonecraft, Mary, 2

yoga, defined, 4
Yogācāra methodology, 63, 86, 121–23, 128–29, 149, 155, 158, 165, 194, 200, 246n1
Yogasūtras of Patañjali, 6, 17–19, 23, 25, 44, 55
yogic cognition, 92, 131, 185
yogic perception: absorbed (*yukta*), 19–21, 24–25, 29–30, 34, 36, 46, 60, 216n53, 232n27, 240n25; black-box theory of, 80, 101, 107–8; Buddhist theory of, 81–93; conception and, 76, 81, 89–92, 94, 103–9, 112–20, 178, 197, 203–4; defined, 3; delimitations and future directions, 203–10; as informative (*saṃvāda*), 90–92, 97, 99, 103, 116, 124, 129–31, 188–90, 243n57, 250n52; intellectual development of, 4–5, 81, 203; introduction to, 1–2; main arguments, 3–6; as nonconceptual, 85–91, 106, 108, 114–16, 122–23, 132–34, 153, 166, 180, 185, 189–91, 205; overview of, 3–8; as self-authenticating, 61, 75, 91–92, 101–2; unabsorbed (*viyukta*), 19–20, 23–25, 28–29, 36, 46, 60; as unmistaken, 90, 97–98, 101, 176, 180, 195; as vivid, 63–64, 89–91, 95, 97, 120, 124
yuj, defined, 3, 4

GPSR Authorized Representative: Easy Access System Europe, Mustamäe tee 50, 10621 Tallinn, Estonia, gpsr.requests@easproject.com

www.ingramcontent.com/pod-product-compliance
Lightning Source LLC
Chambersburg PA
CBHW022039290426
44109CB00014B/910
* 9 7 8 0 2 3 1 2 1 5 5 3 4 *